MEN'S HEALTH TODAY 2005

MEN'S HEALTH TODAY 2005

Get Ahead in Everything You Do

Edited by Deanna Portz, Men'sHealth Books

RODALE

Notice
This book is intended as a reference volume only, not as a medical manual. The information given here is designed to help you make informed decisions about your health. It is not intended as a substitute for any treatment that may have been prescribed by your doctor. If you suspect that you have a medical problem, we urge you to seek competent medical help.

Mention of specific companies, organizations, or authorities in this book does not imply endorsement by the author or publisher, nor does mention of specific companies, organizations, or authorities imply that they endorse this book, its author, or the publisher.

Internet addresses and telephone numbers given in this book were accurate at the time it went to press.

Printed in the United States of America
Rodale Inc. makes every effort to use acid-free ♾, recycled paper ♻.

Book design by Drew Frantzen

ISBN-13 978–1–59486–080–5 hardcover
ISBN-10 1–59486–080–7 hardcover

2 4 6 8 10 9 7 5 3 1 hardcover

RODALE
WE INSPIRE AND ENABLE PEOPLE TO IMPROVE THEIR LIVES AND THE WORLD AROUND THEM

CONTENTS

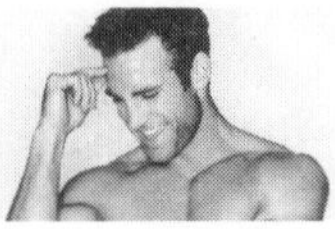

PART FIVE:
YOUNG MAN: ANTI-AGING

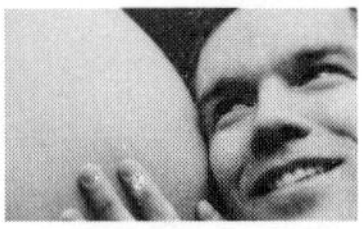

PART SIX:
FAMILY MAN:
FERTILITY AND FATHERHOOD

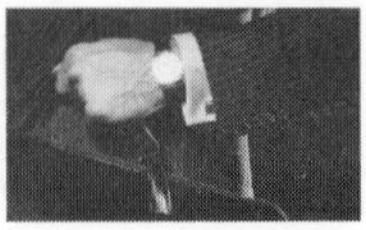

PART SEVEN:
BUSINESS MAN:
WORK AND CAREER

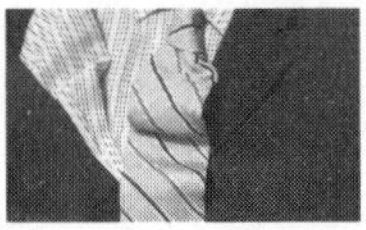

PART EIGHT:
LOOKIN' GOOD, MAN:
STYLE AND LOOKS

Men's Health Today 2005 Staff

EDITOR: Deanna Portz

CONTRIBUTING WRITERS: Daniel Amen, M.D.; Craig Ballantyne, C.S.C.S.; Matt Bean; Jamie Beckman; David Blend; Brian Boyé; Steve Calechman; Adam Campbell; Chris Connolly; Jeff Csatari; Kate Dailey; Douglas Dechert; Kathryn Eisman; Jon Finkel; Jessica Fischbein; Liesa Goins; Brian Good; Jim Gorman; Christina Goyanes; Carter Hays, C.S.C.S.; Samantha Heller, M.S., R.D.; Harry Jaffe; Lisa Jones; James Kennedy; Joe Kita; Chris Lawson; Matt Marion; Sarah Mattaliano; Christopher McDougall; Colin McEnroe; Brooke McIntyre; Michael Mejia, C.S.C.S.; Peter Moore; Hugh O'Neill; Stephen Perrine; Meredith Pharaoh; Scott Quill; Phillip Rhodes; Lauren Russell; David Schipper; Lou Schuler; Heidi Skolnik, M.S., C.D.N.; Ian Smith, M.D.; Ted Spiker; Laurence Roy Stains; Bill Stieg; Allen St. John; Bill Stump; Robert Superko, M.D.; Amy Jo Van Bodegraven; Greta Van Susteren; Elizabeth M. Ward, M.S., R.D.; Donovan Webster; John R. White, Jr., Pharm. D.; Mike Zimmerman

INTERIOR AND COVER DESIGNER: Drew Frantzen

PHOTO EDITOR: Darleen Malkames

PROJECT EDITOR: Marilyn Hauptly

COPY EDITORS: Hope Clarke, Jo Ann Learman

LAYOUT DESIGNER: Jan Greenberg

PRODUCT SPECIALIST: Jodi Schaffer

Rodale Men's Health Group

PRESIDENT, MANAGING DIRECTOR: Tom Beusse

VICE PRESIDENT, *MEN'S HEALTH* EDITOR-IN-CHIEF: David Zinczenko

MEN'S HEALTH AND SPORTS BOOKS EXECUTIVE EDITOR: Jeremy Katz

SENIOR MANAGING EDITOR: Chris Krogermeier

VICE PRESIDENT, ART DIRECTOR: Andy Carpenter

MANAGING ART DIRECTOR: Darlene Schneck

VICE PRESIDENT, PUBLISHER OF DIRECT RESPONSE BOOKS: Gregg Michaelson

SENIOR DIRECTOR, DIRECT RESPONSE MARKETING: Janine Slaughter

DIRECTOR, MEN'S HEALTH DIRECT RESPONSE MARKETING: John Sandklev

SENIOR MANAGER, CONTENT ASSEMBLY & PREP: Robert V. Anderson Jr.

CONTENT ASSEMBLY MANAGER: Patricia Brown

INTRODUCTION

HATS OFF TO YOU

One detail I remember fondly about my dad from my childhood: He wore a lot of hats. Literally. His collection of headgear filled an entire shelf in our family coat closet.

Being the sportsman that he is, he had a specific hat for every purpose: a fishing hat with his license and badges pinned onto it, a bright orange hat with ear flaps he wore for deer hunting, a captain's hat for when he was at the helm of our 18-foot ski boat, a set of Payne Stewart-style golf hats in every color of the rainbow, baseball caps for the two teams he coached—my brother's Little League team and my softball team, and hats emblazoned with the logos of his favorite NFL and major league baseball teams to offer a show of support on game days.

My dad's cap collection made me realize that he doesn't just wear a lot of hats, he also wears a lot of hats in the sense that he fills a slew of roles from husband, father, and handyman to businessman, sportsman, and coach. The truth is, men today wear more hats than men of yesteryear wore wing tips.

No matter which hats you don and doff in a day, *Men's Health Today 2005* gives you the keys to success to fill each role with ease. Here are just a few insights you'll find inside:

- **At work . . .** Do away with distractions, impress your boss, master the art of networking, and find your dream job once and for all.
- **At home . . .** Whip up healthy meals in minutes, protect your family from food poisoning, discover the best type of movies to put her in the mood, and shield your kids from the fastest-growing health threat among children.
- **At play . . .** Perfect your putt, hit the ball out of the park, ace your next volleyball serve, and improve your ball control when playing hoops.

These 295 pages are filled with all the best tips and advice you need to get ahead in everything you do. Because let's face it, you wear a lot of hats in a day. They may say that a woman's work is never done, but I take my hat off to you men. Your plates are full, too!

—Deanna Portz, Editor

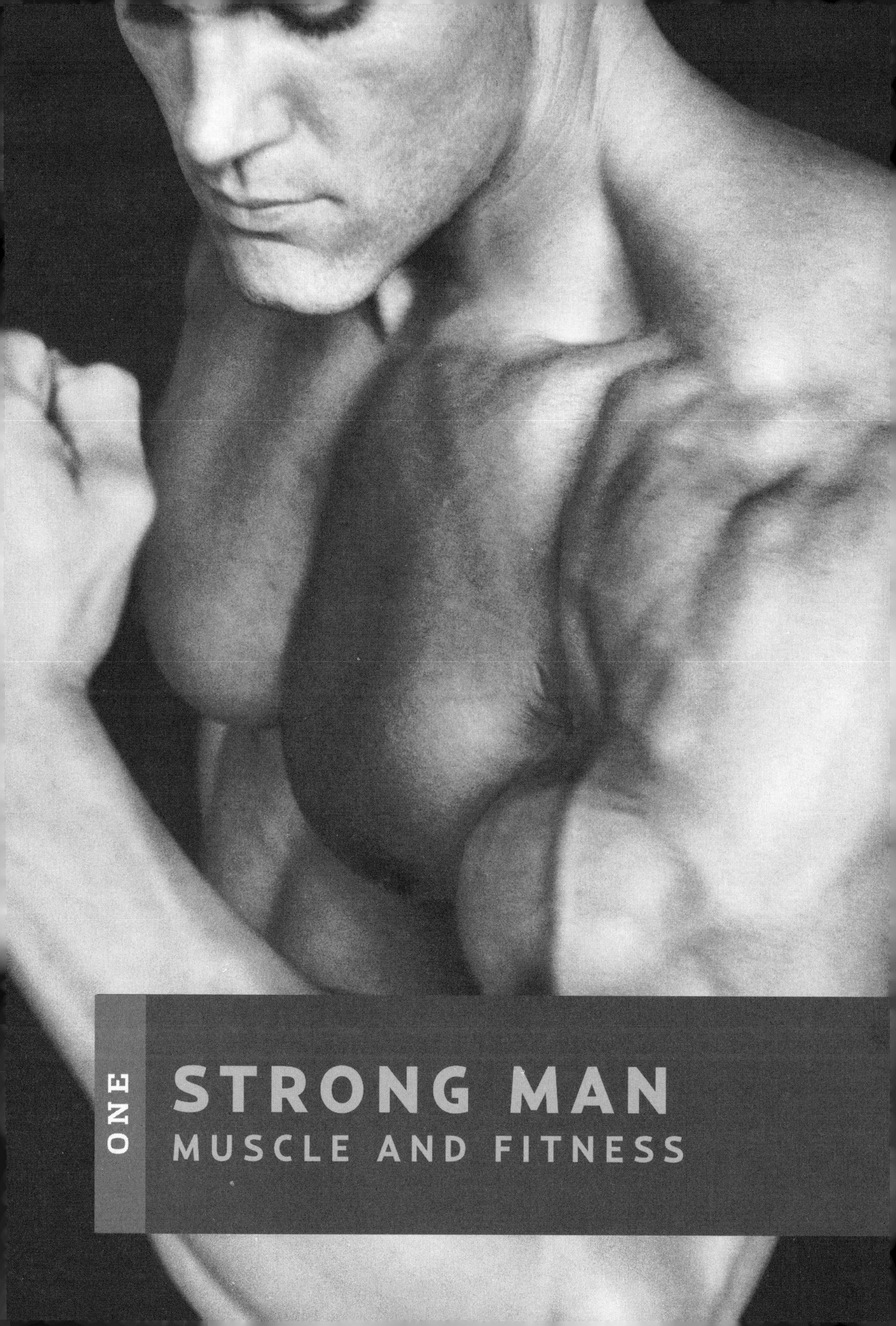

ONE

STRONG MAN

MUSCLE AND FITNESS

MUST READS

The Body You Want

You're just weeks away from more muscle

Whether you yearn for washboard abs, big biceps, or a strong heart, here are 45 of the best tips ever collected on the subject. The only catch is, now you don't have any excuses.

NEVER MISS ANOTHER WORKOUT

Fifty percent of people drop out of their exercise programs within 6 months. Here's how to (finally) stick with yours.

Put your money where your muscle is. A trainer will charge you for an exercise session if you cancel without notice. Treat yourself the same way. Pay a spouse or friend $5 if you miss a scheduled workout. Or take the opposite tack: Pay yourself for every session you attend. Put the money in a fund for a new set of golf clubs, say, or those calf implants you've been eyeing.

Bet on yourself. One study found that people who bet $40 that they could stick with an exercise program for 6 months had a 97 percent success rate. So wager with a workout partner—first man to slack off pays up. Hell, bet a cool grand and you'll never miss a workout again.

Schedule your training. Make appointments for exercise as you do for meetings. If your secretary schedules your business lunches, ask her to schedule your workouts as well. When one needs to be bumped, she can automatically reschedule it for you.

Cross off your workouts. Mark an X on your calendar on the days you exercise. Researchers found that those who used this simple system of tracking workouts made more progress than those who didn't.

Set a 20-minute rule. Make a deal with yourself that even when you're dog tired, you'll do a light workout on your scheduled days. Even if you only

THE MONTH MOST GYM MEMBERS STOP GOING REGULARLY TO THE GYM: March

work up a light sweat or get your heart rate up to 55 to 65 percent of max, most of the time that's enough.

Ask your wife to join you. You'll follow an exercise program better if you work out with your spouse. Nearly half of men who exercise alone quit their programs after 1 year, but two-thirds of those who exercise with their partners stick it out.

Set specific goals. Research shows that people who set goals that are too general ("I want to get in shape") typically don't achieve them. Make sure your goals are specific and challenging, yet realistic. And set a deadline: "Each week I'm going to run 10 minutes longer, and after a month, I want to be able to run 5 miles without stopping."

GET LEANER (AND CLEANER)

Shower before working out. Hot water warms muscles enough to loosen them for exercise.

Blow-dry your feet. To avoid athlete's foot, use a hair dryer to evaporate the moisture from your feet after showering.

THREE MOST POPULAR WORKOUTS

Get fit watching TV. Remember those drinking games from college? You know, someone said "Bob" on *Newhart* and you took a drink? Do the same with exercise and you'll be rippling without missing *Boston Public.*

For instance . . .

The Program	Your Program
The Simpsons	10 pushups every time Homer says, "Doh!"
ER	10 forward lunges whenever a doctor yells, "Stat!"
Any morning show	10 curls whenever the host takes a sip of coffee
America's Most Wanted	10 standing pushups (up against the wall and spread 'em) every time a suspect is cuffed
SportsCenter	10 jumping jacks per smirk (you'll be busy)
Cops	Start pedaling a stationary bike when a pursuit begins. Stop when the perp is apprehended.
The Tonight Show	15 crunches each time Jay Leno laughs at one of his own jokes

Exercise your entire body in 10 minutes. The "four-count squat thrust" works many major muscle groups at the same time. To do it, stand with your feet shoulder-width apart. Quickly drop to a squat so that your knees are touching your chest, and put your hands on the floor in front of you (count one). With your hands still on the floor, shoot your legs to the rear so you're in a pushup position (count two). Draw your knees back to your chest (count three), then explosively push off to stand up again (count four). Perform with continuous motion, each step leading directly into the next. Three sets of 20 will wind you. Works the chest, shoulders, arms, legs, buttocks, and lower back.

Use every machine in the gym. Each type of cardiovascular machine trains your muscles differently. It makes more sense to use each machine for a short time than to spend your entire workout on one. If you have a half hour for cardio, spend 10 minutes each on the treadmill, stairclimber, and stationary bike. Tomorrow opt for the rower, elliptical trainer, and VersaClimber. You'll get a better workout, and it'll be less boring.

MOST AWESOME MOVE

The One-Handed Pushup. Spread your legs as wide as possible and move your arm toward the center of your body. Then simply press up as you would for a normal pushup. If that's too difficult, put your hand on an elevated surface, such as a chair. This reduces the percentage of body weight you have to lift, making the exercise easier. When you can do three sets of eight repetitions with your hand on a chair, you're ready to drop to the floor.

THE BEST AB EXERCISE EVER

Biomechanics researchers at San Diego State University hooked up exercisers to an electromyograph machine and determined that the bicycle maneuver worked the rectus abdominis muscles 150 percent harder than a crunch. Lie on your back, hands behind your head, and crunch your left knee to your right elbow; using a pedaling motion, alternate sides. If your abs are covered by a layer of fat, cut 250 to 500 calories a day from your diet (or 10 to 20 percent of the calories it takes to maintain your current weight). Focus on eliminating refined carbohydrates, such as white bread and pasta. Don't bother working your abs more often. It takes 250,000 crunches to burn just 1 pound of fat—that's about 100 crunches a day for 7 years.

WEIGHT LIFT FOR WEIGHT LOSS

Hit the gym before you hit the road. One of the oldest debates in the gym—right up there with whether women wear thongs for personal pleasure or athletic function—is the question of whether you should do aerobic exercise before or after weight lifting. To find an answer, we hooked a fit guy to equipment that measures calorie expenditure and reveals how many of those calories come from fat. We had him do identical combinations of aerobics and strength training on 2 different days, once doing aerobics first, once hitting the weights first. The weight workout consisted of 15 sets; the aerobic workout was 20 minutes. Here are the results.

Weights, then aerobics
Total calories burned: 371
Calories of fat burned: 107

Aerobics, then weights
Total calories burned: 346
Calories of fat burned: 66

ALL-TIME BEST WEIGHT-LIFTING TIPS

Completely burn yourself out. Partial repetitions, or "burns," consist of pressing a weight only partway up. You do them at the end of your usual set, when you're too tired to do any additional full reps. Burns allow you to go beyond what you'd normally do and place a little more overload on the muscles. Here's what to do: Let's say you've bench-pressed a weight 10 times and you can't do it even once more. Instead of letting the weight down and moving on to the next exercise, slowly lower it just a few inches. Then raise it back to the fully extended position. Often you can squeeze out two or three additional half reps before your muscles completely fatigue. That extra bit of effort builds a sizable amount of strength.

Get Popeye forearms. Find a broomstick that's at least 8 inches long and drill a hole in the center. Thread a 3-foot-long rope through the hole and tie one end to the stick. Attach a 2½-pound barbell plate to the other end of the rope. Now hold the stick at both ends, standing with your feet shoulder-width apart and your arms out in front of you. Your forearms should be parallel to the floor, palms down. Roll the stick so the rope wraps around it. Continue rolling until the weight reaches the stick. Now roll in the opposite direction until the plate is back where it started. Do this exercise three times for a complete forearm workout, adding a pound whenever the exercise becomes easy. Over time, this will give you more than just Popeye-like arms; you'll also get a firmer handshake and a distinct advantage in any sport in which you have to carry or hit a ball.

Power through a pyramid. Pressed for time? In one quick series, you can get your muscles warm, do your exercise, and cool down. It's called the pyramid system of weight lifting. We'll use the curl as an example: Stand at a dumbbell rack and pick up a pair of light weights—say, maybe half of what you'd normally lift for 10 repetitions. Curl them five times. Then, after a short pause, replace them with the next-heaviest dumbbells and do five more repetitions. Continue up the rack until you reach a weight that's too heavy to curl five times. Then begin working your way back down through the weights until the lightest pair of dumbbells becomes a chore. (You'll know you're doing it right if, by the end of the pyramid, you look a little silly straining to lift the tiniest weight you can find.)

Make the easy part hard. There are two parts to every exercise: lifting the weight and lowering it. It's sensible to assume that most muscle building comes from lifting because it seems more difficult, but studies find that the lowering, or negative, phase may actually be more important. Concentrate on slower, better-controlled negative movements. Spend 2 seconds lifting and 4 seconds lowering.

Calculate your max. To determine how much weight you can lift in any one exercise without herniating yourself, do some math. Add 33 percent to the weight you can use for 10 repetitions. If you consistently bench 150 pounds, for instance, your max should be about 200.

Ask someone to scream at you. You'll be able to lift 5 to 8 percent more weight if you receive oral encouragement from a spotter. It could be the difference between a 200-pound and a 215-pound bench press.

Get older, get stronger. The closer you move to the half-century mark, the more your focus should shift toward strength training. If you don't do any resistance exercise, you'll lose about 10 percent of your muscle mass between ages 25 and 50. Between 50 and 80, you lose another 35 percent. Everyone should be lifting weights by midlife. However, don't stop your cardiovascular exercise; it will help ward off heart disease.

BENCH-PRESS MORE

Focus on your triceps, not your chest. With hands shoulder-width apart and elbows tucked close to your body, press the bar up in a straight line from your lower sternum. By pushing the bar in a straight line instead of back toward your head (as most men do), you decrease the distance it moves by about 10 inches. This will enable you to lift more weight.

THE ONLY STRETCH YOU NEED

End every workout with this one move that works 10 muscles: Sit on the floor with your right leg straight in front of you. Bend your left leg and put the sole of your left foot against the inside of your right thigh. (Your legs will look like the number 4.) With your right hand, try to touch either your right ankle or your right big toe. This stretches your right calf, Achilles tendon, hamstring, hip, knee, glutes, lower back, shoulder, and wrist. Hold the position for 30 to 60 seconds, then switch sides.

INCREDIBLE FITNESS TRICKS

Practice sports with a strobe. Buy a strobe light for 25 bucks at an electronics store. Then go into a darkened room and turn it on. Now practice some basic skills. Play catch or putt a golf ball into a practice cup. The strobe causes visual "noise" that makes your eyes work harder to see the ball. In normal light, it'll become much easier to concentrate because your eyes will have grown accustomed to flashes of dark and light. The ball will actually look slower and larger.

Take honey before a workout. Honey is a cheap alternative to pre-exercise sports drinks and carbohydrate gels. Researchers gave people about 3 tablespoons of honey just before their workouts. Turns out that nature's carbohydrate gel was just as good a source of energy as commercially available products. You'd have to slug a liter of a sports drink for the same effect.

Dress as if it's 10 degrees warmer. You should feel slightly chilled when you start exercising in cold weather. If you're cozy, you're overdressed.

Improve your peripheral vision. Here's a trick from former U.S. senator and Knicks star Bill Bradley: As you walk down the street, keep your eyes looking straight ahead. Now rattle off the objects you can see at the very edges of your vision. Bradley claims this exercise helped him develop the kind of basketball skills that other athletes believed were God-given.

Kick in those afterburners. For a jolt of energy late in an event, carry a small water bottle or plastic flask with defizzed cola or strong, sweet coffee. The sugar and caffeine will give you a rocketlike lift when you need it most.

Don't choke. Next time you're facing a tough opponent in any sport, try this mental trick: Focus all your intensity on one aspect of your game. In practice, say to yourself, I will not double-fault, or, He isn't going to beat me to my right. Achieving perfection in one aspect of your game will help you achieve it in everything.

Get rid of a side stitch. To ease a side stitch, push three fingers deep into your belly just below your ribs on the side that hurts, purse your lips tightly, and blow out hard. This releases pressure on the diaphragm.

Control your wind. Whatever your winter outdoor activity, try to head into the wind on your way out so you'll have it at your back on your way home. A tailwind supplies a subtle push when you're tired, thereby preventing you from slowing down and getting chilled.

Serve up a floater. If you want to serve a volleyball better, hit the center of the ball with the heel of your hand. This will make the ball "float" just like a knuckleball.

Be a better jumper. If you're new to skipping rope, do as many jumps as you can, then swing the rope beside you and continue hopping up and down. The motion will build your endurance without the frustration of stumbling over the rope as you get tired.

See the ball like never before. When you step into the batter's box, first focus your eyes on the symbol on the pitcher's cap, then focus on a point in center field, then back to the pitcher's cap. Repeat as many times as you can before the first pitch. It gets the eyes ready to track the ball.

Consult the classifieds. Be wary if you see lots of ads for the same exercise machine in the classified section of the newspaper. This tells you that although a lot of people were seduced by the marketing, many are unhappy with the results.

HOW DO I GET A COVER-MODEL BODY?

Gregg Avedon is one of *Men's Health*'s most popular cover guys. Here are his tips for getting lean and ripped.

Eat frequently. "I eat six to nine meals every day, whether I'm trying to lose weight, add muscle, or maintain. I count snacks as meals, and I try to get at least 20 grams of protein per larger meal."

Supplement at breakfast. "By taking supplements with breakfast, I benefit throughout the day. Plus, it cuts the queasy feeling I get when I take them on an empty stomach. Three essentials: a multivitamin, alpha lipoic acid [a dietary antioxidant], and glutamine [to enhance protein metabolism]."

Push or pull. "Organize your workouts according to pushing and pulling movements. Work your chest, shoulders, and triceps 1 day [pushing]; your legs, back, and biceps the next [pulling]. Do this 4 days a week, exercising each muscle group twice."

Curl like an Olympian. "Use an Olympic barbell [straight, 7 feet long, 43 pounds] for standing biceps curls. It thickens the muscles more than an EZ-curl bar [zigzag]. When curling with dumbbells, touch the inner part of the weight to the outside of your shoulder. This works the outer half of the biceps."

Shake it up midmorning and after a workout. "A protein shake at around 10 A.M. gives me energy, and a shake after each of my workouts helps repair and fortify muscle. My favorite shake contains 22 grams of whey protein and 8 to 12 ounces of water. I eat a couple of pieces of fruit with the shake because I enjoy carbs more that way."

BEST BASKETBALL DRILL

Play blind. For quickness on the court, ball control is more crucial than running speed. You need to have a sense of where the ball is at all times. One way to develop this is a method called "blind dribbling." Start by bouncing the ball while walking up and down the court with your eyes closed. You'll begin to develop a sixth sense of where the ball is; soon you'll be able to change directions quickly and easily without losing the ball. Likewise, shoot 5 to 10 free throws conventionally, then try shooting blindfolded. By practicing without the benefit of vision, you'll learn the mechanics more quickly, since you'll be forced to concentrate more intensely.

BEST GOLF TIPS

Cut the hole in half. Golfers always try to play the longest possible shot from the tee, hoping to smash a 280-yard drive and reduce the length of the next shot. But for duffers, this rarely works. Try this strategy instead: If the hole is longer than 220 yards and shorter than 340 yards, divide the total yardage by two. For example, let's say the hole is 320 yards. Divide by two and you have 160 yards. Can you consistently hit a straight shot 160 yards? If you can, play two 160-yard shots and you'll be on or near the green. If you can't, play two shots of, say, 140 yards and you'll be close enough to chip. If the hole is more than 340 yards, divide the total by three and use the same logic.

Make practice perfect. Ben Hogan, the greatest golfer of his time, would practice his drive by hitting 50 balls in 2 hours. He'd have a purpose for each shot. That's how you should practice. The average guy gets a bucket of balls and hits 50 in 20 minutes. That just reinforces mistakes.

RUN FASTER AND FARTHER

Run in place with dumbbells. Grab a pair of light dumbbells and stand with one foot about 24 inches in front of the other. Now do a smooth and controlled running motion with your arms, keeping your elbows bent 90 degrees and your feet stationary. Continue for 30 seconds, then reverse your stance and repeat. Arm movements are important in locomotion—if you doubt us, try running with your arms straight down at your sides. More powerful arm movements lead to more powerful locomotion. This is why sprinters do a lot of upper-body strength training and why any runner can improve performance with this exercise.

Listen to your feet. To be a better runner, you need quiet feet. If you hear them hitting the ground, you're not running well. You don't want to be pounding the pavement. That's too hard on your joints. Keep your feet close to the ground, using a quick, shuffling stride.

Make the grade 1 percent. If you want to mimic road running on a treadmill, raise the incline to 1 percent before starting your run. Researchers found that this is the degree of treadmill elevation that most closely approximates running outdoors on the road.

SWIM STRONGER AND LONGER

Become a human torpedo. Streamlining is the secret to swimming fast. It involves making your body as long and narrow as possible, and it can trim as many as 10 strokes from one lap in an Olympic-size pool. To make yourself more streamlined, grab a chinup bar before your workout and hang for a while. Position your hands so your thumbs are touching and your palms are facing away from you. Point your toes to the floor. Put your head between your arms so your ears are in front of your biceps, and try to squeeze your shoulder blades together. Hang for 10 seconds, drop off the bar and take a 10-second breather, then hang for 10 seconds more. After a few sessions, increase your hang time to 20 seconds with a 15-second break.

Take a dip. If you've just finished some laps and want to squeeze in some resistance training, stay in the pool and do a few dips. Just by swimming to the edge of the pool and raising your body in and out of the water (as you would on dip bars), you'll exercise your triceps, chest, and back—and also get in some shoulder and forearm work.

STOP A HURT

The recipe for treating a minor muscle pull or strain is pretty simple—rest, ice, compression, and elevation (RICE)—but a lot of guys screw up the elevation part. Unless you've got the injured area above the level of your heart—and preferably above your head as well—you're not minimizing the swelling. And within 24 to 48 hours, try to do some light aerobic exercise. This will deliver fresh blood to the injured site, blast out lactic-acid buildup, and significantly speed recovery time.

Muscles in a Minute

Stay pumped for hours with these quick workouts

By Scott Quill

Patience is for mutual funds and deep-space probes, not muscles. Sometimes we want our bodies to look their best right now.

Maybe you want case-hardened abs for a day on the beach. Or you want your arms to pop at the picnic. Or you need a chest that fills your suit coat at the reunion. We'll tell you how to produce these muscles on deadline, even if you've missed a workout or three.

First, some science. When you lift weights, your muscles contract and apply pressure to the blood vessels running through them. This impedes the normal flow of blood and oxygen (it's an "anaerobic" exercise). When you're finished, blood pressure subsides and backed-up blood and oxygen flood in, temporarily expanding your muscles. Which is why you look good in the locker-room mirror. "That pump you have after a workout is related to an increase in bloodflow," says Jay Hoffman, Ph.D., associate professor of health and exercise science at the College of New Jersey.

You can make that postworkout surge last longer. A recent study published in *Medicine and Science in Sports and Exercise* concludes that doing more reps with less weight provides a longer-lasting pump than fewer reps with more weight. That's the philosophy behind the short workouts that follow, each designed to give you muscle at a moment's notice.

CHEST PUMP

This iron-free workout is ideal "before you jump into the shower before a date," says Scott Rankin, C.S.C.S., a trainer in Toronto.

Perform as many pushups as you can in 1 minute. (Keep count.) Without resting, move into a modified pushup position, your knees on the ground. Do as many repetitions as you can in 1 minute. (Keep count.) Then, hold yourself about 2 inches off the ground for 20 seconds—or as long as you can.

That's one superset. Rest only long enough for the burning in your muscles to subside, then repeat the superset twice. Your goal is to not let the amount of either type of pushup drop by more than five each superset. If you can do more, your rest periods are too long.

ARM PUMP

"Remember that the upper-arm muscles are 60 percent triceps and only 40 percent biceps. You want to work the triceps just as hard as the biceps," says Tim Kuebler, C.S.C.S., a Kansas City–based personal trainer. Rest 4 to 5 minutes between these exercises.

OVEREXTENSION KICKBACK

Grab a light dumbbell in your right hand and place your left hand and knee on a bench. Plant your right foot flat on the floor. Bend forward at the hips so your torso is parallel to the floor. Hold the dumbbell next to your thigh with a neutral grip (palm facing your leg).

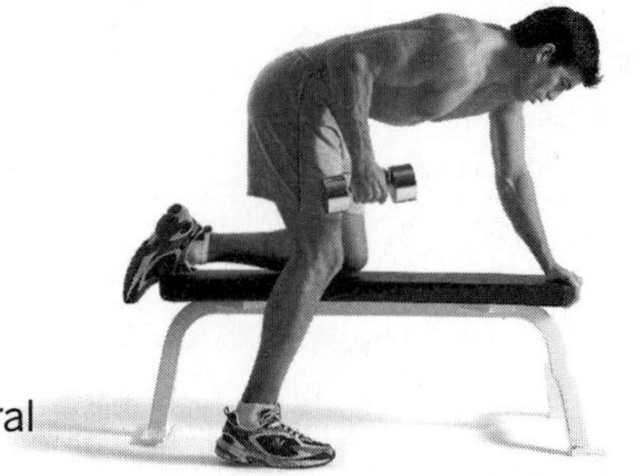

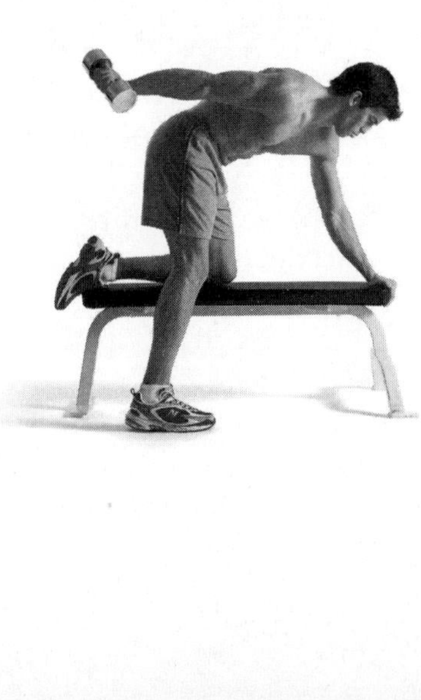

Lift the weight up and back. As the weight clears your butt, slowly rotate your palm up toward the ceiling so that the back of your hand faces your body by the time your arm is straightened. Pause, then slowly return to the starting position. Do three sets of eight repetitions with each arm. Rest 2 to 3 minutes between sets.

BENCH DIP

Place your hands behind you on the edge of a bench and your feet on another bench a few feet in front of you. Ask someone to place a few weight plates on your lap and steady them so they don't fall.

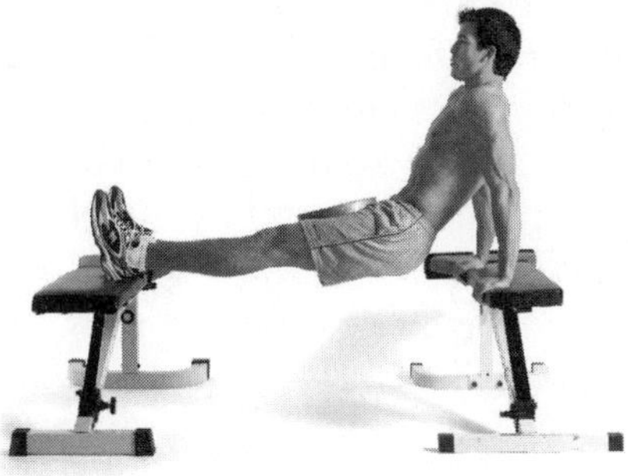

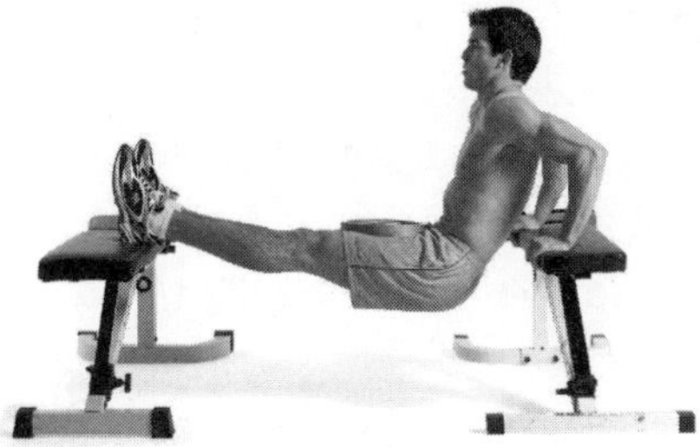

Lower your body until your upper arms are nearly parallel to the floor. Pause, then press back to the starting position. As you fatigue, ask your spotter to remove one weight plate at a time; continue until you can't do any more with only your body weight. Now, place your feet flat on the floor with your knees bent as if you were seated in an invisible chair; lower your body as before, completing as many repetitions as you can.

SUPINATING DUMBBELL CURL

Hold light dumbbells at your sides, palms toward you.

Curl the weights up, rotating your wrists inward 180 degrees by the time the weights reach your shoulders. Reverse this motion as you lower the weights. Do three sets of 8 to 12 repetitions, resting 2 to 3 minutes between sets.

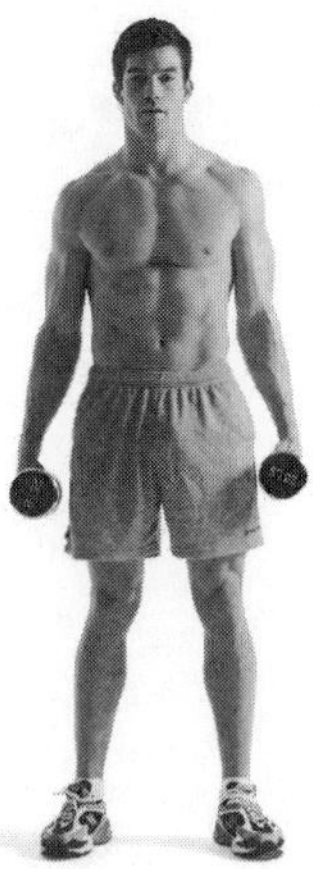

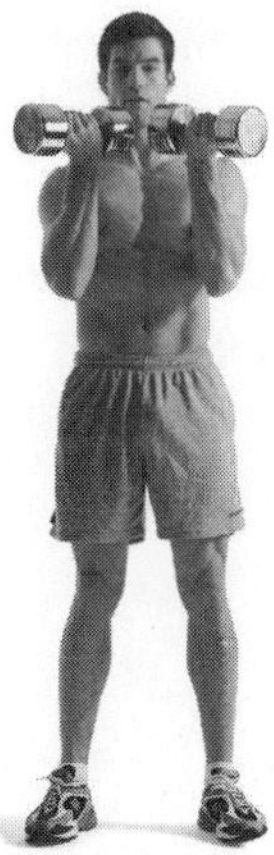

Rest 5 minutes and perform one set of preacher curls. Start with a weight that's about 80 percent of your maximum and do as many repetitions as you can. Remove 10 to 15 percent of the weight and start again without rest. Continue removing weight and curling until you can no longer curl the bar.

AB PUMP

Tire the obliques first so your rectus abdominis—the six-pack—is isolated later, Rankin says. Perform this workout as a circuit, with no rest between exercises. Do three circuits, resting 60 seconds after each.

MODIFIED BICYCLE KICK

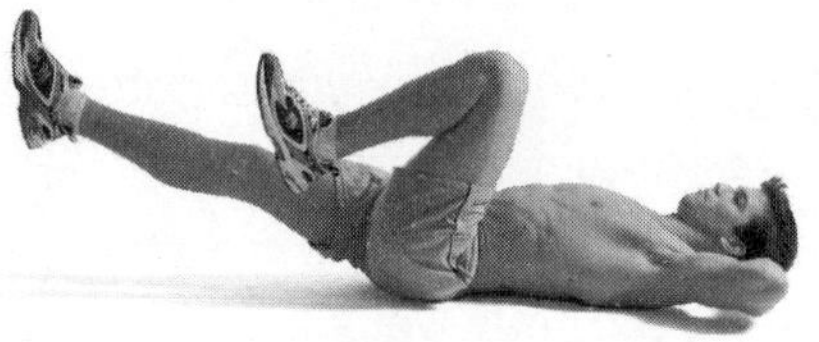

Lie on the floor with your hands behind your head, your right leg straight and off the floor. Bend your left leg so your knee is pulled toward your chest.

Lift your shoulder blades off the floor and take a count of two to touch your right elbow to your left knee. Pause, lower your elbow and shoulder blades back to the floor (again to a count of two), then immediately repeat the move on the other side—bringing your left elbow to your right knee and straightening your left leg. Complete 15 repetitions on each side. Now do 30 conventional crunches.

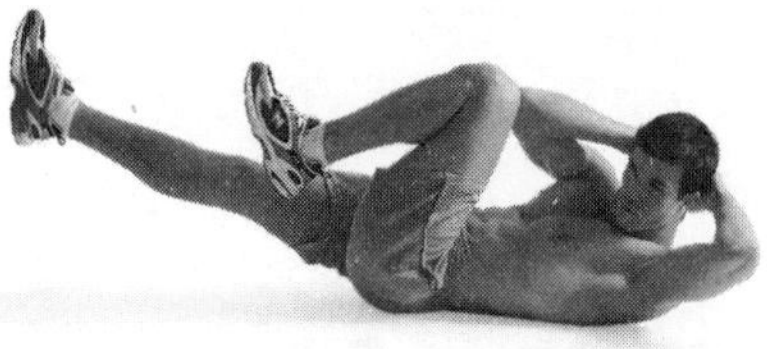

REVERSE CRUNCH

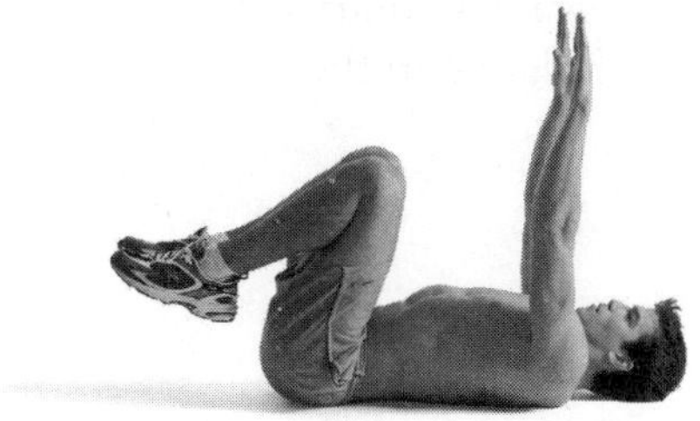

Lie faceup on the floor with your arms straight above you or braced on the sides of a doorway. Bend your knees and lift your heels off the floor and toward your butt.

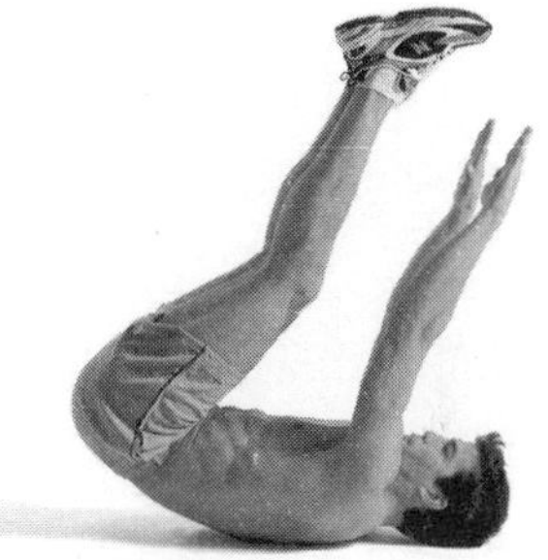

Roll your hips up, bringing your knees toward your chest. As your lower back rises off the floor, straighten your legs, point your toes to the ceiling, and lift your hips. Pause, then slowly reverse the motion. Do 20 repetitions.

ROLLUP

Lie faceup on the floor with your legs straight and your arms at your sides.

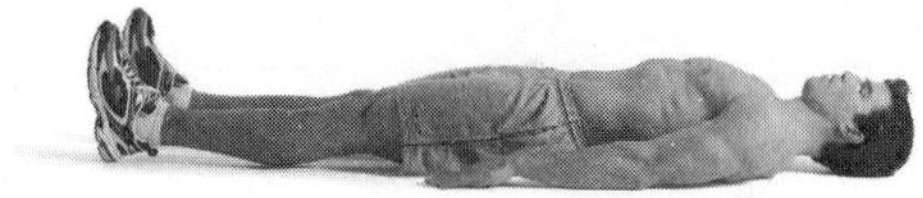

Push your heels into the ground and slowly lift your shoulders and back off the floor. Pause when your upper body is perpendicular to the floor, then slowly lower your body to a count of five. Perform 10 repetitions.

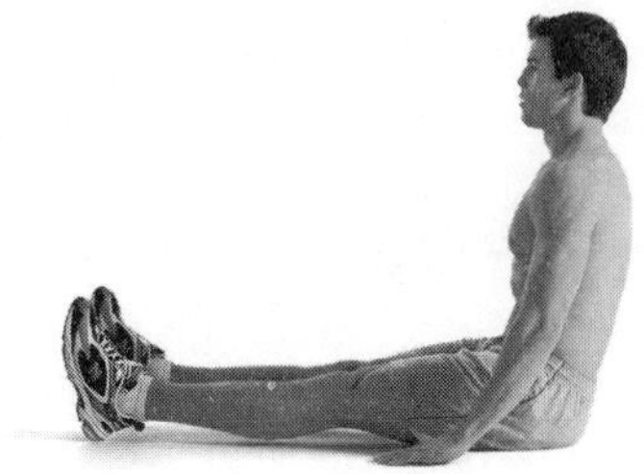

20 Ways to Stick to Your Workout

Fading motivation is the enemy of every great fitness plan. To stoke the fires, top trainers reveal their never-quit, get-fit-quick tricks

By Adam Campbell

You have the right to remain weak. Or fat. Or skinny. But you should know that every workout you miss can and will be used against you to make your muscles smaller and weaker, your belly bigger, and your life shorter. Unfortunately, most Americans are exercising their right not to exercise.

A recent study by the National Center for Health Statistics found that only 19 percent of the population regularly engages in "high levels of physical activity." (That's defined as three intense 20-minute workouts per week.) Another 63 percent—about the same percentage as that of Americans who are overweight—believe that exercising would make them healthier, leaner, and less stressed, but they don't do it. At the root of this problem is motivation, or the lack thereof.

It's the difference between wanting to exercise and actually doing it. That's why the advice you're about to read is priceless. We've filled these pages with the favorite motivational strategies of the top personal trainers in the country. Their livelihoods, in fact, depend on the effectiveness of their tips to inspire their clients to exercise—and to stick with it. After all, statistics don't pay by the hour.

1. Sign up for a distant race. That is, one that's at least 500 miles away. The extra incentive of paying for airfare and a hotel room will increase your motivation to follow your training plan, says Carolyn Ross-Toren, chairwoman of the Mayor's Fitness Council in San Antonio.

2. Make a "friendly" bet. Challenge your nemesis—that idea-stealing coworker or a nonmowing neighbor—to a contest. The first guy to drop 15 pounds, run a 6-minute mile, or bench-press 250 pounds wins. The key: "Make sure it's someone you don't particularly like," says Michael Mejia, C.S.C.S., *Men's Health* exercise advisor. (It's okay if your rival thinks you're best friends.)

3. Tie exercise to your health. Check your cholesterol. Then set a goal of lowering your LDL cholesterol by 20 points and increasing your HDL cholesterol by 5 points. "You'll decrease your risk of heart disease while providing yourself with a very important, concrete goal," says John Thyfault, Ph.D., C.S.C.S., an exercise researcher at East Carolina University. Ask your doctor to write a prescription for new blood work in a month. You'll just have to go to the lab, and the doctor will call you with the results.

4. Switch your training partners. Working out with a partner who will hold you accountable for showing up at the gym works well—for a while. But the more familiar you are with the partner, the easier it becomes to back out of workout plans. "Close friends and family members don't always make the best training partners because they may allow you to slack off or cancel workouts," says Jacqueline Wagner, C.S.C.S., a trainer in New York City. To keep this from happening, find a new, less forgiving workout partner every few months.

5. Compete. Find a sport or event that you enjoy, and train to compete in it. "It adds a greater meaning to each workout," says Alex Koch, Ph.D., C.S.C.S., an exercise researcher (and competitive weight lifter) at Truman State University. Consider training for the World Master's games, an Olympics-like competition for regular guys held in Edmonton, Canada, in July 2005. Events include basketball, rowing, golf, triathlon, and weight lifting. You can register through May 20th at www.2005worldmasters.com.

6. Think about fat. Your body is storing and burning fat simultaneously, but it's always doing one faster than the other. "Understanding that you're getting either fatter or leaner at any one time will keep you body-conscious so you won't overeat or underexercise," says Alwyn Cosgrove, C.S.C.S., owner of Results Fitness Training in Santa Clarita, California.

7. Do a daily gut check. Place your fingers on your belly and inhale deeply so that it expands. As you exhale, contract your abdominal muscles and push your fingertips against your hard abdominal wall. Now pinch. "You're holding pure fat between your fingers," says Tom Seabourne, Ph.D., author of *Athletic Abs*. Do this every day, 30 minutes before your workout, and you'll find that you'll rarely decide to skip it.

8. Join a fitness message board. It'll be full of inspiration from men who have accomplished their goals and are working toward new ones. Our particular favorite: the Belly-Off Club Forum at menshealth.com, where guys post their questions, tips, and success stories to help other men in their quest to lose weight.

9. Strike an agreement with your wife and kids. The rule: You get 1 hour to yourself every day, provided that you use it for exercise (and reciprocate the favor). So there's no pressure to do household chores, play marathon games of Monopoly, or be a doting husband (a fat, doting husband). "Since it's for your health, it's a contract they can't refuse. And that will allow you to exercise guilt-free while acting as a role model for your children," says Darren Steeves, C.S.C.S., a trainer in Canada.

10. Burn a workout CD. Studies have shown that men who pedal stationary cycles while listening to their favorite music will do so longer and more intensely than men who exercise without music. So burn a disc with your favorite adrenaline-boosting songs (maybe something by Limp Bizkit or—if you're over 40—Hot Tuna).

11. Plan your workouts in advance. At the start of each month, schedule all of your workouts at once, and cross them off as they're completed. For an average month, you might try for a total of 16 workouts. If any are left undone at the end of the month, tack them on to the following month. And make sure you have a contingency plan for bad weather and unscheduled meetings. "You're about 40 percent more likely to work out if you have strategies to help you overcome these obstacles," says Rod Dishman, Ph.D., an exercise scientist at the University of Georgia.

12. Squat first. If you have trouble finishing your weight workout, start with the exercises you dread. "You'll look forward to your favorite exercises at the end of your workout, which will encourage you to complete the entire session," says John Williams, C.S.C.S., co-owner of Spectrum Conditioning in Port Washington, New York.

13. Schedule a body-composition test every 2 months. It'll provide you with a clear end date for the simple goal of losing body fat or gaining muscle. "Tangible results are the best motivator," says Tim Kuebler, C.S.C.S., a trainer in Kansas City, Missouri. Your gym probably offers the service for a small fee—just make sure the same trainer performs the test each time.

14. Don't do what you hate. "Whenever you start to dread your workout, do what appeals to you instead," says John Raglin, Ph.D., an exercise psychologist at Indiana University. If you loathe going to a gym, try working out at home. (Check the *Men's Health Home Workout Bible* for ideas.) If you despise the treadmill, then jump rope, lift weights, or find a basketball court. Bottom line: If you're sick of your routine, find a new one.

15. Go through the motions. On days when you don't feel like working out, make the only requirement of your exercise session a single set of your favorite exercise. "It's likely that once you've started, you'll finish," says Rachel Cosgrove,

CHEAP TRICK

Money is a great motivator. Invest in your fitness program by buying these training gadgets, and you'll gain momentum from measuring your workout results.

Gulick Tape Measure. It ensures accurate measurements of your arms, chest, and waist by applying constant tension—6 ounces—to the tape. So it automatically controls the tightness of the tape every time, in contrast to ordinary tape measures, which produce varying results depending on how hard or lightly you pull. $23, performbetter.com

Skyndex I Electronic Fat Kaliper. These electronic skinfold calipers "remember" each measurement and automatically calculate your body fat, unlike standard calipers, which leave the complicated mathematical formulas up to you. $450, performbetter.com

Myo Dynamics Training-Nutrition Manager 2.0. Use this software to analyze your diet and track your strength and endurance progress. It instantly calculates your one-repetition maximum and the total weight lifted each workout—so you always have a number to beat in your next session. It's the perfect tool to help you create attainable goals, a habit YMCA researchers found more than doubles the likelihood that you'll stick with an exercise program. $65, myodynamics.com

C.S.C.S. If you still don't feel like being in the gym, go home. This way, you never actually stop exercising; you just have some gaps in your training log.

16. Start a streak. There's nothing like a winning streak to attract fans to the ballpark. Do the same for your workout by trying to set a new record for consecutive workouts without a miss. "Every time your streak ends, strive to set a longer mark in your next attempt," says Williams.

17. Make your goals attractive. "To stay motivated, frame your goals so that they drive you to achieve them," suggests Charles Staley, owner of edtsecrets.com. For example, if you're a 200-pound guy, decide whether you'd rather bench "over 200 pounds," "the bar with two 45-pound plates on each side," or "my body weight." They're all different ways of saying the same thing, but one is probably more motivating to you than the others.

18. See your body through her eyes. Ask your wife to make like Howard Stern and identify your most displeasing physical characteristic. "It's instant motivation," says Mejia. If she's hesitant, make a list for her—abs, love handles, upper arms, and so on—and have her rank them from best to worst. Make the most-hated body part your workout focus for 4 weeks, then repeat the quiz for more motivation.

19. Buy a year's worth of protein. "If a guy believes that a supplement will help him achieve better results, he'll be more inclined to keep up his workouts in order to reap the full benefits and avoid wasting his money," says Kuebler. Stick with the stuff that really does help: protein and creatine, from major brands like MuscleTech, EAS, and Biotest.

20. Blackmail yourself. Take a picture of yourself shirtless, holding a sign that shows your e-mail address. Then e-mail it to a trusted but sadistic friend, with the following instructions: "If I don't send you a new picture that shows serious improvement in 12 weeks, post this photo at hotornot.com and send the link to the addresses listed below." (Include as many e-mail addresses—especially of female acquaintances—as possible.) "It's nasty, but extremely effective," says Alwyn Cosgrove.

Reach the Next Level

Five fresh ways to bust out of a rut

By Michael Mejia, C.S.C.S.

I was stuck. Thousands of biceps curls for months on end, and nothing. Not even half an inch. My arms had simply stopped growing.

I took the Taoist approach: I quit trying. Instead of doing direct arm work, like curls, I concentrated on my chest, shoulders, and back, hitting them with heavy-lifting sets of chinups, rows, presses, and dips.

That's when it happened. My arms inflated.

Truth is, I hadn't really stopped working my arms. I was working them harder than ever—by association. The exercises I was using for my chest and back were also enlisting my biceps and triceps, stimulating more muscle fibers in different ways than with the arm-isolation exercises.

My realization: Changing the training approach is the trigger for blasting

ARMS WITHOUT CURLS

Most men who want big arms assume they have to do biceps curls and triceps extensions. But those are performed with limited weights. If you do exercises that require lifting more weight and enlisting more muscles, your arms will take care of themselves. Try this workout. Your arms will thank you.

Workout A

SUPERSET 1

Start with a set of chinups, then follow with the close-grip bench press.

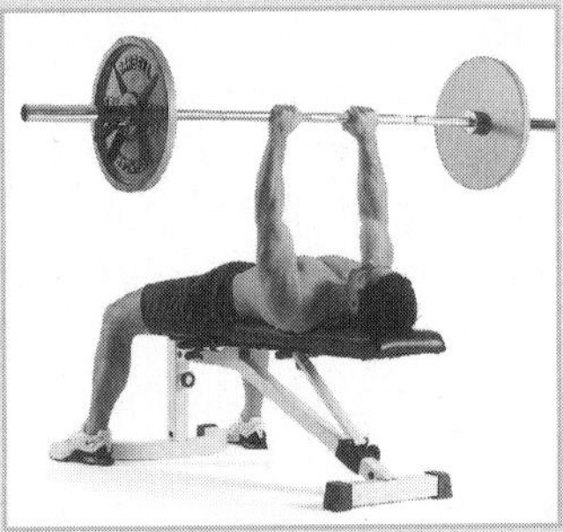

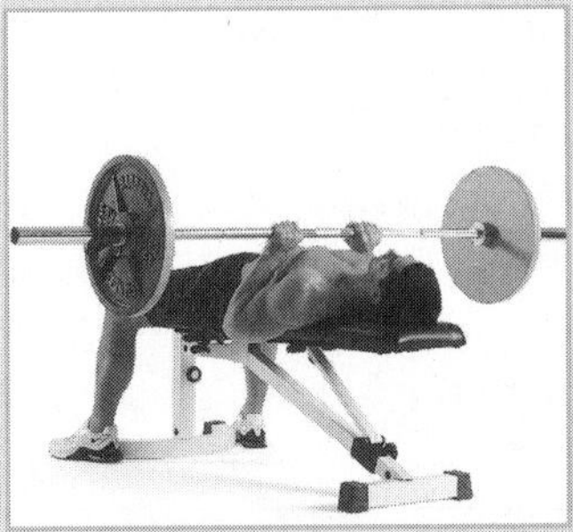

SUPERSET 2

Start with a set of military presses, then follow with the bent-over row.

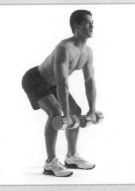

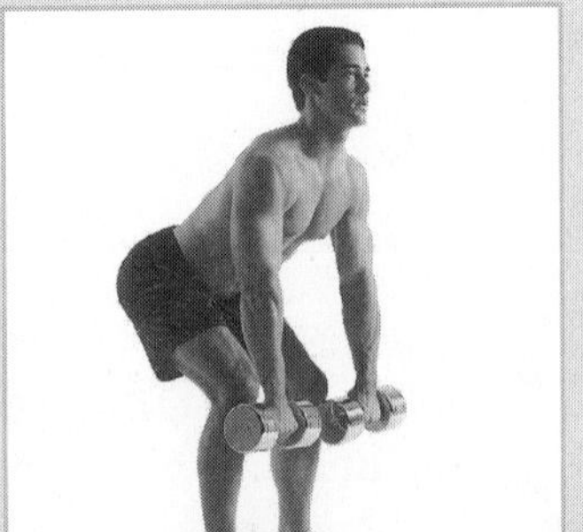

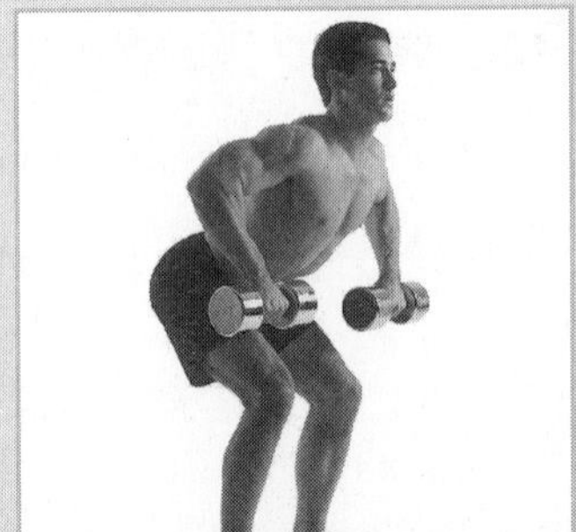

through a frustrating plateau, in either muscle or strength.

Since then, I've experimented with dozens of rut-busting methods. Here I list five of the best. For maximum benefit, use only one technique at a time, for one exercise at a time, every 4 weeks. If you've been lifting consistently for a year or more, you'll change the look of your workout—and of your muscles.

General rules: Alternate between Workout A and Workout B every 4 days. So you might do Workout A on Monday and Workout B on Friday, then Workout A again on Tuesday. Complete four sets of six repetitions of each superset before moving to the second superset. Within each superset, don't rest between different exercises, but rest 90 seconds before starting the next pair of exercises.

Workout B

SUPERSET 1

Start with a set of dips, then follow with the upright row.

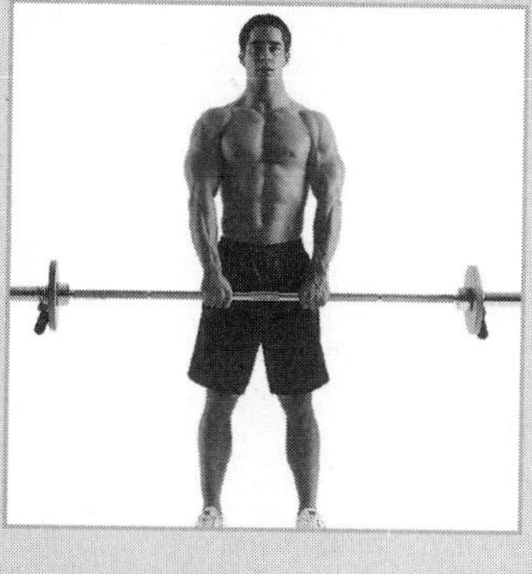

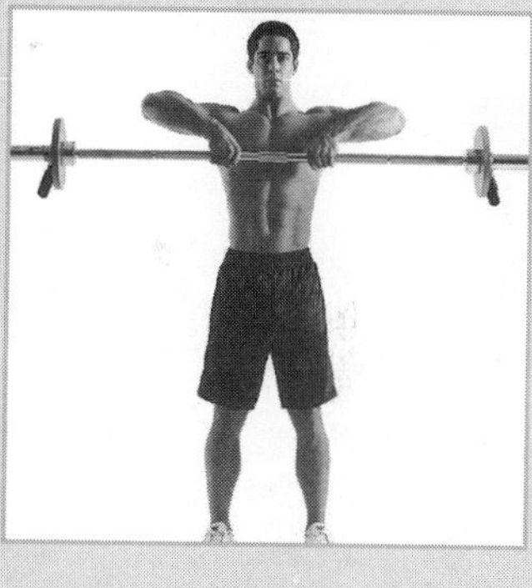

SUPERSET 2

Start with a set of pullups, then follow with the incline press.

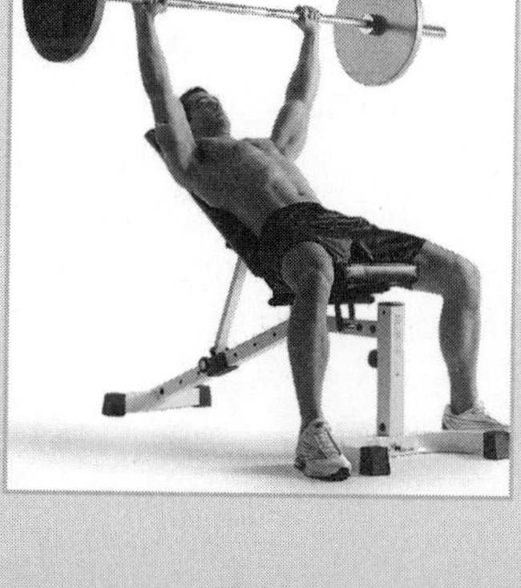

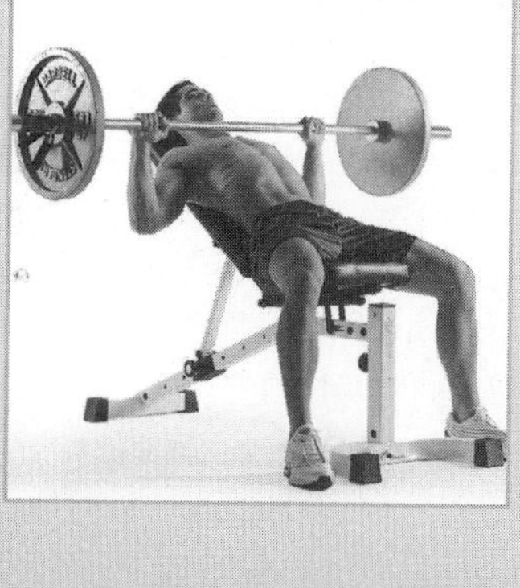

IDENTIFY WEAKNESSES

Every guy, on every lift, has a sticking point: that part of the move at which he's the weakest. Find yours and strengthen it, and you'll be able to lift heavier weights, which will make your muscles work harder and grow faster. Your weak link is easy to locate: It's the point at which your movement starts to decelerate.

The fix: "Partial overloads," an idea from Alwyn Cosgrove, C.S.C.S., a trainer and the owner of Results Fitness Training in Santa Clarita, California. Set a pair of pins in a power rack, level with your deceleration point, so you start at your weak spot. Place the barbell on the pins and perform the exercise in the shortened range of motion. For virtually any lift, follow these guidelines: Do one set of 10 repetitions, lifting about 70 percent of the maximum weight you can lift one time. Rest 3 minutes, then increase the weight by 10 to 20 percent and crank out two more sets of six repetitions.

Example: In the bench press, you'll start at the slow-down point—about two-thirds of the way up, for most men. Each time you complete a repetition, allow the bar to rest on the pins for 2 seconds, then repeat. Wait 3 minutes after each set, then finish with a full-range set of six repetitions.

THINK SMALL

"Most men try to increase the load by too much and stall their training programs as a result," says John Williams, C.S.C.S., co-owner of Spectrum Conditioning in Port Washington, New York. Adding too much weight too fast disrupts your muscles' adaptation process, which should be gradual. A psychotherapist might call it baby steps.

We prefer a much cooler term: microloading. It's the simplest way to see immediate gains when you're stuck in a rut.

The fix: Increase the weight by the smallest amount possible. This guarantees progress. "Psychologically, increasing your weight more frequently is tangible proof that you're making progress," says Williams.

Example: Use 1½-pound PlateMates for dumbbells ($15 at fitnessfactory.com) instead of jumping up in 5-pound increments. On the barbell, use 2½-pound plates instead of the 5- and 10-pounders you'd normally add on.

DO MORE

Hormones regulate almost every physiological process in the body. Stimulate the release of hormones through exercise and you'll improve body composition and performance, says Jeff Volek, Ph.D., R.D., an exercise-and-nutrition researcher at the University of Connecticut.

The fix: Start hormones flowing by doing more total sets and repetitions and limiting rest periods to 60 seconds. But restrict this to a single exercise, and switch moves every 4 weeks to avoid overtaxing your body.

Example: Decide if you're going for size or strength. For size, do five sets of 10 repetitions with a weight that's 55 to 65 percent of the amount you can lift one time. For strength, do five sets of five repetitions with a weight that's 85 to 90 percent of that amount.

LIFT LIGHT

Small blood vessels called capillaries deliver oxygen, amino acids, and hormones to your muscles, helping them recover—and grow—faster. Research has shown that heavy weight training decreases capillary density.

The fix: Do high-repetition sets with light weights (25 percent of the amount you can lift once) on your days off, targeting whatever muscle group is lagging. "It'll increase the number of capillaries in your working muscles, allowing better nutrient transfer," says Chad Waterbury, a strength coach in Arizona.

Examples: Perform a total of 100 repetitions with the light weight. So if your triceps are lacking, continue to do your normal workout 1 or 2 days a week. But you'll also do 100 repetitions of a triceps exercise on the other 5 days. Use a weight that's about 25 percent of the heaviest amount you can lift one time. Do four sets of 25 repetitions or two sets of 50 repetitions, spaced throughout the day.

MOVE FASTER

When you lift weights slowly, your body uses only whatever muscle fibers are necessary. As those fibers fatigue, others take their place, while the first ones recover and wait to return to action—it's sort of a tag-team effort. So if you're doing 10 slow repetitions, a fiber might work for the first three or four repetitions, be replaced by another, and then recover to contribute on the final two or three repetitions of your set. This limits the number of muscle fibers you're using, unless you're lifting near maximal weights.

The fix: Lift light weights fast. "Trying to move a weight as fast as you can forces your body to recruit more muscle fibers," says Craig Ballantyne, C.S.C.S., owner of workoutmanuals.com. This will help you improve strength quickly, while challenging your muscles in a different way than with heavy weights.

Example: For exercises like the bench press, use a weight that's about 40 to 55 percent of the heaviest weight you can lift one time. Do six to eight sets of three to five repetitions, resting for 60 seconds between sets.

NEED TO KNOW

Muscle Made Easier

Australian scientists may have found the ultimate muscle-building combo. A new study reports that men taking a combination of creatine and whey experienced greater muscle growth than men taking any other supplement. Researchers divided 31 male weight lifters into four groups and gave them either creatine and whey, creatine and carbohydrates, whey alone, or carbs alone. After 11 weeks, the men taking the creatine and whey were leaner and stronger and had larger muscle fibers—a key factor in determining how big your muscles look.

More Powder to You

Speaking of creatine, researchers at the Medical College of Wisconsin recently reviewed more than 500 studies on creatine supplementation published over the past 40 years. Their findings: Men under the age of 36 who take creatine for just 2 to 3 months may be able to boost their maximum bench press by 15 pounds and their squat by 21 pounds, on average.

The bad news? Creatine's strength-boosting benefits taper off as you get older. And not all creatine is created equal. When ConsumerLab.com, an independent research company, evaluated the purity of 10 brands of creatine, it found that liquid formulations often contain less creatine than listed on the label. One brand actually had 1 percent less than what it claimed. What's more, some also contained creatinine—a degraded form of creatine—and dicyandamide—an impurity with unknown effects, says Richard Kreider, Ph.D., chairman of the exercise and sport nutrition laboratory at Baylor University. Stick with the powdered form; it tested best for content and quality. Try mixing it with sweetened iced tea. Glucose carries creatine to your muscles 20 to 40 percent more efficiently than water does, says Kreider.

AVERAGE PERCENTAGE BY WHICH YOUR AMOUNT OF BODY FAT COULD INCREASE IF YOU QUIT EXERCISING FOR JUST 8 MONTHS: 8.6

The Cost of Skipping Your Workouts

Missed a workout or two? Here's what falling off your fitness routine could cost you over the next 9 months.

You get . . .	Research shows . . .	You pay . . .
Viagra	Men who don't work out have an increased risk of developing erectile dysfunction.	$135
A good tailor (to adjust your suits to your expanding waistline)	Weight loss achieved through exercise can reduce abdominal fat more successfully than diet alone.	$40
SmartSet CD/clock radio (you'll need extra help waking up)	Men who don't exercise have more trouble falling and staying asleep.	$80
2 sick days	Those who exercise less are more likely to contract upper respiratory tract infections.	$296
Wednesdays on the couch with Dr. Headshrink	A workout is a good way to fight stress and anxiety.	$3,240
Swopper ergonomic chair	Sitting in this chair will help you deal with back pain; aerobic exercise relieves pain all over your body, including your back.	$500
E.R. visit	Skip your daily workout and your bones won't get the protective benefit of exercise, putting you at risk for fractures.	$159
Gym dues	If you're not using the gym, it's wasted money.	$296
TOTAL		$4,746

A Dose of Exercise

Think of your workout as powerful medicine. Scientists at the University of Pennsylvania found that rapid bloodflow evidently fights inflammation in your arteries like a high dose of glucocorticoids, a steroid.

Inflammation is a prime suspect in heart disease. Flowing blood triggers receptors in the cells in the lining of your blood vessels, activating anti-inflammatory properties. Summing up: Inflammation bad, exercise good. Got it? Now go.

Sweat Away Stress

A new study from the University of Missouri confirms what we've been telling you for years: High-intensity exercise is one of the best ways to reduce stress and anxiety. Researchers found that people who engaged in strenuous exercise for more than 30 minutes had significantly less anxiety than individuals who pushed themselves with less intensity for a shorter period of time.

Don't Let It Bug You

The Centers for Disease Control and Prevention is warning sports teams about an antibiotic-resistant staph infection that has been plaguing athletes. "Athletes are at a particular risk because of close contact and increased incidence of broken skin," says Dan Jernigan, M.D., chief of epidemiology at the CDC, who notes that the infection is passed through shared equipment and close-contact sports. Though there have been no reported cases of staph infection spread through gyms, wipe down equipment before using it and wash your hands thoroughly after a workout.

FAST FIXES

Take the "work" out of "workout" and maybe you'd set foot in the gym more often. Besides, you have enough work to do. So change the way you approach exercise. Think of it as recess, like when you were set free on the playground as a kid. These 12 tips will help put you into this new mind-set. They make your workouts less work, so you'll get the most out of your fitness program and stick with it for the long haul.

1. Be a morning person. Bright light in the early morning may boost your testosterone levels. So spend those early hours with the fish instead of Matt and Katie. (Cloudy morning? Fluorescent lights accomplish the same thing.) Researchers at the University of California at San Diego school of medicine found that early-morning light raised levels of luteinizing hormone (LH) by 70 percent. This is exciting because LH can help hike testosterone levels—and that's exciting because higher testosterone levels can help build muscle, cut fat, and lift your mood. Researchers haven't determined whether increasing LH automatically triggers a surge in testosterone, but it can't hurt.

2. Start the week out right. Never miss a Monday workout. "Exercising on the first day of the week sparks a chain reaction in your workout program," says Jim Annesi, Ph.D., author of *Enhancing Exercise Motivation*. You'll be establishing a behavior pattern. Since our mind is wired to keep a chain reaction going, your Monday workout sets the tone for the week.

3. Set yourself up for success. The best way to reach your goals: Make failure impossible. Break down your larger goal into components. "If you're hitting the smaller goals that all lead to achieving your long-term goals, you stay motivated," says Mark Nutting, C.S.C.S., owner of Metamorph Fitness in Northport, Maine. Making progress, Nutting says, means you're less likely to get discouraged or quit.

4. Check your meds. It isn't only illegal drugs like cocaine and steroids that increase the risk of midworkout injury—many common prescription medications for men don't mix with exercise. But don't just go off the meds

PERCENTAGE BY WHICH THE AVERAGE MAN'S TESTOSTERONE LEVEL DECREASES EACH YEAR AFTER AGE 40: 1

or stay on the couch. Instead, consult this cheat sheet, created with the help of researchers from the school of pharmacy at the University of Missouri at Kansas City.

Drug: Cialis, Levitra, Viagra (erectile-dysfunction drugs)

Possible side effect: A drop in blood pressure that may leave you feeling dizzy and nauseated during a strenuous workout

Strategy: Wait at least 6 hours after taking erectile-dysfunction drugs before working out.

Drug: Crestor, Lescol, Lipitor, Mevacor, Pravachol, Zocor (cholesterol-lowering statins)

Possible side effects: Muscle aches and weakness, making it difficult to lift heavy weights or complete all your reps and sets

Strategy: If muscle weakness or pain is severe or persists for more than 3 days after a workout, ask your doctor about CoQ10, a supplement that may lessen symptoms.

Drug: Diuretics (fluid-reducing drugs for high blood pressure)

Possible side effect: Muscle cramping caused by loss of potassium

Strategy: You may need a potassium supplement. See your doctor if muscle cramping is more painful or lasts longer than usual.

Drug: Avelox, Cipro, Levaquin (fluoroquinolone antibiotics)

Possible side effect: Increased risk of rupturing an Achilles tendon while running due to the drug's effect on cartilage

Strategy: Spend 15 minutes warming up on a treadmill (at 3 mph or less) before beginning your run. Go to your doctor if you notice any inflammation or tenderness.

Drug: Celexa, LuVox, Paxil, Prozac, Zoloft (SSRI antidepressants)

Possible side effects: Temporary drowsiness and dizziness, making it dangerous to perform exercises requiring balance

Strategy: Until your body adjusts, do leg presses instead of squats and perform shoulder presses seated instead of standing.

Drug: Beta-blockers (drugs for high blood pressure)

Possible side effect: Decreased heart rate, making it more difficult to perform cardiovascular workouts or weight training

Strategy: Plan to work out at a lower intensity, and avoid getting up quickly from exercise equipment.

5. Get juiced before a workout. University of Florida researchers found that a combination of vitamin E, omega-3 fats, and flavonoids helps muscles repair themselves quickly after intense lifting or long runs. In a 2-week study, those men who took a daily supplement containing the three compounds had 50 percent less muscle inflammation after performing heavy arm curls than those who took a placebo. Load your diet with fish for omega-3s, and almonds and fortified cereals for vitamin E. These two nutrients need time to be absorbed. But you can have the flavonoids—try citrus fruit, grapes, and grape juice—right before your workout.

6. Work the crowd. Hate a crowded gym? Quit your complaining—having people around can boost your bench press. Researchers found that men are able to bench-press an average of 41 pounds more with spectators than when they lift alone. "An audience can motivate guys," says Matthew Rhea, Ph.D., lead author of the study, published in the *Journal of Strength and Conditioning Research.* The researchers studied 15 men performing their one-rep maximums—the kind of heavy lifting that builds strength. Moreover, Rhea said, working out in a busy gym might shake off the staleness of your usual solitary session. Just don't show off—many injuries occur when lifters try to do too much.

7. Get a deal. Don't belong to a gym? The New Year's a great time to join—it's recruiting season for health clubs, which want their share of newly resolved members. "Gyms can see up to a 100 percent increase in new membership and are usually offering their best discounts," says Dave Reiseman, a spokesman for Gold's Gym International. To get the best deal anytime of year . . .

Play the field. Talk to the staffs at two or more clubs. "You may have to look around to find the perfect fit," says Reiseman. See if your favorite will match another gym's promotion, suggests Richard Ned Lebow, author of *The Art of Bargaining.*

Bring friends. "Member referrals are huge," says Reiseman. "We take good care of the members who take care of us." A group of coworkers, friends, or family can drive a better bargain as a group, Lebow says.

Get covered. Find out what discounts you qualify for. And see if your insurance provider might offer a fitness benefit.

Don't commit. Some gyms offer cheap short-term packages. Why not join four gyms for 3 months at a time rather than one for 12?

Think big. Speak to a manager or owner—he or she will have more power to give you a deal.

Ignore swag. Bargain for freebies that actually help you reach your goals—like a free training or nutrition session, not a T-shirt or water bottle.

8. Get up for your workout. Lots of exercises that men perform sitting down would be more beneficial if done standing up. Sitting down—at machines or with free weights—doesn't work your abdominal muscles enough. This can lead to weakness in your back and abs and sometimes to injury, says Stephen Holt, C.S.C.S., a personal trainer in Maryland.

So stand up for lateral raises, shoulder presses, biceps curls, and French presses (overhead triceps lifts). Maybe you don't have the core strength to do these properly. But if you just sit there, you'll never build that strength.

9. Lighten the load. Try a "back-off" set after a heavy weight-lifting session. Use a weight that's about 30 to 50 percent of the most you can lift one

THE NUMBER OF PROTEIN GRAMS PER KILOGRAM (2.2 POUNDS) OF BODY WEIGHT THE AVERAGE WEIGHT LIFTER NEEDS FOR OPTIMAL MUSCLE GROWTH: 2

time, and complete as many repetitions as you can for one last set. Researchers in Japan found that men who used this approach increased their levels of a hormone that signals your body to burn fat and build muscle. Don't go lower than 30 percent. In the study, the men performed five sets with a weight that was 90 percent of the most they could lift one time. For the back-off set, dropping the weight to 20 percent of their maximum diminished the effects.

10. Take it easy. You don't have to exercise at a high intensity to increase your metabolism, build strength, or feel energized. Moderate activity yields these same rewards without exhausting a person, says Steve Edwards, Ph.D., a professor of sports psychology at Oklahoma State University. Exercise at a moderate intensity (breathing slightly harder than at rest) and you're making progress. You'll get a little endorphin high from even the lightest workout. "If you have a better response to exercise, then you'll be more likely to engage in it again," says Edwards.

11. Run for it. There's a bit of the weight lifter inside any runner who includes wind sprints in his workout. Running recruits mostly slow-twitch muscle fibers, and weight lifting mostly fast-twitch. But Kyle Tarpenning, Ph.D., researched this correlation in a 20-year study published in *Medicine and Science in Sports and Exercise,* and says that running intervals—repeated sprints with rest between—maintains muscle quality and helps increase the quantity of both types of leg-muscle fibers, from youth into your 80s. Tarpenning recommends mixing 1 or 2 days of interval training per week with a couple of days of steady distance work.

12. Get enough protein. Don't skimp on the protein powder in your postworkout shake. A study in the *Journal of Nutrition* showed that people who ate 60 percent less protein than another group had 81 percent less "protein synthesis"—the production of protein that stimulates muscle growth. Biochemical pathways in muscle cells stay quiet when protein intake is low, suggests lead author Irwin Brodsky, M.D.

OUR FINAL ANSWERS

Running On Empty

Am I better off eating before or after exercising?

—N.G., Las Vegas

A vigorous workout is the best way to burn calories and build muscle and endurance, but you can't exercise vigorously on an empty tank. Trying to work out on "empty" will limit the time and power of your workout and sabotage any weight-loss efforts, says Heidi Skolnik, M.S., C.D.N., nutritionist for the New York Giants. A harder exercise session (alternating high-intensity with endurance training) will yield greater results than skipping a meal.

If you work out at the crack of dawn, eat enough beforehand to get your blood-sugar level back on track after the overnight fast—a piece of fruit or some toast should work. Then eat a more substantial breakfast with protein and fiber after your workout. The same goes for a midday session: Have something light—nuts or cheese and crackers—for energy before and a sensible lunch after. If you plan to hit the gym after work, schedule a snack around 4:30. The calories will give you an energy boost for your end-of-the-day burn-off.

Make Your Muscles Think

I've been curling the same weight for weeks now. How can I step it up a notch?

—H.R., Menomonee Falls, Wisconsin

Shake up your workout with a technique called offset training, in which you curl a dumbbell with one hand and a lighter one with the other. You choose a weight that allows you to perform at most eight repetitions with one hand, and a dumbbell that's about 15 to 20 pounds lighter for the other hand. You'll hot-wire your brain-to-muscle connection—the key to fast strength gains.

Here's how it works: Right before you curl a dumbbell, your brain estimates the number of muscle fibers that need to fire and recruits them for duty. But when you're using the offset technique, your brain has to send two different signals simultaneously, which forces it to work harder to communicate with your muscles.

The result: The pathways between your brain and your muscles become more efficient, since they have to learn to deliver more messages at the same time. So when you switch back to matching weights, you should actually be able to lift more, says Carter Hays, a National Strength and Conditioning Association–certified personal trainer in Houston. If you work out 3 days a week, swap in an offset dumbbell routine on one of those days.

Two-in-One Chest Exercise

What can I do besides bench presses to make my chest bigger?

—P.G., New York City

Surprise your muscles. "The key to adding mass to any large muscle group, such as the chest, is varying the type of stress you put on it," says Michael Y. Seril, NSCA-C.P.T., owner of Michael Seril Fitness, a personal-training company in Orange County, California. "Try combining these two movements into one exercise," he says. It's sort of a "press-fly." The bonus: You'll save time, because you'll be doing more work with less rest between exercises.

Lie faceup on a bench, holding dumbbells with an underhand grip at the sides of your chest. Press the weights straight up (1) and rotate them until your palms are facing each other (2). Keeping your elbows slightly bent, lower the dumbbells outward in an arc until they're at chest height (3). Use your chest to pull them back up, following the same route in reverse. Lower the weights back to the starting position. That's one repetition. Perform three or four sets of 8 to 12 repetitions.

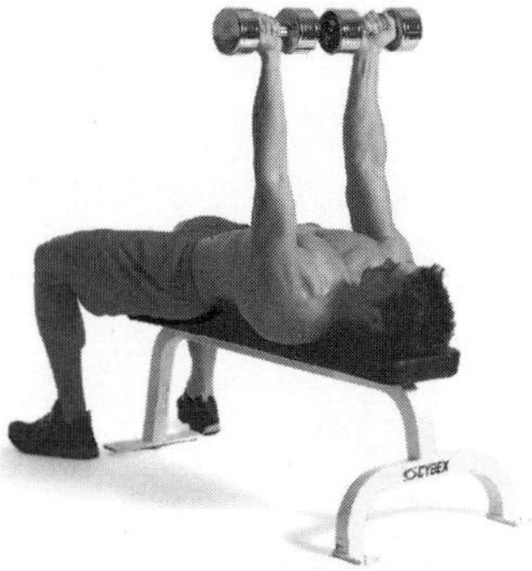

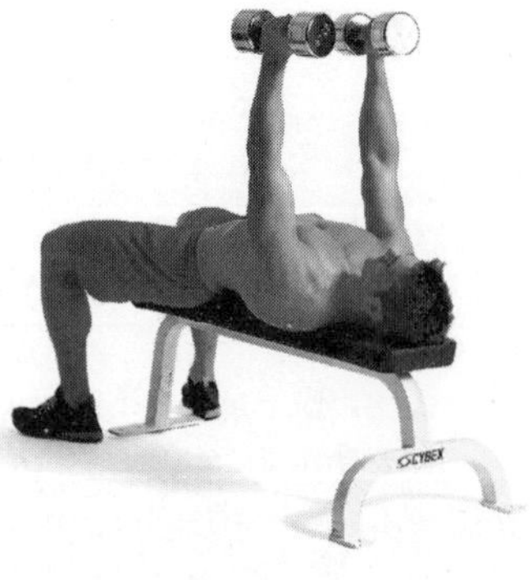

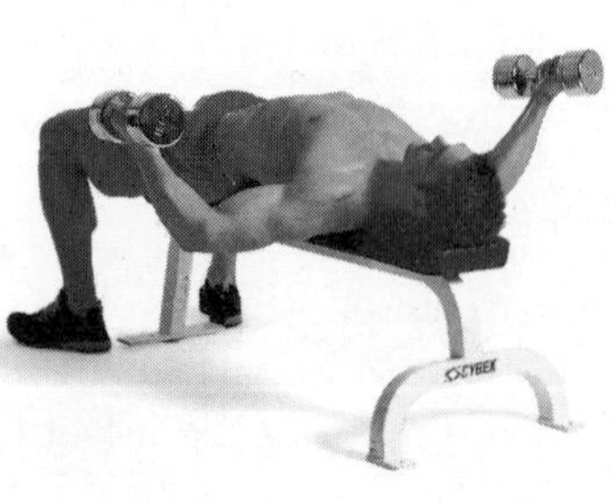

Tame the Twitch

My muscles sometimes spasm after a workout. Is that a good sign?

—R.W., Fort Myers, Florida

It's a good sign—that you're dehydrated or that you didn't stretch enough after your workout. The causes behind spasms are obscure, says Ken Baldwin, Ph.D., professor of physiology at the University of California at Irvine. But it probably has to do with a combination of sodium loss and dehydration, which makes the muscles more sensitive to nerve stimuli. To avoid the twitch, make sure you warm up by doing a short set without weights, advises Samantha Heller, M.S., R.D., a senior clinical nutritionist and exercise physiologist at NYU medical center. End your workout by stretching the largest muscles you just worked, such as your chest and back. One way to do it: Hang from a pullup bar and turn your body left and right. Hold each turn for 10 to 15 seconds. You can avert a more extreme form of postworkout tightening—cramps—by guzzling a sports drink.

Stretch Your Limits

Is there a quick way to tell if I'm stretching enough?

—C.M., Schenectady, New York

Try the overhead squat test, says Joe Dowdell, owner of Peak Performance in New York City. Hold a broomstick overhead with both hands, arms straight, feet shoulder-width apart. Squat slowly as if you're sitting on a stool, and pay attention: If your feet rotate outward or come off the ground, or if your knees buckle inward or your back hyperextends, you have range-of-motion limitations or muscle weaknesses or both, says Dowdell. If your arms fall forward, there could be range limitations in the shoulders or a lack of thoracic spinal extension. For better flexibility, try the following stretches.

NUMBER OF INCHES BEYOND HIS TOES THE AVERAGE GUY CAN REACH WHEN SEATED WITH HIS LEGS FORWARD ON THE FLOOR: 1.5

For the back of your body: Assume the upside-down-V position, with your hands flat on the floor, legs straight, and butt raised toward the ceiling. Push your heels to the floor and hold for 20 to 30 seconds. Repeat twice.

For the front of your body: Lie faceup on a Swiss ball, feet flat on the floor and knees bent 90 degrees. Extend your hands over your head and reach for the floor. Shoot for two reps of 20 to 30 seconds each.

Hit the Road

I want to cycle to build my cardiovascular endurance. Should I buy a road bike or a mountain bike? And how much should I spend?

—S.D., Allentown, Pennsylvania

A road bike is your heart machine. *Bicycling* magazine fitness columnist Selene Yeager explains why: "Because of the demanding terrain, mountain biking is more of a stop-and-go activity, like interval training. It's punishing. With road cycling, you can build cardiovascular endurance without beating the crap out of yourself." Expect to spend between $700 and $1,300. You could easily shell out more, but it'd be like getting a Porsche for your 16th birthday—way more juice than you need. The absolute best entry-level road bike is the K2 Mach 3.0 ($1,300, k2bike.com). It has reliable components and some high-end perks, like a lightweight carbon-fiber fork, according to our friends at *Bicycling*. Go ahead and drop $20 on a CatEye (cateye.com) handlebar computer, too. It's the easiest way to log your time and distance and track your progress. Start with this 4-day-a-week program:

Monday....................60 minutes at moderate intensity

Wednesday..............45 minutes of hills or sprints
(four to six sprints of 30 to 60 seconds each)

Friday......................60 minutes at moderate intensity

Saturday..................1 to 2 hours of leisurely riding

Save Your Breath

I have asthma but love to play sports. How dangerous is this, really?

—L.G., Newton, Massachusetts

A recent study looked at the dangers of asthma and exercise and found that in a very small number of cases, exercise-induced asthma attacks can be fatal.

(Most asthma deaths occurred during basketball.) But this doesn't mean asthmatics should take up chess as their most challenging physical activity. Check with your doctor at least once a year to make sure your asthma medications are current. Keep an inhaler nearby. And rest during a game to make sure you remain beneath the attack threshold. Determine what your tolerance level is and learn to accept it. Pushing yourself, even for a short time, can bring on an attack.

Don't Sweat It

How can I squeeze in a lunchtime workout and not sweat like a pig during my 1:30 meeting?

—R.K., Killeen, Texas

On the night before your workout, put on Certain Dri antiperspirant ($6, drugstore.com) before you hit the sack. Your pores will absorb it at night, and a morning shower won't affect its action. "It's an over-the-counter medication that contains a significant percentage of aluminum chloride [which is the active ingredient in antiperspirants]," says Barry A. Solomon, M.D., assistant professor of dermatology at SUNY–Health Science Center in Brooklyn.

If you want to improve the performance of your usual antiperspirant, add a second dose. A recent study found that applying antiperspirant at night and again in the morning increases the product's effectiveness by 20 percent.

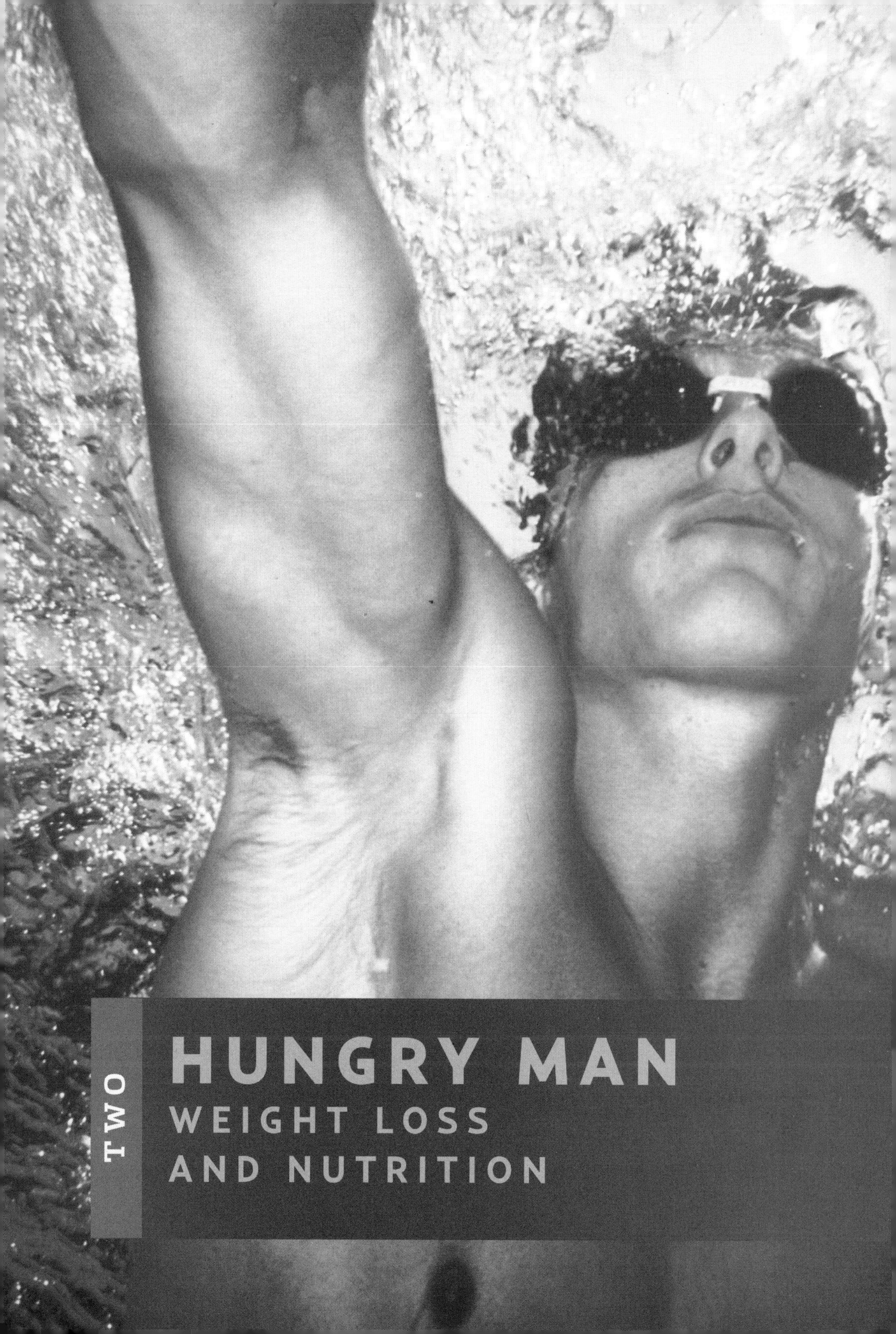

TWO

HUNGRY MAN

WEIGHT LOSS AND NUTRITION

MUST READS

The Lowdown on the Low-Carb Craze

When a weight-loss theory becomes a marketing tool, the food manufacturers gain profits and America gains weight. Here's how to defend yourself

By Stephen Perrine

The keys to my salvation lie glistening in their own grease.

Tinged orangey red, their skins all puckered and pimply, their little bones jutting akimbo from the plate, they're as plump with promise as they are with flavor. They promise a streamlined body, a circulatory system unmolested by cholesterol, and a lifetime of freedom from the hard choices I once thought critical for maintaining a healthy lifestyle. They're buffalo wings, as hot and spicy and greasy as I remember from college, with their inevitable accoutrements of snappy celery and globulous blue cheese. But no carrots, the other crudités that sometimes accompany such a platter.

Because carrots are evil, or haven't you heard?

My cabdriver has heard. "What is this about the carbohydrates?" she asks in an Eastern European accent when she overhears me talking about the Atkins diet. "I am on the Atkins. I lose weight, but now I gain it back."

The people sitting at the next table at dinner have heard, too. Maybe that's why they've come to this dingy T.G.I. Friday's in midtown Manhattan, to sample its Atkins-approved menu. They can choose foods that are either low in carbohydrates or low in something called "net carbs." The menu ranges from steaks to cheese dips to the "Cheeseburger Cheeseburger," of which the menu copy conspiratorially notes, "You try hard to pass on the ketchup. We'll keep the bun in the kitchen."

The greasy wings and the bunless burgers are the newest weapons in the hands of a nation at war with itself. With more than 60 million Americans qualifying as obese—more than 20 percent over their optimal body-mass index—our country is eating itself to death and desperate for a way out. And we've chosen low-carb eating as the magical answer—one that allows us to consume all the food we want, as long as it's low in carbohydrates.

But a lot of nutrition experts warn that in the rush toward low-carb eating, marketers, consumers, and the government itself are ignoring science, the law, and plain common sense. And, like many once-promising offensives in the war on obesity, the low-carb diet is a weapon we're about to turn on ourselves.

ANATOMY OF A DISASTER

We've been here before—about 10 years ago, in fact. The last time a diet craze swept the country, it ushered in more than 3,000 new food products on the wings of just three simple words: Eat less fat. And yet, in the ensuing decade, the number of overweight Americans increased by 15 percent, according to the National Center for Health Statistics, and the average American man's waist size increased by an inch and a half. Weight management became even more difficult because the supermarket became more confusing, and the three simple words that were supposed to squeeze us back into our wedding suits let us down terribly.

And it's about to happen all over again. "Consumers think carb-free is calorie-free, which it's not," says Leslie Bonci, a spokeswoman for the American Dietetic Association (ADA). "They think someone's giving them permission to eat that food. And what's going to happen is, we're going to see people start to gain weight."

In January of this year, more than 400 people who work in the food industry gathered at the Adam's Mark hotel in Denver for the first-ever *Low-Carbiz* Summit to learn how they could profit from the new craving for low-carbohydrate foods. What they heard at the start was a warning from Fred Pescatore, M.D., a protégé of Dr. Robert Atkins, the original low-carb guru: "We can't be like low-fat," he said. "We can't be just a fad."

And then, for 2 days, they learned ways to turn the low-carb craze into exactly that. In between snacking on low-carb foods and drinking Bacardi and diet cola (the official adult beverage of the low-carb movement), conference-goers attended sessions like "Low Carb for the Nondieter" and "The Scientific Case *against* Low Carb: Know What the Industry's Detractors Are Saying and How to Respond."

If you eat the typical American diet, it makes sense to cut down on carbs. To eat more protein. To limit saturated fat and eat the mono- and polyunsaturated kinds. We ought to be at the dawn of a new era in which everyone knows what's good and what's bad, what makes us fat and what keeps us thin.

But the truth about low-carb diets is that they work, just not in the way their supporters claim. See, any diet that requires you to cut out a certain number of foods—fats, carbs, whatever—works in the short term for one reason: because it causes you to consume fewer calories. "Weight loss is not based on how much carbohydrate one eats or how much fat one eats or how much protein one eats," argues Santhay Bowmen, Ph.D., a researcher in the Nutrient Data Laboratory at the United States Department of Agriculture

(USDA). "It is independent of the micronutrient composition of the diet. If you eat less energy than you expend, then you lose weight." And that's the simple truth, whether you're eating only meat, or only grapefruit, or only Cracker Jack.

In the typical American diet, a lot of our calories come in the form of refined carbohydrates—including sugar, milled grains, and the sugar substitute high-fructose corn syrup, or HFCS. And there's no denying that they're bad for you. Refined carbs offer all the calories of their less-refined cousins, whole-grain breads and cereals, but with many important nutrients—in particular, fiber—stripped out of them. According to USDA data, the typical American eats roughly 50 teaspoons of natural and artificial sugar every *day*—that's 147 pounds of sweet stuff a year.

In this scenario, cutting out carbohydrates—at least certain carbohydrates—makes sense. Low-carb diets decrease calorie consumption in two ways: first, because they force you to cut out easy-to-eat junk foods—obvious ones, like potato chips, candy, and pretzels, and less obvious ones, like white bread and bagels and fruit-juice blends. Cutting down on these empty calories is a plan with which few could argue.

But the other way low-carb diets work is by making eating a little less convenient. You can always toss a bagel into your briefcase as you head out the door; sliding in a serving of steak and eggs to nosh on the way to work is a little more complicated. That's great if you're looking to shave a few calories—and hence a few pounds. If you can't take it with you, you can't eat it on the way.

This protein lust is turning into a windfall for chicken, pig, and cattle ranchers. According to a *LowCarbiz* survey, 59 million Americans are on low-carb diets. Sales of eggs increased 18.5 percent from 2002 to 2003, while bacon was up 9.8 percent and lunchmeat up 3.8 percent, according to ACNielsen.

But it's not so great for companies selling grain-based foodstuffs. Sales of white bread, cookies, and cereals dropped about 3 percent in the same calendar year, according to ACNielsen. Packaged-food manufacturers needed to get their lard-asses on the low-carb bus. And now that they have, the bus has started listing in a very dangerous direction.

WHO MOVED MY CHEETOS?

The low-carb craze is a very simple idea that's gone terribly awry. And part of the blame belongs to an assemblage of statistics called the glycemic index.

The glycemic index is a list created by Canadian researchers that ranks foods according to how they react inside the body. Popular diet books like *Atkins for Life* and *The South Beach Diet* (the latter published by *Men's Health*'s parent company, Rodale) use the glycemic index to delineate which foods are good for weight management and which are bad.

The theory works like this: Food is digested by the body and turned into glucose, or blood sugar. Blood sugar is regulated by the hormone insulin, which is manufactured in the pancreas. Insulin is your body's air traffic controller: It tells the glucose where to go—to the muscles to be stored (in the form of glycogen) for quick energy, to the brain for thinking power, to all the body's cells for proper maintenance and function.

Foods that have a low glycemic index (GI)—mostly proteins and fats—are digested slowly. That's good, because a slower digestion rate means that your blood sugar remains relatively stable and cells are nourished with the right amount of energy. But foods that have a high GI are digested quickly, and they can cause a sudden spike in blood sugar. That's bad, because when glucose spikes dramatically, insulin takes the extra blood sugar your body doesn't need and turns it into body fat. Then your blood sugar level plummets, and you get hungry again.

That's why the glycemic index is a pretty good indicator of which foods will lead to increased calorie consumption and obesity. But the glycemic index isn't perfect. Carrots have a high GI. But they're very low in calories, so you'd have to eat a bushel to touch off an insulin spike.

Joanne Ikeda, R.D., of the department of nutritional sciences at the University of California at Berkeley, points out another flaw: "The glycemic index is fine if all you eat is one food. But we don't do that—we eat a mixed diet. That's where the glycemic index falls apart."

It fails in other ways, too. The more fat (and hence, the more calories) a high-carb food packs, the lower its GI ranking, because fat slows the digestion process. You could make room for Cheetos and ice cream on your list of low-GI foods. And some high-GI foods, such as bananas and oranges, are low in calories and high in vitamins and other nutrients, and belong on your plate.

So what we're saying here is, eat lots of fruits and vegetables and whole grains. It's a simple sentence that would seem like common sense in any other era. But today, it seems like heresy. Because, rather than explain all these complex permutations, many diet moguls simplify things into one easy, three-word mantra: Cut out carbs.

And tens of billions of dollars are in play here. "Flour consumption per capita has dropped 1 to 2 pounds in the past 3 years," says Dale Eustace, a professor of grain science and industry at Kansas State University. That could translate to as much as $1.6 billion per year of lost revenue for agribusiness (based on statistics from the USDA). If that trend continues, food manufacturers may face some lean financial times. No wind for Cap'n Crunch's sails. No wax for Chef Boyardee's mustache.

And that's why the food industry has invented and embraced the net carb.

THE CARBOHYDRATE WITCH HUNT

What, exactly, is a "net carb"? Is it . . .

1. The carbs found in seafood, shellfish, and other foods caught in nets?
2. The total number of carbohydrate units left in a food once you subtract fat, protein, moisture, and "ash," then subtract fiber, maltitol, glycerin, erythritol, and other forms of sugar alcohol?
3. The total units of carbs that actually affect the body once you consume them?

If you're a representative of Atkins Nutritionals, the arm of the Atkins empire that both packages its own foodstuffs and licenses Atkins's scarlet A to restaurants and other food marketers, the answer is both 2 and 3.

But not according to many other food researchers, some of whom believe net carbs are one of the worst dietary hoaxes ever played on the American public. "You just twist the food composition a bit by taking some of the starch and sugar out and adding some of the sugar alcohols and maltodextrins, and then [a manufacturer] can say, 'I, the food processor, have given you a low-carb food,'" says Manfred Kroger, Ph.D., professor of food science at Penn State University. "Lower than before, but maybe only by a small percentage. It's the same game the cigarette companies play when they say, 'We're going to give you a low-tar and low-nicotine cigarette.' You can make this claim by reducing the nicotine by only a small percentage."

The idea behind net carbs is that you need to be concerned only with foods that trigger an insulin spike. Fiber, which for the most part passes through the body without being absorbed, doesn't jolt blood sugar or insulin levels. And the other common low-carb stand-ins—maltitol, glycerin, and erythritol—are sugar alcohols. According to low-carb marketers, including Atkins, fiber and sugar alcohols don't raise blood sugar levels.

Atkins-brand foods didn't even list total carbs on their labels until the FDA seized company products in 2001 for failure to comply with food labeling law. In response, Atkins listed all these other forms of carbohydrates but added the term "net carb." The rationale: Subtract fiber and sugar alcohols, and only what's left—the net carbs—counts, says Colette Heimowitz, vice president of education and research for Atkins Health and Medical Information Services. The other carbs don't matter.

Except they do. Sugar alcohols are sweeteners made with hydrogenated starch molecules, and, like any other food, they come with their own calorie counts. Erythritol carries less than 1 calorie per gram, while maltitol—one of the most commonly used sugar alcohols—carries about 2 per gram. (Table sugar weighs in at about 4 calories per gram.) That's why the FDA requires that they be listed on all food packaging. "The number on the government-mandated nutrition label is right, not the box in the corner from the manufacturer saying don't count those carbs, those sugar alcohol calories," says Larry Lindner, executive editor of the *Tufts University Health & Nutrition Letter*. "They're calories; they go to your belly."

What they do once they're inside you, however, is a matter of some concern. Sugar alcohols seem to have different effects on some people than on others. A review of literature in the *Canadian Journal of Diabetes* found that chocolate bars sweetened with maltitol raised blood sugar levels as high as chocolate bars sweetened with table sugar.

In other individuals, however, some sugar alcohols seem to pass through the digestive system undigested. This would appear to be a good thing, until you consider the result: High levels of undigested sugar alcohols settle in the gastrointestinal tract, causing diarrhea or flatulence.

"This is a trick siblings have played on each other for years. If they have a greedy little brother, they give him diabetic candy [which is flavored with sugar alcohols]. And sure enough, if the little 5-year-old takes an overload, he has diarrhea for the next 2 days," says Kroger. Even if you're willing to trade a little more stomach upset for a little less stomach, you might be left wondering, How can a food company market a product packed with calorie-laden carbohydrates and yet claim it's only the "net carbs" that matter?

They can do it because there aren't any FDA rules governing such a thing. Manufacturers can put "2 net carbs!" or "2 net superfats!" or "2 net poo-poo flava!" on their labels if they can define it and show a consistent formula by which they've arrived at such a figure. "The food label could become a zoo. A company could subtract carbs that don't cause tooth decay or fats that don't raise blood cholesterol," says Bonnie Liebman, nutrition director for the Center for Science in the Public Interest (CSPI). Such claims are allowed under FDA rules because they don't address anything the FDA deems relevant. In its eyes, "net carbs" is scientifically meaningless—but that's not the way it's marketed.

LICENSE FOR GLUTTONY

Think back to the two reasons low-carb diets worked in the first place: Number one, they eliminated foods that were high in carbohydrates. Number two, they made snacking less convenient, because the foods that are easiest to grab (those offered by vending machines or drive-thrus) are loaded with carbohydrates. By whacking out a wide range of junk foods, they suppressed calorie intake and triggered weight loss.

But what if all those once-verboten foods suddenly came in low-carb versions, with all of the convenience and caloric load of their old selves but with an unofficial stamp of approval? That's exactly what's happening today, in a replay of the low-fat craze. Ten years ago, dieters gobbled up low-fat ice creams and cakes and brownies and got fatter because, in order to make low-fat foods taste palatable, manufacturers had to load them up with extra sugar. The fat content was lower, but the calories remained the same—and the more calories you take in, the more weight you gain. Worse, because the foods carried the "low-fat" label, consumers figured they had a license to pig out—no fat, no foul.

Today, dieters are gobbling up the new lines of low-carb ice creams and cakes and brownies with much the same abandon. Low-carb–branded snack and beverage sales have tripled in the past 3 years, according to Information Resources, a sales and marketing research group. The firm also estimates that the average low-carb dieter spends $85 a month on specialized products, for a total market of $15 billion in 2003 and an estimated $25 billion to $30 billion this year. Big players like Unilever and Anheuser-Busch, and restaurants like Subway, Don Pablo's, and Burger King have all introduced low-carb products.

And so, in a nation already under siege by a crisis in obesity, fat's new offensive is coming on two fronts.

First, there are the low-carb and Atkins-approved meals now being offered by major restaurant chains and mom-and-pop greasy spoons alike. Those chicken wings offered by T.G.I. Friday's, for example, are sold as an appetizer for the weight conscious. Yet there is no difference between these wings and the wings that have been the favorite food of fat men for years. (T.G.I. Friday's refused to provide an official calorie count for its appetizer, but a typical order of wings would carry about 1,000 calories for 24 pieces—and remember, that's an appetizer.) Even the Atkins folks are concerned that casual diners are misreading "low-carb" as "diet." Regarding those buffalo wings, Heimowitz says, "They're for people following a low-carb diet. They're not for people trying to cut calories and fat. The worst thing you can do is eat a high-fat food [like wings] and then eat a high-carb food."

Second, there is the new breed of "carb-aware" packaged foods, like CarbSmart ice cream and Carb Control yogurt. In many cases, these products carry as many calories as or more calories than their original formulations, or use other labeling tricks to masquerade as healthier choices. For example, Thomas's multigrain bagels have 300 calories per serving and 57 grams (g) carbs; Thomas's carb-counting bagels have 140 calories and just 23 g carbs. That looks like a great substitution, until you realize the carb-counting bagel is only a little more than half the size, by weight, of the original. Eating the same amount of both foods leaves the consumer about even. The words "carb-counting" indicate that this is a diet food.

And it's not.

THE FDA TO THE RESCUE! (MAYBE. EVENTUALLY. WHO KNOWS?)

Although their numbers have dropped dramatically, from 2,076 in 1996 to 1,052 in 2003, you can still find plenty of foods that carry the "low-fat" or "reduced-fat" label. That's because in 1994, the FDA issued a ruling specifying that "low-fat" means 3 g or less per serving amount, and "reduced fat" or "less fat" is at least 25 percent less than the full-fat version of that food.

"When the FDA issued its guidelines, two things happened," says Lynn Dornblaser, director of consulting services for Mintel, a market-research company. "Fringe products went off the market, and others were reformulated to fit the FDA guidelines."

The FDA has yet to issue guidelines defining the terms "low-" and "reduced-carbohydrate," so these terms shouldn't appear on product labels. But they do. At Giant, a typical suburban grocery store in eastern Pennsylvania, contraband nutritional claims are everywhere. Among the most obvious offenders was "Bella Vita Low Carb Pasta with 80 percent less carbs." And Sipper Sweets offered "low-carb" lemonade and cocoa, among other beverages.

Even terms that aren't against the law, like "net carbs," aren't always properly presented. "There's a lot of label fraud out there," says Will Lederman, COO of Keto Foods, a low-carb food manufacturer. "For example, a low-carb pasta that's selling very well right now claims to contain 10 net carbs, but our testing in a third-party lab found 33."

Many of these products slide under the radar because the FDA's inspection process isn't broad enough. Typically, the FDA checks compliance by sending agents to a manufacturer's headquarters unannounced and randomly selecting three of the company's products to analyze. If the manufacturer is found to be in violation, the FDA's Division of Enforcement Programs issues a warning letter. But despite the widespread appearance of "low-carb" labels, in 2003, the FDA issued only two warning letters to manufacturers who were using these terms to describe their products—one for a "reduced-carb" bread and one for a candy bar called Pure De-lite Chocolate Bar. In the case of Pure De-lite, the company used the claims "low-carb" and

PERCENTAGE MORE LIKELY AN OVERWEIGHT MAN IS TO BE HOSPITALIZED FOR CHRONIC HEARTBURN THAN A NORMAL-WEIGHT MAN: 22

"only 1.1 carbs!" on its packaging, even though the candy contained maltitol and about 20 g total carbohydrates.

But even if the FDA inspected every single product on the market, manufacturers could still skirt the issue in several ways. First, there's the "net carbs" approach. Second, manufacturers can use words that imply reduced carbs, such as "carb conscious" or "carb wise." And finally, even if you can't market a food as low-carb, you can still sell it as "part of a low-carb lifestyle."

And the food manufacturers can market any food—even pure sugar, if they like—using these claims. "As a result, we have a lot of products on the market that are lower in carbohydrates than the original versions, but not that much lower," says Dornblaser.

Eager to cash in on the craze, grocery retailers are following suit. Giant, for example, has a program that awards stars to products it deems "carb friendly," including such standard fare as shrimp, peanut butter, cream cheese, and spinach—products that common sense would deem low-carb anyway but that Giant hopes to move in greater quantities. Other grocers are creating low-carb aisles, and some cater exclusively to the carb-conscious consumer. One such retailer, Pure Foods, has two stores in its franchise and had plans to roll out more in 2004, carrying products like shrimp and spinach as well as the pastas, candy bars, and bagels that proclaim their merits with the "low-carb" or "net carbs" labels.

It may be only a few more months before the government steps in to clear up the confusion. On March 11 of last year, ConAgra Foods, Kraft Foods, and the Grocery Manufacturers of America, a trade group representing more than 140 food manufacturers, filed a petition with the FDA, asking the administration to clarify and legitimize four nutritional claims, including "carbohydrate-free" and "low-carbohydrate." The FDA accepted the petition and has begun the rule-defining process, which includes giving public advocacy groups an opportunity to register their comments. A committee of FDA advisors likely will decide on the proposed regulation and issue its recommended guidelines sometime this year.

But it's hard to predict how long the process may take. "We submitted a petition to have trans fats listed some time ago, and they just got around to it," says CSPI's Liebman. "It's been almost a decade."

And even if the FDA does rule, that ruling will have no direct effect on restaurants touting the "net carbs" claim, on diet moguls pushing a butter diet, or on consumers who want to believe that their dietary salvation lies in the meatiest, greasiest, fattiest foods they can get their sticky fingers on. In 2003, for example, dieters sent sales of one low-carb treat soaring more than 27 percent. The product: fried pork rinds.

For now, the diet wars rage on, and all of us—marketers and consumers alike—are getting fat off the spoils.

Big Fat Secret

A poisonous fat is lurking in thousands of processed foods, and you probably don't even know it's there

By Samantha Heller, M.S., R.D.

Twist the top cookie of the Oreo to the right, the bottom to the left, and pull apart. Now, before you scrape that sweet cream filling into your mouth with your top teeth as you've done hundreds of times since you were 5, take a good look at some very bad fat.

It's called trans fat, and chances are you've never heard of it because until just recently, companies weren't required to list it on their labels. Trans fat is simply vegetable oil infused with hydrogen. It's used in thousands of common prepared foods, from frozen waffles to Oreo cookies, french fries to bran muffins. Vegetable oil seems innocent enough, until you learn that the hydrogenation process turns it into one evil fat. It's a fat that's difficult to digest, so it increases the amount of bad cholesterol in your blood and can dramatically boost your risk of heart disease. If saturated animal fats are unhealthy, trans fats are far worse. They can weaken your immune system. They can cause diabetes. You're almost better off eating butter and bacon.

Harvard scientists estimate that trans fats may contribute to more than 30,000 premature deaths each year. So why did it take so long for the FDA to change its regulations and force companies to reveal the amount of trans fats in their products? In a word: fear.

The food and edible-oil industries are worried that if we ever find out exactly how many killer fats are actually in some foods, we'll stop buying them—costing their companies millions, and possibly billions, of dollars each year.

TRANS FAT 101

The trans fat story begins in the 1950s, when scientists first made the link between saturated fat, cholesterol, and heart disease. After the discovery, manufacturers scrambled to find a way to cut saturated fats. Their immediate solution: a decades-old process called partial hydrogenation. Vegetable oils are combined with hydrogen and heated to extreme temperatures. As the molecules in the oil warm up, they bond with the hydrogen, creating a new, man-made structure called a trans fatty acid. The result is the transformation of liquid to solid—vegetable oil into Crisco.

Suddenly, hydrogenated oil was an out-of-the-box hit. Restaurants liked it because they could fill their fry vats with the stuff and keep it hot all day without smoking up their kitchens. Hydrogenated fats were also cheaper than butter and had a longer shelf life, so burger shops could not only use the same oil over and over in their fryers but also buy the stuff in bulk, leaving it on a shelf in the back without worrying about spoilage.

If hydrogenated oils were a home run for the fast-food industry, they were a grand slam for the burgeoning junk-food industry. Trans fats made potato chips and crackers crispier than ever and gave manufacturers a way to add the great taste of fat to places it had never been before—like Oreo cookie filling.

While normal vegetable oils would have slowly leaked out of mass-produced cookies and chips, leaving a greasy mess behind, trans fats were different. Since trans fat molecules turn solid at room temperature, manufacturers were now able to lock fat into their food, giving it an injection of fat—and flavor—that couldn't be dabbed away.

Combine this with the longer shelf life of foods made with hydrogenated oil rather than butter, and it's no wonder trans fats are considered one of the

YOU WANT TRANS FATS WITH THAT?

The Institute of Medicine recommends cutting as many grams of trans fats as you can from your diet. With this in mind, check out how these popular guy foods rate.

Food	Trans Fat (grams)
1 chicken pot pie	8
2 biscuits	8
1 large order of french fries	7
1 cinnamon roll	6
6 fish sticks	5
1 order of nachos with cheese	5
1 Tbsp stick margarine	5
6 Oreos	4
1 waffle	4
9 Tater Tots	4
1 small movie-theater popcorn (4 c)	3½
1 slice apple pie	3
1 pack cheese-and-cracker sandwiches	3
2 homemade chocolate-chip cookies	3
5-piece chicken tenders	2½
1 brownie	2½
1 jelly doughnut	2
1 cup Chex party mix	2
1 hamburger bun	less than 1
1 slice cheese pizza	less than 1

triggers that helped the junk-food market explode. Today, the FDA estimates that most supermarkets carry more than 42,000 products containing partially hydrogenated vegetable oil as one of their primary ingredients.

But all that fat has a price.

ANATOMY OF A KILLER

Since trans fats don't occur widely in nature, your body has a much harder time processing them than it does other types of fat. So, while you may stop thinking about your morning doughnut the second you shake the crumbs off your tie, the trans fats in that doughnut linger on inside your body. Their first target? Your heart.

"Besides increasing the number of LDL [bad] cholesterol and triglyceride particles in the bloodstream, trans fats also lower your HDL [good] cholesterol," says Bruce Holub, Ph.D., a professor of nutrition at the University of Guelph in Canada. "Trans fats also increase blood levels of a compound called lipoprotein a. The more of this lipoprotein you have in your system, the greater your risk of developing heart disease," he says.

In an 80,000-person study, Harvard researchers found that getting just 3 percent of your daily calories from trans fats increases your risk of heart disease by up to 50 percent. To put that in perspective, 3 percent of your day's calories totals about 7 grams (g) of trans fat—which is roughly the amount in a single order of fries. But you don't eat french fries? You're still at risk. Even healthy Americans, researchers estimate, eat between 3 and 10 g of trans fats a day.

The damage doesn't stop with your heart, either. A diet high in trans fatty acids is also a major risk factor for diabetes. And it's no bit player: When Harvard researchers reviewed all the previously published data on trans fats, they found that men and women with the highest daily intakes of trans fats were also the most likely to develop diabetes.

Combine these disturbing studies with reports that trans fats may actually promote muscle loss and could even increase your risk of cancer, and it's no wonder the Institute of Medicine recently took a radical step, recommending that all Americans drastically reduce their intake of foods made with hydrogenated or partially hydrogenated oils. A consensus: Trans fats are so unhealthy that there is no safe upper limit of consumption.

PERCENTAGE OF AMERICANS WHO CLEAN THEIR PLATES NO MATTER HOW MUCH FOOD THEY'RE SERVED: 30

Naturally, food manufacturers using trans fats in their products were less than thrilled with the decision.

WHAT THE FOOD INDUSTRY DOESN'T WANT YOU TO KNOW

The Center for Science in the Public Interest—a consumer advocacy group—first began petitioning the FDA to add trans fats to food labels way back in 1993. After years of back-and-forth discussion between the two groups, they nearly reached agreement in 1999.

But as soon as the FDA announced its prospective change, groups like the Grocery Manufacturers of America—the world's largest food and beverage association—kicked into overdrive. Desperate to protect its members, the group began submitting alternate proposals to the FDA, thereby hampering efforts to pass the regulation.

After the Institute of Medicine's condemnation of trans fats early in 2003, the FDA stepped up regulation efforts again. Before the ink was even dry on a new proposal, manufacturers were up in arms again, claiming that new regulations may frighten consumers.

Finally, after months of debate, the FDA gave in, passing a regulation in July 2003 that forces companies to list trans fats as a separate entry on food labels. But companies are free to phase in the change, meaning you won't see trans fats listed on all ingredient labels for many years.

THE TRANS FAT YOU NEED

With all the evidence against trans fats, there's now data showing that at least one distant member of the trans fat family may actually be good for you. The compound in question—conjugated linoleic acid (CLA)—is a naturally occurring fat found primarily in beef and dairy products like milk, yogurt, and cheese.

Consider it the white sheep of the black-hearted trans fat family. CLA has no relation to partially hydrogenated oils, but the structure of the molecules in CLA is similar enough to that of trans fats that scientists place them both in the same category.

Although research is in its earliest stages, a number of promising studies suggest that CLA may help people lose weight, as well as help fight off cancer, diabetes, and heart disease—the very diseases brought about by the bad hydrogenated trans fats.

"If we're not careful, it's possible that CLA could get lumped in with all the other trans fats on food labels," says CLA expert Martha Belury, Ph.D., R.D., professor of nutrition at Ohio State University. "If this happens, people who try to cut all the trans fats out of their diets could end up avoiding some very important and beneficial foods."

DIAMONDS IN THE ROUGH

Partially hydrogenated oils are everywhere. You can't eliminate them from your diet, but if you pick the right brands of the foods you love, you can dramatically reduce the amount you're taking in on a daily basis.

If you want . . .	Pick this trans fat–free option
A candy bar	Dove dark chocolate bar
Cereal	Kellogg's Frosted Mini Wheats or Post Premium Raisin Bran
Cheese spread	Cheez Whiz Light
Cookies	Archway fat-free cookies or Pamela's Gourmet cookies
Corn chips	Tostitos Natural yellow corn chips
Crackers	Wheatables original reduced-fat crackers
Fish sticks	Van de Kamp's Crisp & Healthy breaded fish sticks
French fries	McCain Shoestring 5-minute French-Fried Potatoes
Frozen waffles	Kellogg's Special K fat-free waffles
Margarine	I Can't Believe It's Not Butter Fat Free spread or Smart Balance Light spread
Popcorn	Air-popped popcorn
Potato chips	Ruffles Natural sea-salted, reduced-fat chips
Potpies	Amy's organic potpies
Stuffing	Butterball One-Step seasoned stuffing

WHAT YOU CAN DO . . .

Until all companies start listing trans fats on their labels, here are some things you can do on your own to keep these fats out of the foods you eat.

. . . At the grocery store

Check the ingredient list for the words "hydrogenated" or "partially hydrogenated." The higher these ingredients are on the label, the more trans fats the food likely contains—with some exceptions, of course. Peanut butter, for example, can contain trace amounts of hydrogenated oil. But there's not enough trans fat to have a negative effect.

Decode the food label. Three Oreo cookies contain 7 g of fat. Of that fat, 1.5 g is saturated, 0.5 g is polyunsaturated, and 3 g is monounsaturated. Add these fats together, subtract 5 from 7, and you can estimate that each serving contains 2 g of trans fats.

Buy margarines that are free of trans fats, like Smart Balance Light. (Some cholesterol-lowering spreads still contain trans fats, so be careful.) Or at least opt for squeeze margarine, which has less trans fat than the stick variety.

Watch out for misleading labels. Products that are cholesterol-free, low-cholesterol, free of saturated fat, or vegetarian can still contain trans fats. But if a label says a food is fat-free, it's also trans fat–free.

Buy natural or organic brands. They're less processed and more likely to be trans fat–free.

. . . At home

Use milk instead of nondairy creamer in your morning coffee. Two cups of coffee could add more than a gram of trans fat to your diet.

Spread jelly instead of margarine on toast.

Pick high-protein breakfasts like eggs or Canadian bacon instead of waffles. If you want carbs, go for fat-free cereal.

Make a wrap with a tortilla or stuff a pita with lunchmeat instead of using bread.

Flavor vegetables with olive or sesame oil or butter-flavored spray instead of margarine.

Coat pans with nonstick spray instead of using margarine.

Snack on baked chips or chips fried in olive oil instead of vegetable shortening. (Check the ingredient list to be sure.)

Mix it up. Biscuits, cakes, and cookies made from a mix have fewer trans fats than their refrigerated or store-bought counterparts.

. . . At a restaurant

Ask what kind of oil the chef uses. You want to hear olive oil, not shortening.

Order foods that are baked, broiled, or grilled—not fried.

Skip the mayo when ordering a sandwich or burger. Pick mustard or ketchup instead.

Blot oil from fries as quickly as possible. Either spread the fries over a napkin, or dump them into the bag your order came in and shake it around to absorb the excess grease.

Avoid breads, which may be filled with trans fats. Pick a baked potato instead of a biscuit, or soup or salad instead of a roll.

For dessert, choose ice cream, frozen yogurt, or sorbet over cakes, cookies, or pie. Or pick angel food or sponge cake. Both are usually made with egg whites, flour, and sugar and contain very little fat.

HOW MUCH MORE FOOD PEOPLE SERVE THEMSELVES AT HOME, COMPARED WITH 20 YEARS AGO: 2 TIMES

When Dinner Is Dangerous

Our First World food supply is often cursed with Third World cleanliness—and the results can be pretty gruesome. Here, a rogue's gallery of the 10 dirtiest foods on our plates

By Jim Gorman

On October 6, 2003, Jeff Cook took his family out to dinner at Chi-Chi's Restaurant in the Beaver Valley Mall, north of Pittsburgh. When his chicken-and-steak fajitas arrived at the table, they were accompanied by the obvious—sautéed peppers, onions, sour cream—and the invisible—a helping of hepatitis A. Cook, 38, healthy and energetic on that autumn evening, died of acute liver failure a month later.

Hepatitis A may have been the disease that ended up sickening 575 Chi-Chi's patrons and employees—and killing three—but a batch of green onions was the carrier. Dirty food. The Centers for Disease Control and Prevention estimates that every day, 200,000 Americans contract food poisoning. But Philip Tierno, Ph.D., a microbiologist at New York University medical center and author of *The Secret Life of Germs*, pegs the true eat-'em-and-weep rate at around 800,000 a day. "Everyone in this country will have at least one incident of sickness this year attributable to a foodborne virus, bacteria, or toxin," Tierno says. Except that most of us won't know what hit us; we'll chalk up the usually mild symptoms—nausea, diarrhea, cramping—to "that stomach flu that's going around."

Scientists currently know of only one 100 percent foolproof way to prevent food poisoning: Stop eating. Or, almost as effective, obsess over every morsel you bring to your mouth and whether it might be staring back at you. But assuming you'd rather not die of slow starvation or, worse, live like Nick Nolte, we present you with a third, saner solution: Identify and sanitize the 10 dirtiest foods.

After considering incidence of outbreaks, relative danger of the dirt, and how often the carrier is found on our forks, we came up with a list of the edibles most likely to send your day spiraling down the crapper. We then assembled simple strategies for decontaminating the prime suspects—from the supermarket to the supper table—without worrying yourself sick. And what if, as with Jeff Cook, someone else does the cooking? We'll also tell you how to spot a dirty restaurant. Add it all up and what we're giving you is a recipe—for clean living.

CHICKEN

The dirt: Never mind cigarettes; the Surgeon General should slap a warning label on chicken. The USDA recently reported that a typical serving of chicken can contain 3.6 to 5.2 micrograms of arsenic, which is used as an antibiotic in their feed to prevent bacterial infections. But in humans, it's been linked with nervous system disorders and respiratory, skin, and bladder cancers. And recent nationwide testing by Consumers Union, the advocacy group behind *Consumer Reports,* notes that of the 484 raw broilers examined, 42 percent were infected by *Campylobacter jejuni,* and 12 percent by *Salmonella enterides.* (See "The Dirt Decoder," below.) The latest USDA research notes similar *Salmonella* levels. Now add in the fact that we each consume about 70 pounds of chicken a year—more than our intake of beef, pork, or turkey—and it's a wonder broilers don't come with barf bags.

THE DIRT DECODER

Nine bugs that can make eating a gut-wrenching experience

***Campylobacter jejuni* (bacteria):** The second leading bacterial cause of foodborne illness in the United States.

Symptoms: Fever, diarrhea, and nausea for 7 to 10 days.

***Clostridium perfringens* (bacteria):** Delay refrigerating leftovers and *Clostridium* can flourish.

Symptoms: Cramps and diarrhea usually lasting less than 24 hours.

***Cryptosporidium* (parasite):** Eighty percent of the U.S. population has been infected by it.

Symptom: Diarrhea usually lasting 2 to 4 days.

***E. coli 0157:H7* (bacteria):** Once limited to meats but now showing up throughout the food chain.

Symptoms: Commonly diarrhea but can also include vomiting and severe cramps.

***Listeria monocytogenes* (bacteria):** One of the deadliest pathogens. Can kill infants and the elderly.

Symptoms: Nausea, vomiting, and diarrhea, as well as flulike symptoms.

Norovirus: Causes one-third of all stomach viruses.

Symptoms: Mild nausea, vomiting, and diarrhea usually lasting 1 to 3 days.

***Salmonella enterides* (bacteria):** Close cousin to typhoid. Found throughout the food chain.

Symptoms: Nausea, vomiting, cramps, diarrhea, and fever usually lasting for 1 to 2 days.

***Shigella* (bacteria):** Accounts for less than 10 percent of all foodborne illnesses in the United States.

Symptoms: Diarrhea, cramps, and sometimes vomiting. It can take 3 days for symptoms to develop.

***Vibrio vulnificus* (bacteria):** Found in all U.S. coastal waters.

Symptoms: Cramps and vomiting within 16 hours of ingestion.

At the supermarket: Look for birds labeled "free range." Close quarters in the henhouse give bad bugs the chance to spread, as do high-volume processing operations. Free-range chickens, which are given more room to roost and are usually slaughtered in smaller numbers, present a potentially safer option. For example, Ranger chickens, a free-range brand sold in the Pacific Northwest, came up negative for *Salmonella* and *Campylobacter* in Consumers Union's tests.

At home: First, bypass rinsing your raw bird in the sink, and instead put it directly into a baking dish or pan. This shortcut reduces the odds of sullying counters and other foods, says Janet B. Anderson, R.D., director of the Safe Food Institute in North Logan, Utah. If you used a cutting board, clean it (and the knife) with a mild, dilute bleach solution. As for your heat treatment, cook breasts and other cuts until the temperature hits 180°F. (If it's a whole bird, take the temperature in the thickest part of the thigh.) "Poking the chicken or judging by juice color is risky," says Anderson.

DINNER, WITH RESERVATIONS

How to tell if food poisoning is on the menu

Eat at home, and you control the risks of food poisoning. Dine out, and your fate is in someone else's hands—a scary prospect when you don't know where those hands have been. But since is isn't always easy to tell whether a restaurant is likely to serve its special on a petri dish, we asked Theodore J. Gordon, director of Washington D.C.'s team of 16 restaurant inspectors, what he looks for when he dines out.

Soap and towels. "Walk into the men's room. Is there soap, hot water, towels? If not, walk out," says Gordon. If you can't wash your hands adequately, neither can the cook staff who are about to manhandle your food.

Clean bathrooms. "Is there water on the floor? Are the trash cans overflowing? If the bathrooms are dirty, then 90 percent of the time the kitchen is equally bad or worse," says Gordon.

Spotless kitchen. "If you can see into the kitchen, do you see grease dripping from the filters?" asks Gordon. "If anything looks bad or smells bad, then it is bad." This includes the wait staff.

Nonstick tables. "Tables should be cleared promptly," says Gordon. "If the table's been cleaned and there's a sticky residue, then that's an indication of poor sanitation."

Clean rags. "Look at the busboy's rag. Is it filthy? That's a bad sign," says Gordon.

Temperature extremes. Beware lukewarm food, especially at salad bars and buffets. "Pork chops should be heated to 140°F. If food is supposed to be cold, then it should feel cold," says Gordon.

GROUND BEEF

The dirt: Even a little ground chuck can make you upchuck. When USDA inspectors last tested hamburger meat, they looked at 563 sources nationwide and discovered *Clostridium perfringens* in 53 percent of the batches, *Staphylococcus* in 30 percent, and *Listeria monocytogenes* in 12 percent. Interestingly, the USDA found no trace of *Escherichia coli 0157:H7*, a.k.a. *E. coli*. Despite this finding, if slaughterhouse safeguards fail (and they sometimes do), *E. coli* could potentially pop up in your next patty.

At the supermarket: Choose ground cow that's been nuked. "Find a grocery store that sells irradiated ground beef," says Donald W. Schaffner, Ph.D., an extension specialist in food science at Rutgers University. The package will bear the words "treated by irradiation." Schaffner gives the safety of the treatment a glowing review: "The amount of induced radioactivity is 200,000 times smaller than the level of radioactivity naturally present in all foods."

At home: Add fresh oregano to your burgers and meat loaf. When researchers at Kansas State University mixed a variety of common household spices into ground beef to test their antibacterial properties, oregano tested as one of the best at wiping out *E. coli*. Use at least 1 tablespoon per pound of meat. Just as important, flatten your patties—thick burgers will char on the outside before the interior reaches the required 160°F.

GROUND TURKEY

The dirt: Potentially one of the foulest of the fowl. A USDA survey showed that the odds are better than one in four that your ground gobbler contains *Listeria, Campylobacter, Clostridium,* or some combination of the three. What's more, in a separate study by the FDA and the University of Maryland, 24 percent of the ground turkey sampled came back positive for *Salmonella*. And some of that *Salmonella* was resistant to antibiotics.

At the supermarket: Hunt for organic turkey. Most commercial turkey processors pump up their birds with antibiotics, a practice that may have encouraged the rise of resistant bacteria. Organic outfits, on the other hand, say no to drugs. When you reach the checkout, insist that the turkey be slipped into its own plastic bag and then placed in a meat-only shopping bag. This rule applies to beef and chicken, too. Otherwise, meat drippings might contaminate other groceries.

At home: "Change your mind-set about poultry. Start by thinking of it as being contaminated," says Schaffner. Immediately retire to the dishwasher any platter that has come in contact with raw ground turkey. (Use the hottest setting.) Serve cooked turkey burgers (180°F) on a clean plate. And wipe up any spillage with a paper towel instead of a sponge. "The sponge is the most dangerous item in the house because of the organisms potentially living in it," says Tierno.

RAW OYSTERS

The dirt: Oysters' power as an aphrodisiac is overblown, but their power as a diarrheic when slurped raw is not. These filters for ocean waste can contain the norovirus (a pathogen notorious for nixing ocean cruises), *Campylobacter*, and *Vibrio vulnificus*. University of Arizona researchers who studied oysters from so-called certified-safe beds discovered that 9 percent were contaminated with *Salmonella* bacteria. Still hungry? "We found *E. coli* in 100 percent of Gulf Coast locations, and in high amounts," says Lynn Joens, Ph.D., the study author.

At the supermarket: Buy from the same beds that a chef stakes his reputation on. Sandy Ingber, executive chef and seafood buyer for Grand Central Oyster Bar in New York City, buys Blue Point, Chincoteague, Glidden Point, Narragansett Bay, Pemaquid, and Wellfleet oysters in the winter months. During summer, he buys Coromandel oysters from New Zealand. The reason for the seasonal shift: More than three-quarters of outbreaks involving raw oysters occur in the Northern Hemisphere's warm-water months.

At home: Very simple: Eat only thoroughly cooked oysters. If you must slurp, do so only after following the buying advice above.

EGGS

The dirt: Which is dirtier, the chicken or the egg? The chicken, by a long shot, or so it seems at first. More widespread pasteurization has reduced the rate of *Salmonella* contamination in eggs to only 1 in 20,000. But that still leaves more than two million hazardous eggs in circulation each year. Food poisoning linked to eggs sickens an estimated 660,000 people annually and kills 300. "Often, dishes made at restaurants are from pooled eggs," which increases the risk, says Schaffner. "It's really a matter of statistics. Eat an egg sunny-side up and your risk of salmonella is 1 in 10,000. Eat an undercooked omelette made from a mix of 100 eggs, and the risk is significantly higher."

At the supermarket: Check the egg cartons. You're looking for one word—"pasteurized"—and four numbers—the expiration date. Then remove each egg and look for cracks; germs can enter after pasteurization.

At home: Ignore the egg keeper on the refrigerator door. Instead, keep the eggs in their carton and stow it in the coldest part of your fridge (usually the back of the lowest shelf). Then, after you crack one open, wash your hands. In her study of household food preparation, Utah State's Anderson reports that 60 percent of people failed to wash their hands after handling raw eggs. Finally, cook your eggs thoroughly (or, if they're an ingredient in a dish, to 160°F).

CANTALOUPE

The dirt: File this under "Who knew?" When the FDA sampled domestically grown cantaloupe, it found that 3.5 percent of the melons carried *Sal-*

monella and *Shigella,* the latter a bacteria normally passed person to person. Among imported cantaloupe, 7 percent tested positive for both bugs. And because you eat melons raw, the bacteria go right down your gullet. That's a big part of the reason why, from 1990 to 2001, produce in general has sickened as many people as have beef and poultry combined.

At the supermarket: Dents or bruising on the fruit can provide a path in for pathogens. But don't think precut cantaloupe is safer. "I've been in several supermarkets where the produce was cut by personnel who didn't wash their hands after handling eggs and other items," says Anderson.

At home: Because cantaloupe grows on the ground and has a netted exterior, it's easy for *Salmonella* to sneak on, and once on, it's hard to clean off. Scrub the fruit with a dab of mild dishwashing liquid for 15 to 30 seconds under running water. And make sure you buy a scrub brush that you use exclusively to clean fruits and vegetables; otherwise it could become cross-contaminated.

PEACHES

The dirt: Being pretty as a peach comes at a price. The fruit is doused with pesticides in the weeks prior to harvest to ensure blemish-free skin. By the time it arrives in your produce department, the typical peach can be coated with up to nine different pesticides, according to a USDA sampling. And while apples tote a wider variety of pesticides, the sheer amount and strength of those on peaches sets the fuzzy fruit apart. On an index of pesticide toxicity devised by Consumers Union, peaches rank highest.

At the supermarket: Fill your plastic produce bag with peaches that wear a "USDA Organic" sticker. And since apples, grapes, pears, and green beans occupy top spots on the Toxicity Index, too, you may want to opt for organic here as well. Just know that organic produce also contains some pesticide residues, but in minuscule amounts.

At home: Wax on, wax off. "A lot of produce has a natural wax coating that holds pesticides, so wash with a sponge or scrub brush and a dab of mild dishwashing detergent. This can eliminate more than half of the residues," says Edward Groth III, Ph.D., a senior scientist with Consumers Union. Got kids? Play it extra safe, and wash and pare peaches, apples, and pears.

PREPACKAGED LETTUCE

The dirt: Don't look now, but the lettuce on a burger could cause you more grief than the beef. Outbreaks of *E. coli* sickened 36 people in San Diego in September 2003 and sent 29 people reeling in eastern Washington in July 2002. In both cases, prepackaged lettuce was to blame. And according to the Center for Science in the Public Interest, lettuce accounted for 11 percent of reported food-poisoning outbreaks linked to produce from 1990 to 2002, and "salad" accounted for 28 percent.

At the supermarket: Prepackaged salad mix is not inherently more hazardous than loose greens or a head of lettuce. It's the claims of being "triple washed" that lull consumers into complacency. "Just because something is wrapped in cellophane doesn't mean it's free of pathogens," says J. Glenn Morris, M.D., chairman of epidemiology and preventive medicine at the University of Maryland school of medicine.

At home: Rinse salad greens one leaf at a time under running water before eating. Beware of cross-contamination, too. "People know it's risky to put salad in the same colander they washed chicken in," says Anderson, "but they think nothing of touching a towel used to wipe up poultry juice, then making a salad."

COLD CUTS

The dirt: Germs don't take a number in the deli; cold cuts have been labeled at "high risk" of causing listeriosis by a joint team of researchers from the USDA, FDA, and CDC. While only 3 percent of the deli meats sampled contained *Listeria* at the point of purchase, the bacteria's rapid growth rate on cuts stored even under ideal conditions concerned researchers. Combine that with the fact that cold cuts are, well, eaten cold, and you've got trouble; *Listeria* thrives at refrigerator temperatures that stun other foodborne pathogens.

At the supermarket: Turns out the most likely source of *Listeria*-contaminated cold cuts is the deli slicer. Without regular cleaning, the blade can transfer bacteria from roast beef to turkey to pastrami and back. But aside from asking the clerk to stop and clean the slicer before handling your order, the best you can do is avoid delis that are obviously dirty and stick with those that are annoyingly busy. Meats that rotate through a deli quickly have less opportunity to bloom with *Listeria.*

At home: From now on, skip the sniff test and trash whatever meat you haven't eaten in a week. When you're ready to build your sandwich, slather on the mustard. Researchers at Washington State University killed off 90 percent of three potent pathogens—*Listeria, E. coli,* and *Salmonella*—within 2 hours of exposing them to a mustard compound.

SCALLIONS

The dirt: Scallions play a bit part in most dishes, but a little goes a long way, as evidenced by the massive hepatitis A outbreak at that Chi-Chi's last October. Dirty scallions have also triggered small hep A outbreaks in Georgia, North Carolina, and Tennessee. Other bugs known to have grabbed a ride on green onions include the parasite *Cryptosporidium, Shigella,* and the ever-present *Salmonella.* In FDA tests, U.S.-grown scallions carried *Salmonella* or *Shigella* in 3 percent of samples, nearly twice the number detected in imported samples.

At the supermarket: Forget trying to weed out U.S. or Mexican scallions. Given current labeling laws, grocers are under no obligation to list the country of origin of any produce item. More important, buy refrigerated scallions; room temperature can trigger a bacterial explosion.

At home: Turn on your faucet full force to blast away visible dirt. As you rinse, remove the outer sheath to expose lingering microorganisms, but realize that any step short of thorough cooking is only a partial solution. "More and more, pathogens are entering produce like scallions at a cellular level," says Caroline Smith DeWaal, director of food safety at the Center for Science in the Public Interest.

Take the Guesswork Out of Grocery Shopping

We scoured the supermarket and picked the 125 best foods for guys. Now all you have to do is pull up a plate

By Brian Good

Space isn't the final frontier. There's also the supermarket. Except instead of searching for new solar systems, signs of intelligent life, or lingering extraterrestrial evidence of the Big Bang, we scan the aisles for something infinitely more elusive: a great low-calorie ice cream.

Well, plant a flag, because you've landed in the right place. We've discovered said ice cream (chocolate-fudge brownie, at that), along with more than 100 other foods that taste so good and are so good for us that they've earned our highest honor: the Munchie Award. The list of winners includes such notables as DiGiorno for Best Frozen Pizza—Round; Edy's for Best Ice Cream—Vanilla; and Uncle Ben's for Best Frozen Breakfast—period. Oh, sure, they can't actually hop down from their shelves, stroll up to a podium, and thank the academy (that's us). But that's for the best, since otherwise it might be a little awkward when it comes time to shove one of the winners into the microwave.

THE BEST PANTRY FOODS

Best Baked Beans

Bush's Best Vegetarian. Fat-free with a sweet, smoky flavor. Per 1/2 cup: 130 calories, 6 grams (g) protein, 24 g carbohydrates, 0 g fat, 6 g fiber

Best Salsa

Tostitos Party Bowl. Restaurant salsa for multiperson dunking. Per 2 Tbsp: 10 calories, 0 g protein, 2 g carbohydrates, 0 g fat, < 1 g fiber

Best Canned Fruit

Dole Tropical fruit salad. Three vitamin-packed fruits—papaya, pineapple, and guava—in one convenient can. Per 1/2 cup: 80 calories, < 1 g protein, 20 g carbohydrates, 0 g fat, 1 g fiber

Best Peanut Butter

Peter Pan Whipped. Lower in calories and creamier than regular PB, but nearly as much monounsaturated fat. Per 2 Tbsp: 140 calories, 6 g protein, 5 g carbohydrates, 12 g fat (2.5 g saturated, or sat., fat), 2 g fiber

Best Tuna

Starkist Tuna Creations. No draining (it comes in a foil pouch) and three different flavors. Per 2 ounces of herb and garlic: 80 calories, 13 g protein, 0 g carbohydrates, 3 g fat (0 g sat. fat), 0 g fiber

Best Canned Vegetable

Taylor's sweet potatoes. All the benefits of beta-carotene without the brown-sugar glaze—or the extra calories. Per 2 potatoes: 90 calories, 1 g protein, 22 g carbohydrates, 0 g fat, 3 g fiber

Best Tomato Soup

Campbell's Ready-to-Serve Creamy. No high-fructose corn syrup, just pure liquid lycopene. Per cup: 130 calories, 3 g protein, 26 g carbohydrates, 1.5 g fat (1 g sat. fat), 2 g fiber

Best Canned Soups

Progresso. A just-like-homemade hat trick.

Beef: Grilled Steak. Per cup: 120 calories, 10 g protein, 13 g carbohydrates, 3.5 g fat (1 g sat. fat), 1 g fiber

Chicken: 99% Fat Free Chicken Noodle. Per cup: 90 calories, 7 g protein, 13 g carbohydrates, 1.5 g fat (0 g sat. fat), less than 1 g fiber

Vegetable: Basil Rotini Tomato. Per cup: 120 calories, 5 g protein, 22 g carbohydrates, 1.5 g fat (0 g sat. fat), 2 g fiber

Best Canned Tomatoes

Contadina Recipe Ready Diced Tomatoes Primavera. All the ingredients for the primavera in pasta primavera. Per 1/2 cup: 60 calories, 1 g protein, 13 g carbohydrates, 0 g fat, 2 g fiber

Best Pasta Sauce

Ragu Rich & Meaty Mama's meat sauce. Chunks of ground beef, thick sauce, and the spices to pull it all together. Per 1/2 cup: 130 calories, 7 g protein, 8 g carbohydrates, 8 g fat (2 g sat. fat), 2 g fiber

Best Refried Beans

Old El Paso Fat-Free. Thanks to a mix of salt, onion, garlic, chili peppers, and other spices, these beans only *taste* refried. Per 1/2 cup: 100 calories, 6 g protein, 18 g carbohydrates, 0 g fat, 6 g fiber

Best Instant Mexican Meal

Old El Paso seasoned ground beef with taco sauce. A heat-and-eat meat. With this seasoned, fully cooked ground beef, you can make instant tacos and burritos that are healthier than the kind you get at restaurants. Or you can spoon it on tortilla chips and then top everything with lettuce, tomatoes, and fat-free sour cream. Per 1/2 cup: 90 calories, 6 g protein, 5 g carbohydrates, 5 g fat (2 g sat. fat), 0 g fiber

THE BEST SNACKS

Best Regular Pretzel

Rold Gold Honey Wheat Braided Twists. Per 2 ounces: 220 calories, 4 g protein, 47 g carbohydrates, 2 g fat (0 g sat. fat), 2 g fiber

Best Flavored Pretzel

Rold Gold Honey, Mustard and Onion pretzel pieces. Per 1/3 cup: 150 calories, 2 g protein, 20 g carbohydrates, 7 g fat (1 g sat. fat), 1 g fiber

Best Plain Cracker

Triscuit Reduced Fat whole-wheat crackers. Per 7 crackers: 120 calories, 3 g protein, 21 g carbohydrates, 3 g fat (0.5 g sat. fat), 3 g fiber

Best Potato Chip

Low Fat Kettle Krisps. Per ounce: 110 calories, 3 g protein, 22 g carbohydrates, 1.5 g fat (0 g sat. fat), 2 g fiber

Best Multigrain Chip

SunChips original flavor. Per 11 chips: 140 calories, 2 g protein, 19 g carbohydrates, 6 g fat (0.5 g sat. fat), 2 g fiber

Best Tortilla Chip

Garden of Eatin' Black Bean tortilla chips. Per 13 chips: 140 calories, 3 g protein, 18 g carbohydrates, 7 g fat (0.5 sat. fat), 4 g fiber

Best Corn Snack

Original Corn Nuts. Per 1.7-ounce bag: 210 calories, 4 g protein, 34 g carbohydrates, 8 g fat (1 g sat. fat), 4 g fiber

Best Cheese Cracker

Kraft Reduced Fat Cheddar Cheese Nips. Per 31 crackers: 130 calories, 3 g protein, 21 g carbohydrates, 3.5 g fat (1 g sat. fat), less than 1 g fiber

Best Cheese Puff

Quakes Nacho Cheese Baked Corn Rings. Per ounce: 120 calories, 2 g protein, 20 g carbohydrates, 4 g fat (0.5 g sat. fat), 1 g fiber

Best Cookie/Cracker Combo

Quaker Crisp'ums Cinnamon Sugar Crisps. Per 1.15-ounce package: 150 calories, 2 g protein, 24 g carbohydrates, 5 g fat (1 g sat. fat), 1 g fiber

Best Chocolate Cookie

Pepperidge Farm Double Chocolate Nantucket cookies. Per cookie: 140 calories, 2 g protein, 18 g carbohydrates, 7 g fat (3 g sat. fat), 1 g fiber

Best Sandwich Cookie

Teddy Grahams BearWiches. Per 2 cookies: 130 calories, 1 g protein, 19 g carbohydrates, 5 g fat (1 g sat. fat), 0 g fiber

Best Plain Popcorn

Orville Redenbacher's Butter Light popcorn. Per cup: 20 calories, less than 1 g protein, 4 g carbohydrates, 1 g fat (0 g sat. fat), less than 1 g fiber

Best Flavored Popcorn

Pop-Secret Honey Butter popcorn. Per cup: 35 calories, less than 1 g protein, 4 g carbohydrates, 2.5 g fat (0.5 g sat. fat), less than 1 g fiber

THE BEST CONDIMENTS

Best Steak Sauce

London Pub. A-1 is grade B compared with this sauce's tart vinegar-and-onion flavor and low sugar content. Per Tbsp: 10 calories, 0 g protein, 3 g carbohydrates, 0 g fat, 0 g fiber

Best Soy Sauce

Kikkoman Lite. About 50 percent less BP-raising sodium than regular soy sauce, but 99 percent of the flavor. Per Tbsp: 10 calories, 1 g protein, 1 g carbohydrates, 0 g fat, 0 g fiber

Best Spice

Mrs. Dash Salt Free Grilling Blends Mesquite. Can't grill? Broil. But first, sprinkle this mix on all your meat. Per 1/4 tsp: 0 calories, 0 g protein, 0 g carbohydrates, 0 g fat, 0 g fiber

Best Jam or Jelly

Smucker's Low Sugar preserves. Low sugar means you actually taste the fruit. Per Tbsp: 25 calories, 0 g protein, 6 g carbohydrates, 0 g fat, 0 g fiber

Best Dressings

Five great excuses to eat more salad.

Thousand Island: Kraft Light Done Right. Per 2 Tbsp: 60 calories, 0 g protein, 9 g carbohydrates, 2 g fat (0 g sat. fat), 0 g fiber

Italian: Newman's Own Dynamite Lite. Per 2 Tbsp: 30 calories, 0 g protein, 3 g carbohydrates, 2 g fat (0 g sat. fat), 0 g fiber

Ranch: Wishbone Just 2 Good Parmesan Peppercorn. Per 2 Tbsp: 45 calories, 0 g protein, 6 g carbohydrates, 2 g fat (0 g sat. fat), $<$ 1 g fiber

Blue Cheese: Kraft Light Done Right Roka. Per 2 Tbsp: 70 calories, $<$ 1 g protein, 3 g carbohydrates, 6 g fat (1 g sat. fat), 0 g fiber

French: Wishbone Just 2 Good. Per 2 Tbsp: 45 calories, 0 g protein, 7 g carbohydrates, 2 g fat (0 g sat. fat), less than 1 g fiber

Best Mustards

Sweet: French's Sweet Onion. Classic yellow made less sharp with sweet onion. Per tsp: 10 calories, 0 g protein, 2 g carbohydrates, 0 g fat, 0 g fiber

Spicy: Jack Daniel's Horseradish mustard. It isn't spiked with Jack, but it has a kick. Per tsp: 5 calories, 0 g protein, 0 g carbohydrates, 0 g fat, 0 g fiber

Best Barbecue Sauce

Dinosaur Bar-B-Que Roasted Garlic and Honey. Just tomato sauce, mustard, honey, brown sugar, spices, and great flavor. Per 2 Tbsp: 35 calories, 1 g protein, 8 g carbohydrates, 0 g fat, 0 g fiber

Best Relish

Mt. Olive No Sugar Added. One of the few relishes without covert calories. Per Tbsp: 4 calories, 0 g protein, 1 g carbohydrates, 0 g fat, 0 g fiber

Best Sandwich Spread

Hellmann's Bacon and Tomato Twist Light mayonnaise. A smoky bacon flavor that reinvents any sandwich. Per Tbsp: 50 calories, 0 g protein, 1 g carbohydrates, 5 g fat (1 g sat. fat), 0 g fiber

Best All-Purpose Hot Sauce

Mc.Ilhenny Co. Tabasco Green Pepper. Use it to doctor anything into edibility. Per tsp: 0 calories, 0 g protein, 0 g carbohydrates, 0 g fat, 0 g fiber

Best Mayonnaise

Kraft Fat-Free. Still the best of the lower-calorie mayonnaise bunch. Per Tbsp: 10 calories, 0 g protein, 2 g carbohydrates, 0 g fat, 0 g fiber

Best Syrup

Maple Grove Farms Sugar Free. Pour it on; the real maple taste is there, but the calories aren't. Per 1/4 cup: 10 calories, 0 g protein, 4 g carbohydrates, 0 g fat, 0 g fiber

THE BEST WORK FOODS

Best Breakfast to Eat over Your Keyboard

Chex Morning Mix. We like the cinnamon mix; it has almonds, cranberries, and raisins. Per pouch: 130 calories, 2 g protein, 24 g carbohydrates, 3.5 g fat (0.5 g sat. fat), 1 g fiber

Best Stashable Drink

Horizon Organic Reduced Fat chocolate milk. Spoil-proof moo. Per 8 ounces: 180 calories, 8 g protein, 28 g carbohydrates, 4.5 g fat (3 g sat. fat), 0 g fiber

Best Instant Soup

Nile Spice Red Beans & Rice. A low-fat, high-fiber, Louisiana-style soup. Per cup: 170 calories, 10 g protein, 35 g carbohydrates, 1 g fat (0 g sat. fat), 10 g fiber

Best Snack Bag

Seneca Crispy Cinnamon sweet-potato chips. Seven chips provide your recommended daily intake of beta-carotene. Per ounce: 150 calories, 1 g protein, 16 g carbohydrates, 9 g fat (1 g sat. fat), 4 g fiber

Best Dried Fruit

Blackbird Food Co. Fruit Crunchies. Almost all the nutrients of fresh fruit, but without the hassle. Per cup: 100 calories, 2 g protein, 18 g carbohydrates, 1 g fat (0 g sat. fat), 2 g fiber

Best High-Energy Snack

PowerBar Energy Bites. The whole oats, soy protein, and glucose will carry you to quitting time. Per bag of peanut-butter bites: 210 calories, 8 g protein, 32 g carbohydrates, 5 g fat (1 g sat. fat), 1 g fiber

Best Fruit Cup

Dole Fruit Bowls sliced peaches. More of what we want—peaches—and less of what we don't—sugary syrup. Per cup: 120 calories, < 1 g protein, 29 g carbohydrates, 0 g fat, 2 g fiber

Best Hard Candy

Creme Savers Sugar Free. The same flavor as regular Creme Savers. Per 5 candies: 45 calories, 0 g protein, 13 g carbohydrates, 1.5 g fat (1 g sat. fat), 0 g fiber

Best Chocolate Bar

Dove dark. Contains levels of disease-fighting flavonoids similar to those of chocolate used in studies. Per 1.3-ounce bar: 200 calories, 2 g protein, 22 g carbohydrates, 12 g fat (7 g sat. fat), 2 g fiber

Best Microwavable Soup Cups

Not quite dinner, but enough to hold you over.

Beef: Chef Boyardee beef stew. Per container: 150 calories, 8 g protein, 19 g carbohydrates, 5 g fat (2 g sat. fat), 2 g fiber

Chicken: Dinty Moore chicken and dumplings. Per container: 200 calories, 12 g protein, 25 g carbohydrates, 6 g fat (2 g sat. fat), 1 g fiber

Best Meal for When You're Working Late

Dinty Moore American Classics roast beef and gravy with mashed potatoes. Shelf-stable meat that tastes better than it sounds. Per package: 240 calories, 24 g protein, 24 g carbohydrates, 5 g fat (2 g sat. fat), 2 g fiber

Best Instant Macaroni and Cheese

Kraft Easy Mac Original. The bachelor staple made nukable. Per pouch: 250 calories, 7 g protein, 38 g carbohydrates, 8 g fat (2.5 g sat. fat), < 1 g fiber

Best Yogurts

You can go low-cal (Dannon) or extra fruit (Stonyfield). Either way, store a few in the office fridge.

Low-Sugar: Dannon Light 'n Fit. Per 6 ounces: 90 calories, 6 g protein, 17 g carbohydrates, 0 g fat, 0 g fiber

THE LIFETIME ACHIEVEMENT AWARD GOES TO . . .

Hormel Chili. We honor their chili for outstanding service to the stomachs of American men since 1935. Their recipe for success? Beef, beans, tomatoes, spices, and a willingness to experiment. You can now choose from eight different variations on the meat-and-bean theme, including Tabasco-flavored and our healthy favorite, turkey with beans; 1 cup contains 17 g protein, 5 g fiber, and just 3 g fat (1 g saturated fat). The only serious misstep: vegetarian chili. By our book, chili minus the meat isn't worth a hill of beans.

Regular: Stonyfield Farm Organic. Per 8 ounces: 150 calories, 8 g protein, 30 g carbohydrates, 0 g fat, < 1 g fiber

THE BEST DRINKS

Best Iced Green Tea

Honest Tea Green Dragon. In a Rutgers University study of green teas, this brew had one of the highest levels of phenols, potent disease-fighting compounds. Per 8 ounces: 30 calories, 0 g protein, 9 g carbohydrates, 0 g fat, 0 g fiber

Best Iced Black Tea

Tazo. Made with just a bit of cane sugar to cut the bitterness of the tea without hiding the flavor. Per 8 ounces: 35 calories, 0 g protein, 10 g carbohydrates, 0 g fat, 0 g fiber

Best Vegetable Juice

Spicy Hot V8. Still the best. We went with spicy over regular, since the bite makes the drink a bit less boring. Per cup: 50 calories, 1 g protein, 10 g carbohydrates, 0 g fat, 2 g fiber

Best Bottled Smoothie

Stonyfield Farm. Contains no high-fructose corn syrup and has a just-blended taste. Flavors: Peach, raspberry, strawberry, wild berry, and tropical fruit. Per serving: 240 calories, 9 g protein, 44 g carbohydrates, 3 g fat (2 g sat. fat), 2 g fiber

Best Iced Coffee

Folgers Jakada mocha coffee latte. Think Starbucks Frappuccino with a stronger coffee flavor, fewer calories, and less fat. Per 10.5 ounces: 180 calories, 5 g protein, 33 g carbohydrates, 3.5 g fat (2 g sat. fat), 0 g fiber

Best Soft Drink

Natural Brew Outrageous ginger ale. Made with Jamaican and Chinese ginger, plus a shot of cane juice; you get hot and sweet with every swallow. Per 12 ounces: 170 calories, 0 g protein, 42 g carbohydrates, 0 g fat, 0 g fiber

Best Chocolate Drink

Hershey's. Tied tastewise with Yoo-hoo, Hershey's gets the nod for being free of high-fructose corn syrup. Per cup: 130 calories, 2 g protein, 29 g carbohydrates, 1 g fat (0 g sat. fat), 0 g fiber

Best Single-Serving Orange Juice

Tropicana Pure Premium. The original not-from-concentrate OJ. Down one a day to boost your HDL cholesterol. Per 14 ounces: 190 calories, 3 g protein, 43 g carbohydrates, 0 g fat, 0 g fiber

Best Low-Calorie Juice

Ocean Spray Light Ruby Red grapefruit juice. Sweetened with Splenda, for close to two-thirds fewer calories per glass. Bonus: Ruby red grapefruit is a source of lycopene. Per cup: 40 calories, 0 g protein, 10 g carbohydrates, 0 g fat, 0 g fiber

Best Bottled Juice

Welch's grape juice. One of the only grape juices made from Concord grapes, a flavonoid-rich variety that can help prevent blood clots and reduce your risk of heart disease. Per cup: 170 calories, 0 g protein, 42 g carbohydrates, 0 g fat, 0 g fiber

Best Drink for After You Mow the Lawn

Crystal Light lemonade. Studies show that citrus-flavored, noncarbonated drinks like this one are best at quenching thirst. They might just be right. Per 16 ounces: 10 calories, 0 g protein, 0 g carbohydrates, 0 g fat, 0 g fiber

THE BEST FREEZER FOODS

Best Frozen Breakfast

Uncle Ben's Ham, Egg & Peppers Breakfast Bowl. A few minutes in the microwave and you get hot, high protein (17 g), and a heck of a lot like homemade. Per bowl: 230 calories, 17 g protein, 22 g carbohydrates, 9 g fat (4.5 g sat. fat), 3 g fiber

Best Shrimp Dinner

Gorton's Fried Rice Shrimp Bowl. Selenium-packed shrimp and just 2 g fat. (It is high in sodium, so don't eat it every day.) Per bowl: 320 calories, 11 g protein, 67 g carbohydrates, 2 g fat (0.5 g sat. fat), 2 g fiber

Best Round Pizza

DiGiorno Spicy Chicken Supreme. The perfect balance between fat and flavor. Our tasters loved the garlic-and-pepper-spiked chicken. Per $^1/_6$ of pizza: 320 calories, 17 g protein, 40 g carbohydrates, 10 g fat (4.5 g sat. fat), 3 g fiber

Best Single-Serving Pizza

Healthy Choice Solos Supreme French Bread. Portion-controlled pizza that, thanks to 8 g fiber, will fill you up. Per pizza: 360 calories, 20 g protein, 58 g carbohydrates, 5 g fat (1.5 g sat. fat), 8 g fiber

Best Ice-Cream Sandwich

Eskimo Pie Sugar-Free. A ringer for the original, but with a third fewer calories. Per sandwich: 160 calories, 4 g protein, 27 g carbohydrates, 4 g fat (2 g sat. fat), < 1 g fiber

Best Ice Creams

Chocolate: Healthy Choice No Sugar Added Chocolate Fudge Brownie. Rich and creamy, with a hit of chocolate syrup and moist brownie chunk every third or fourth bite. Per 1/2 cup: 120 calories, 3 g protein, 21 g carbohydrates, 2 g fat (1 g sat. fat), 1 g fiber

Vanilla: Edy's Grand Light. A strong vanilla-bean flavor that beat out some full-calorie contenders. Per 1/2 cup: 100 calories, 3 g protein, 15 g carbohydrates, 3.5 g fat (2 g sat. fat), 0 g fiber

Best TV Dinners

Beef: Stouffer's Homestyle Dinners Slow Roasted beef and gravy. Just like real CIY (carve-it-yourself) roast beef. Plus, it comes with mashed—skins-on—potatoes. Per package: 400 calories, 24 g protein, 41 g carbohydrates, 16 g fat (4.5 g sat. fat), 9 g fiber

Chicken: Stouffer's Homestyle Dinners Chicken Monterey with rice and whipped sweet potatoes. Most chicken dinners skimp on—go figure—the chicken. This version satisfies with five or six large chunks. Per package: 580 calories, 29 g protein, 68 g carbohydrates, 21 g fat (7 g sat. fat), 4 g fiber

Turkey: Stouffer's Homestyle Entrées roast turkey breast with gravy, stuffing, and mashed potatoes. Turkey tenderloins and paprika-spiced mashed potatoes give you the flavor of Thanksgiving without the just-stuffed feeling. Per package: 300 calories, 16 g protein, 34 g carbohydrates, 11 g fat (3 g sat. fat), 2 g fiber

Fish: Weight Watchers Smart Ones Tuna Noodle Gratin. The creamy sauce and bread crumbs make this taste richer than it really is. Bonus: Tuna is a good source of omega-3s. Per package: 270 calories, 14 g protein, 38 g carbohydrates, 7 g fat (2.5 g sat. fat), 3 g fiber

Italian: Uncle Ben's Three Cheese Ravioli Pasta Bowl. Topped with mozzarella, a three-cheese ravioli that blows away the canned kind. Per package: 380 calories, 21 g protein, 55 g carbohydrates, 7 g fat (4 g sat. fat), 6 g fiber

Best Frozen-Fruit Bar

Edy's Whole Fruit No Sugar Added fruit bar. Unlike the sickly sweet Popsicles you remember, these are made with fruit juice and bits of real fruit (strawberry, tangerine, or raspberry). Per bar: 30 calories, 0 g protein, 7 g carbohydrates, 0 g fat, 0 g fiber

Best Frozen Sandwich

Lean Pockets chicken fajita. The crust is more croissant than tortilla, but it packs a payload of guilt-free cheese (only 7 g fat each). Per fajita: 260 calories, 11 g protein, 38 g carbohydrates, 7 g fat (2.5 g sat. fat), 3 g fiber

MAXIMUM PERCENTAGE OF CALORIES IN YOUR DIET THAT SHOULD COME FROM SUGAR: 10

Best Frozen Smoothie Mix

VIP Ready to Blend Cherry Berry Blizzard. A five-fruit smoothie in under 10 minutes. Per 8 ounces: 170 calories, 2 g protein, 38 g carbohydrates, 1.5 g fat (0 g sat. fat), 3 g fiber

Best Frozen Burger

Aqua Cuisine salmon burger. Skip the fish fry and grill these babies. Each lemon-and-dill-flavored patty is ultralean—made with just salmon, bread crumbs, and spices—and contains more than 1,000 milligrams of heart-healthy omega-3 fatty acids. Serve on an Arnold Country Wheat Sandwich Roll with a dab of French's Sweet Onion mustard. Per patty: 140 calories, 16 g protein, 3 g carbohydrates, 7 g fat (1.5 g sat. fat), 0 g fiber

THE BEST MUSCLE FOODS

Best Flavored Water

Fruit 2 O Natural Lemon water. Gatorade too sweet? Plain water too plain? Meet the perfect compromise. Per serving: 0 calories, 0 g protein, 0 g carbohydrates, 0 g fat, 0 g fiber

Best Protein Shake

Nitro-tech Chocolate Swirl shake. Muscle-building whey protein disguised as dessert. Per 11 ounces: 190 calories, 40 g protein, 6 g carbohydrates, 1.5 g fat (0.5 g sat. fat), 0 g fiber

Best Energy Bar

Honey Stinger. Oatmeal-cookie crunch with honey for long-lasting energy. Per Rocket Chocolate bar: 190 calories, 10 g protein, 28 g carbohydrates, 4.5 g fat (2.5 g sat. fat), 2 g fiber

Best Fruit Snack

Stretch Island Fruit Leather. You can gnaw on nine flavors, including raspberry and mango. Per Tropical Fruit bar: 45 calories, 0 g protein, 11 g carbohydrates, 0 g fat, 1 g fiber

Best Snack in a Tube

Skippy Creamy Peanut Butter Squeeze Stix. These have all the perks of peanut butter—protein, monounsaturated fat—in a convenient, stow-away tube. Per tube: 140 calories, 6 g protein, 5 g carbohydrates, 12 g fat (2.5 g sat. fat), 2 g fiber

Best Meal Replacement

Snapple a Day. A drinkable multivitamin that's fortified with fiber. Per bottle Tropical Blend: 210 calories, 7 g protein, 43 g carbohydrates, 0 g fat, 5 g fiber

Best String Cheese

Kraft Polly-O String-Ums Lite mozzarella. With 8 g protein per stick, this is a great postlift snack. Per stick: 60 calories, 8 g protein, less than 1 g carbohydrates, 2.5 g fat (1.5 g sat. fat), 0 g fiber

Best Sports Drink

Gatorade Ice. The sugar in Gatorade is primarily glucose—the carbohydrate most readily used by the body for energy. Other sports drinks? High-fructose corn syrup. Per 8 ounces: 50 calories, 0 g protein, 14 g carbohydrates, 0 g fat, 0 g fiber

Best Sports Gel

PowerBar. Eighty percent complex carbs and 20 percent simple carbs for energy now and later. Per serving: 110 calories, 0 g protein, 28 g carbohydrates, 0 g fat, 0 g fiber

And the other winners are . . .

Best Bread: Milton's Multi-Grain
Best Tortilla: Tumaro's Honey Wheat
Best Bun: Arnold Country Wheat sandwich roll
Best English Muffin: Thomas Honey Wheat
Best Cold Cereal: Atkins flakes with almond
Best Hot Cereal: Quaker Instant Oatmeal Express Cinnamon Roll
Best Eggs: Egg-lands Best Eggs
Best Whole Wheat Pasta: Hodgson Mill spaghetti with flaxseed
Best Spinach Pasta: Davinci fusilli
Best Instant Meal: Tyson seasoned beef-sirloin roast
Best Instant Chinese Meal: Chef's Choice beef stir-fry
Best Instant Italian Meal: Simply Simmered chicken marinara
Best Precooked Chicken: Louis Rich Southwestern strips
Best Chicken Sandwich Meat: Butterball Sandwich Starters Mesquite
Best Turkey Lunchmeat: Hillshire Farm Deli Select oven-roasted turkey breast
Best Beef Lunchmeat: Hillshire Farm Deli Select oven-roasted cured beef
Best Chicken Lunchmeat: Healthy Choice oven-roasted chicken breast
Best Ham Lunchmeat: Hormel Canadian Bacon Style lunchmeat
Best Sliced Cheese: Borden 2% Milk Reduced-Fat American
Best Sausage: Casual Gourmet red-bell-pepper-and-basil chicken
Best Pizza Topping Hormel turkey pepperoni
Best Shredded Cheeses: Kraft Free Cheddar, Sargento Light Mexican, Kraft Reduced Fat Parmesan
Best Hot Dogs: Healthy Choice Low-Fat beef, Louis Rich Bun-Length turkey
Best Side Dish: Lipton Thai sesame noodles

The Top 10 Supplements for Men

Your drugstore carries thousands of bottles of colored pills. These are the ones you actually need

By Elizabeth M. Ward, M.S., R.D.

The greatest moment in the history of supplements came on September 1, 1998. That's when a sportswriter challenged Sammy Sosa on how he could compete with the androstenedione-assisted Mark McGwire. In reply, Sosa uncorked a shocker: He owed it all—wink—to Flintstones vitamins. Coincidence or not, after Sosa bunny-hopped and blew a kiss to the pill makers, the market soared, with $17 billion in sales in 2000.

So that you spend your share wisely, we asked shrewd judges of vitamin talent to name a supplement all-star team for men. Judge your strengths and weaknesses, and pencil in a lineup that will work for you.

BORON TO PROTECT YOUR PROSTATE

Men with the highest boron intakes are 65 percent less likely to develop prostate cancer than men with lower levels, studies show. American men have one of the lowest boron intakes in the world.

How much? 3 milligrams (mg) a day. It doesn't just fight cancer: USDA researchers found that this is the best dosage to improve memory and concentration.

Tip: It's not in every store, but GNC carries it. If you can't find it, eat raisins and almonds.

CALCIUM TO LOSE WEIGHT AND STRENGTHEN BONES

Most men don't get the recommended 1,000 mg of calcium a day (a cup of milk has 300). Men with the highest calcium intakes weigh less on average than men consuming less calcium.

How much? Aim for 1,200 mg calcium citrate—half in the morning, half at night, to maximize absorption. Avoid coral calcium, which can be full of impurities.

Tip: If you already eat three servings of dairy a day, you won't need the excess calcium. There's a risk you may exceed the maximum intake of 2,500 mg.

CHROMIUM TO WARD OFF DIABETES

You may know it as a muscle-building supplement, but if you're overweight or diabetes runs in your family, "taking chromium is one of the best things you can do to help keep insulin levels where they belong," says Richard Anderson, Ph.D., a researcher with the USDA. Chromium improves

MULTIPLE CHOICE

Looking for a good multivitamin? Swallow one of these

You still need to take a multivitamin. It's one of the best ways to reduce your risk of a number of ills, including heart disease, stroke, and diabetes. Our favorite? Centrum Silver, which contains 100 percent of your recommended intake of 16 core nutrients, along with additional doses of 15 other disease fighters—such as lycopene, lutein, and selenium. (Ignore the "for adults 50+" on the label—it's great for men of all ages.) An added bonus: Unlike other multis, Centrum Silver is free of iron—a mineral that can increase some men's risk of heart disease and Parkinson's disease. Our backup choice, One A Day Men's Health Formula, comes close, with higher doses of some of the basics but without a few of the extras in Centrum Silver.

the body's sensitivity to insulin, making it easier to keep blood sugar levels under control.

How much? 35 micrograms (mcg) a day. Check the label for "chromium picolinate," the form that studies have found to be the most effective.

Tip: If you already have diabetes, ask your doctor if you should take 200 mcg, Anderson says.

COENZYME Q_{10} TO BOOST ENERGY

Your body produces coenzyme Q_{10}; it helps cells manage your body's energy supply. But as you get older, production decreases. The only way to get back up to youthful levels is by taking a supplement. Recent studies suggest that coenzyme Q_{10} may fight cancer, Parkinson's disease, and Huntington's disease and may thin the blood to help prevent heart disease. Q_{10} is also packed with free-radical-fighting antioxidants, which can slow the signs of aging.

How much? Researchers recommend 100 mg a day. You won't find Q_{10} in a multivitamin or get any useful quantity from food.

Tip: If you're taking statins, which can reduce Q_{10}, consider upping your intake to 200 mg.

CREATINE TO BOOST MUSCLE AND MEMORY

Researchers at the Medical College of Wisconsin found that men taking creatine for just 2 to 3 months increased their maximum bench presses by an average of 15 pounds and their squats by 21 pounds. Australian researchers say memory and intelligence test scores improved after just 6 weeks of creatine use.

How much? 5 grams (g) a day. Mix it with whey in a protein shake for maximum benefit.

Tip: Some men don't respond to creatine by itself. Mixing it with large amounts of sugar can help turn nonresponders into responders.

FOLIC ACID TO CUT ALZHEIMER'S RISK

Folic acid helps prevent clogged arteries and improves bloodflow to the brain by keeping down levels of homocysteine, an amino acid that increases your risk of blood clots. High homocysteine levels are associated with early warning signs of Alzheimer's, such as dementia and memory loss. Researchers in Sweden found that Alzheimer's patients are more likely to have folic acid deficiencies. Getting enough folate also helps prevent heart disease and colon cancer and keeps sperm vigorous.

How much? 500 mcg a day, which could help lower homocysteine levels by 18 percent or more. Food sources include citrus fruit, beans, and fortified breads and cereals.

Tip: Certain heartburn medications, such as Tagamet, can deplete levels of folic acid.

GLUCOSAMINE TO GREASE YOUR JOINTS

You don't have the same amount of cartilage in your joints that you had at 19—maybe you've noticed. To reverse the damage and actually rebuild cartilage, take glucosamine, made from the shells of crabs and lobsters. In a 3-year study of 200 people with joint problems published in the *Lancet*, glucosamine reduced joint pain and stiffness by up to 25 percent and helped prevent the progression of osteoarthritis in the knees. The *British Journal of Sports Medicine* says that 88 percent of people with joint problems reported less pain after 12 weeks of treatment.

How much? 1,500 mg a day. Brands that combine glucosamine with chondroitin are fine.

Tip: Rubbing a cream made with glucosamine on a sore joint may relieve pain, according to an Australian study.

OMEGA-3S TO PROTECT YOUR HEART

Omega-3 fatty acids keep blood pressure and triglyceride levels low and the heart beating regularly. They make blood slicker, reducing the risk of clots and blocked arteries. Studies show that men with the highest omega-3 levels have the lowest risk of dying of heart disease.

PERCENTAGE LESS LIKELY YOU ARE TO DEVELOP HEART DISEASE IF YOU TAKE A DAILY VITAMIN: 21

How much? For healthy guys, 1,000 mg a day. Those with heart problems may need 2,000 to 4,000 mg. But check with your doctor—too much can increase your risk of catching a cold.

Tip: Our favorite is Omega Brite, an especially pure brand that comes in 500-mg gelcaps, so you're not popping pills all day. Take omega-3s with meals so you don't burp up a fish scent.

SELENIUM TO FIGHT OFF CANCER

"No other single nutrient appears to prevent cancer more effectively than selenium," says Gerald F. Combs, Ph.D., director of the USDA's Grand Forks Human Nutrition Research Center. It basically forces cancer cells to self-destruct. Combs's studies have linked increased selenium consumption to a decreased risk of cancers of the prostate, colon, and lungs, among others. One caveat: If you've ever had skin cancer, you may want to avoid taking selenium supplements. A recent study of 1,300 people with histories of skin cancer from the Roswell Park Cancer Institute in Buffalo, New York, found that individuals taking selenium were 25 percent more likely to develop malignant skin-cancer tumors than people not taking the supplement. Research into the link is ongoing.

How much? 200 mcg a day—more when you're sick. Research on mice, done at the University of North Carolina, suggests that low levels of selenium

CHEW ON THIS

Thinking of stealing your kids' vitamins? They're not as complete as "adult" multivitamins, but they can't hurt. "If you don't currently take a multivitamin and your diet is already decent, these candy vitamins are a good way to fill in holes and ensure that you're getting the right levels of all the most basic nutrients," says *Men's Health* magazine nutrition advisor Mary Ellen Camire, Ph.D. Below, we rate five kids' chewable vitamins.

Children's Choice Gummi Bear multivitamins. Just seven nutrients. Taste: Tart and chalky.

Flintstones Complete chewable vitamins. Well-rounded, with 100 percent of the adult levels of 15 vitamins and minerals. Taste: A pleasant reminder of childhood.

L'il Critters Vita Worms. 100 percent of adult levels of nine vitamins and minerals. Taste: Just like regular gummy worms.

Sweet Essentials Daily Supplement Malted Milk Balls. Good source of vitamins C, D, and E and six other nutrients. Taste: Yummy.

VitaBall Vitamin gumballs. You have to chew for 10 minutes to release adequate levels of 11 vitamins and minerals. Taste: Awful.

may make it easier for viruses to mutate, worsening symptoms of the flu.

Tip: Nature's selenium supplement is the Brazil nut, which has 100 mcg per nut.

VITAMIN E TO SLOW THE EFFECTS OF AGING

This is one of the most potent antioxidants. "Vitamin E may help reduce the risk of certain eye diseases, heart disease, cancer, even Alzheimer's disease," says Jeffrey Blumberg, Ph.D., professor of nutrition at Tufts University. Bonus: Studies show it also reduces muscle damage after exercise.

How much? Up to 400 international units (IU) a day, since most people get just a fraction of that from their diets. (A typical multivitamin has 45 IU.) You can also increase your intake by eating more nuts and oils.

Tip: Buy natural vitamin E (d-alpha tocopherol) rather than synthetic (dl-alpha tocopherol), which is harder for the body to put to use.

NEED TO KNOW

Toast Your Health

Science has confirmed what Mom always told you: Don't skip breakfast. In a Harvard study of nearly 3,000 men and women, researchers found that eating breakfast every day reduces your risk of obesity, diabetes, and heart disease by 35 to 50 percent. "Eating breakfast daily, especially whole-grain cereals and fruits, may help keep your body's metabolism and hormones at optimal levels for controlling appetite and minimizing disease risk," explains Mark Pereira, Ph.D., the study author.

Your morning meal is in fact the most critical when it comes to weight loss. University of California at Berkeley scientists found that people who ate a grain-based breakfast had an average body-mass index (BMI) of 25.88, about 2 points lower than that of the bacon-and-egg addicts. While fat and fiber levels certainly affected the study's outcome, eating habits may be equally important, says Coralie Brown, one of the study authors. Because cereal and other grain-based meals are usually easier to prepare than meat-and-egg breakfasts, you're less likely to skip them and wind up overeating later in the day.

The Where and When of Weight Loss

There are reasons you can eat all the right foods and get plenty of exercise but still not have your ideal body. The problem may not be what you're eating or how much but rather when and where all that eating is taking place. As we've already mentioned, skipping breakfast is one reason. Eating most of your meals in restaurants is another. Researchers at the University of Massachusetts analyzed the eating habits of 500 men and women and found some interesting connections between the way guys eat and our risk of becoming overweight.

PERCENTAGE DECREASE IN RISK OF DYING OVER A 5-YEAR PERIOD IF YOU EAT JUST ONE BOWL OF WHOLE-GRAIN CEREAL (SUCH AS BRAN FLAKES OR OATMEAL) A DAY: 27

Habit	Changes Your Risk of Obesity by . . .
Eating at least one midday snack	−39 percent
Eating dinner as your biggest meal of the day	+6 percent
Waiting more than 3 hours after waking up to eat breakfast	+43 percent
Eating more than a third of your meals in restaurants	+69 percent
Going to bed hungry (3 or more hours after your last meal or snack)	+101 percent
Eating breakfast away from home	+137 percent
Not eating breakfast	+450 percent

Grab an Ice-Cold One

Instead of loosening your belt before a big meal, chug a tall glass of ice water to boost your metabolism. German scientists report that people who drank 17 ounces of water increased their metabolic rate by 30 percent for up to an hour and a half. Part of the increase came from thermogenesis, a process in which the body burns calories in order to digest food or liquid; cold consumables require more energy. The rest is due to your nervous system's response to a full stomach. Bonus: "In men, stored fat provided the fuel for the heightened metabolic rate," says researcher Jens Jordan, M.D.

Get Skinny by Dipping

Next time you eat out, don't butter your bread; dip it in olive oil instead. Not only is the monounsaturated fat in olive oil better for your heart than the saturated fat in butter or the trans fat in margarine, but it's also better for your waistline. Researchers at the University of Illinois gave 341 people eating in an Italian restaurant six slices of bread along with equal amounts of either olive oil or butter. While diners who were given the olive oil consumed more fat on each slice of bread than those who were given butter, the olive oil group ultimately ate nearly 25 percent less bread. Dippers also took in significantly fewer calories over the course of the meal than their butter-eating counterparts.

Supplement Your Weight Loss

According to a recent study review, only two weight-loss supplements show promise as fat burners. The first is conjugated linoleic acid (CLA), which was found to reduce body fat by 2.8 to 3.8 percent. "It's believed to work by inhibiting an enzyme that breaks down fat for absorption," says Thomas Lenz, Pharm.D., a coauthor of the study. The second is pyruvate, an enzyme that helps manipulate fat metabolism. It helped cut body fat by up to 12 percent when combined with exercise. But as impressive as those results are, don't overdo it, Lenz cautions. More is not better when it comes to dosage. "You should take the same dosage for the same amount of time that was tested," he says. For CLA, that means 3 grams (g) daily for 12 weeks, and for pyruvate, 6 g daily for 6 weeks.

Are You Getting Enough?

Nutrients, that is. According to the USDA, which analyzed the diets of thousands of men, the average guy is woefully low on certain important dietary vitamins and minerals—even if he takes a multivitamin supplement. Most men need to focus on getting more folate and vitamin E—key nutrients for heart and immune-system health. They also need to bone up on calcium (see more on that in the next item).

Why Dairy Is Queen

Americans still aren't getting enough dairy, according to a new National Dairy Council report. Most men, in fact, consume only half the recommended three servings a day. This shortfall weakens bones and can cause weight gain, since the calcium in milk and cheese also helps keep guys lean. A recent study from the University of California at Davis shows that dairy foods may help curb your appetite. Researchers found that when men ate meals that were low in all forms of fat except dairy, their levels of a satiating hormone called cholecystokinin (CCK) rose by 20 percent. Lead study author Barbara Schneeman, Ph.D., speculates that the lipid structure of dairy fat or as-yet-undiscovered components in dairy foods caused the spike. "Not all dairy products must be fat-free to be useful [for weight loss]," she says. Even a small amount—a pat of butter, a slice of Cheddar—will boost your CCK level.

Another Soy Warning

On the heels of research linking soy-rich diets to Alzheimer's and abnormally high estrogen levels comes another, equally disturbing finding. A new study published in the *Journal of Urology* suggests that eating soy may alter male reproductive organs, triggering sexual dysfunction. The data comes from a very preliminary series of trials conducted on rats. The study's authors say it's too early to alter your diet based on their research, but men should be aware of this potential new risk, especially since the rats' sexual dysfunction lasted long after they transitioned back to a diet lower in soy.

A Zinger from Zinc

Forty-seven thousand men can't be wrong. That's the number of men National Institutes of Health researchers studied to determine that supplementing with zinc may raise the risk of advanced prostate cancer. The study showed that men who consumed more than 100 milligrams (mg) of zinc per day had over twice the risk of advanced prostate cancer, compared with those who took in less. Why? Excess zinc may interfere with the protection provided by other nutrients. "For example, zinc may counteract the tumor-protective effects of selenium," says Michael Leitzmann, M.D., one of the study authors. Look for a multivitamin that contains no more than 11 mg zinc, the recommended daily allowance for men.

Take It Easy on the Tums

Your addiction to antacids may cause food allergies, say Austrian researchers. In a study of 153 people, 25 percent developed signs of food allergies after taking antacids like Tums, proton-pump inhibitors like Prilosec, or h-2 inhibitors like Zantac for 3 months. Along with blocking stomach acids, antacids also block the action of the digestive enzyme pepsin. "Since the food can't be degraded, the immune system assumes it's dangerous and attacks it," says study author Erika Jensen-Jarolim, M.D. If you're on any of these meds for a diagnosed condition, fine. But don't pop pills instead of avoiding foods that cause heartburn and indigestion.

Stomach Saver

If you get stomach cramps or bloating after eating olestra or Olean, be extra careful which low-fat foods you buy from now on. The FDA is allowing food manufacturers to remove olestra warning labels. So the only way you'll know if something contains olestra will be to check the ingredient list.

We'll Drink to That

We've told you dozens of times that drinking alcohol can reduce your risk of having a heart attack, but according to a new study, it's how frequently you drink—not how much—that may be the key to avoiding the big one. In a study of 38,000 men, researchers found that guys who drank three or four times a week were 68 percent less likely to have a heart attack than men who drank less than once a week, regardless of the type or amount of alcohol they consumed.

Fill Up on Fiber

A high-fiber diet may reduce your risk of colon cancer after all. European researchers found that men with the highest daily intakes of fiber also had a 40 percent lower risk of developing colon cancer. And a recent government study of 40,000 Americans reports similar findings.

Harvard physicians may have figured out why a high-fiber diet may reduce your risk of some cancers. In trials, researchers found that cancer cells contain high levels of a protein called interleukin-6. To test the hardiness of the protein, the researchers treated it with a compound called butyrate, which is produced when the body breaks down fiber. Surprisingly, the butyrate reacted with the interleukin-6, preventing the growth of cancer cells. To boost butyrate in your body, eat more whole-grain bread, oatmeal, and baked beans.

Smoke Screen

If you still smoke despite everything we've told you over the years, then at least try to eat more fish and drink more iced tea. Irish researchers found that a compound in fish can help reduce damage to the lungs caused by smoking. In studies, smokers who were given a daily dose of 1.5 grams of taurine—the amount found in a single serving of fish—had healthier lungs than those who were getting less of the substance. In addition, preliminary research from India found that black tea contains compounds that also may help counteract the lung damage caused by smoking. More research is expected.

The Daily Rind

An orange a day keeps the neurologist away. Australian scientists report that eating an orange daily is associated with a 19 percent reduction in the risk of stroke, as well as reductions of 40 to 50 percent in the risk of stomach, mouth, and larynx cancers. "The benefit probably comes from nutrients such as vitamin C and folate, plus the concentration of antioxidants," says study author Katrine Baghurst, Ph.D. For example, a single orange contains 170 different phytochemicals. When buying, pick oranges that feel heavy for their size. Don't go by color; even ripe ones may have a green tinge.

Go Organic

Organic fruits and vegetables can contain up to 50 percent more disease-fighting antioxidants per serving than regular produce, University of California researchers found. Look for the "USDA Certified Organic" label.

FAST FIXES

There's probably a reason you eat the foods you do. Because your mom made them for you. Or because they come in the EZ-open pouch. But if you keep eating the way you always have, you'll never improve on the body you've got. And the prognosis—on the mom diet, at least—isn't good. Look at your dad. That's why we're providing you with 15 sneaky ways to turn ordinary foods into nutritional superpowers. Same foods, better results. And nobody needs to be the wiser. Just think of these food strategies as the cork in your bat, the glue on your glove, your own personal, syringe-wielding East German Olympic swim-team coach. Only difference is, each one is simple, nutritionally sound, and perfectly legal in all 50 states.

1. Whey your options. Add a cup of ricotta cheese to your fruit smoothie. Ricotta is a soft, mild cheese that's made almost entirely of whey, the liquid that separates from curd during the cheese-making process. Whey contains cysteine, an amino acid that helps produce a cancer-fighting antioxidant called glutathione. When Ohio State University researchers treated prostate cells with whey protein, glutathione levels jumped by 64 percent.

2. See red. Got leftover tuna salad? Stuff it into a red bell pepper instead of sandwiching it between two slabs of Wonder bread. Red peppers and other red-fleshed fruits such as tomatoes, watermelons, and ruby-red grapefruit are high in lycopene, a phytochemical that can reduce the risk of prostate cancer by 20 percent. Bake the pepper and you'll make it even more potent; heat makes lycopene easier for your body to absorb.

3. Hit the sauce. Think of salsa as a vegetable, and eat it as often as you can. "Just take a fish fillet, pour salsa over it, and throw it in the oven—you've got an instant healthy meal," says Cynthia Sass, M.P.H., R.D. In addition to containing lycopene from the tomatoes, salsa has no fat, only 4 calories per tablespoon, and as little as 70 milligrams (mg) of sodium.

AMOUNT OF CANCER-FIGHTING LYCOPENE LOST FROM TOMATO JUICE AND SPAGHETTI SAUCE IF YOU STORE THEM FOR A YEAR: 0

PERCENTAGE BY WHICH A MAN WITH TOTAL CHOLESTEROL OVER 200 MAY LOWER HIS RISK OF HEART DISEASE BY EATING A HANDFUL OF ALMONDS EVERY DAY: 10

4. Switch syrups. Move over, Aunt Jemima: A better syrup has come to take your place at the breakfast table. "Sorghum syrup is produced in much the same way that molasses is made from sugarcane, and it's one of the best, most concentrated sources of dietary antioxidants—period," says Cheryl Forberg, R.D., author of *Stop the Clock! Cooking.* Like grits, sorghum syrup is more widely available in the South. But you can find it at specialty-food stores all over the country.

5. Spread the wealth. You could buy your own produce stand in order to keep up with the National Cancer Institute's recommended nine daily servings of fruits and vegetables. Or you could just buy your fruit in a jar. One tablespoon of unsweetened fruit spread (not sugary jelly or jam) on your morning bagel counts as one of the day's servings, says David Grotto, R.D., director of nutrition education at the Block Center for Integrative Cancer Care in Evanston, Illinois. Look for brands with a high vitamin content, like Crofters Organic.

6. Supplement with herbs. More oregano makes for a more powerful pizza. A tablespoon of fresh oregano (not the dried, bottled kind) has a higher antioxidant yield than an entire apple, according to USDA researchers, who measured the antioxidant levels of 39 common herbs. Bonus: Calorie counts for most herbs and spices are nonexistent. The same can't be said for other pizza toppings, like, say, sausage.

7. Be crafty with broccoli. Power up your mac and cheese by stirring in a cup of chopped steamed broccoli. When you eat cruciferous vegetables—such as broccoli, cauliflower, kale, and brussels sprouts—your body produces a chemical compound called 3,3'-diindolylmethane that inhibits prostate-cancer cell growth by up to 70 percent, according to Leonard Bjeldanes,

NUMBER OF TEASPOONS OF SALT THAT EQUATES TO 2,400 MILLIGRAMS OF SODIUM —YOUR RECOMMENDED MAXIMUM DAILY ALLOWANCE: 1

Ph.D., professor of nutritional sciences and toxicology at the University of California at Berkeley. "I eat a large serving of them three to five times a week," he says. You should, too.

8. Get a fruit fix. That muck on the bottom of most yogurts has more fructose—as in high-fructose corn syrup (HFCS)—than it has fruit. In addition to unnecessarily inflating the calorie count, HFCS can significantly increase blood levels of triglycerides, raising your risk of heart disease. Opt for plain yogurt instead and toss in some raisins or dried pineapple chunks. Dehydrated fruit offers all the health benefits of regular fruit, just concentrated.

9. Go to seed. Risk an encounter with patchouli-scented Birkenstock wearers and buy a bag of ground flaxseed at the health-food store. Add 3 or 4 tablespoons of it to cereal or oatmeal. Ground flaxseed contains omega-3 fatty acids, fiber, and compounds called lignans—the nutrients that can reduce your risk of colon and prostate cancers, heart disease, and age-related vision loss. "You can consume flaxseed as an oil," Grotto says, "but the oil contains more calories and fewer lignans, even in products that boast high lignan content."

10. Feel like a nut—sometimes. Nuts may have shed their unhealthy reputation, but that's still no reason to . . . well, go nuts, cautions Sass. To keep their high calorie content in check, she suggests adding a golf ball–size serving of slivered almonds to cereal and steamed vegetables. Almonds are a rich source of vitamin E, which may reduce the risk of Alzheimer's disease by up to 70 percent, according to a National Institute on Aging study. And their naturally high content of vitamin E, monounsaturated fat, arginine, and fiber helps lower your total and LDL (bad) cholesterol, say researchers from Loma Linda University.

11. Turn over a new leaf. Banish iceberg lettuce from your sandwiches and salads; it has about as much nutritional value as it has taste. "Spinach gives you more bang for the buck," says Forberg. A cup of spinach is an excellent source of folate (58 micrograms), which may help reduce your risk of heart attack.

12. Choc one up. It may sound weird, but try dropping a couple of chunks of chocolate into your pot of chili. Your chili will taste better (trust us), and you'll feel better, knowing that the flavonoids and polyphenols in chocolate can lower your risk of heart disease by 20 percent and keep LDL (bad) cholesterol from oxidizing into an artery-damaging form. Dark or semisweet chocolate has more of the beneficial compounds than other types do.

13. Sow your oats. In recipes that call for crumbled crackers (such as burgers or meat loaf), bait and switch with an equal amount of rolled oats. "Oats contain soluble fiber, and that's been shown to reduce cholesterol," says Grotto. "Oats also contain glucans, which have been shown to enhance natural killer cells—a type of white blood cell that bolsters immune function."

14. Add meal to your meal. Add cornmeal to watery soup to transform it into a hearty, healthier stew, says Forberg. Cornmeal contains an antioxidant called zeaxanthin, which helps preserve vision by increasing the concentration of macular pigment in your eyes. Cornmeal also contains starch that will thicken the soup broth, which is why you should whisk or stir a small handful of it in very slowly (otherwise, the soup may get lumpy).

15. Mash in milk. Whole milk helps make mashed potatoes fluffy. Unfortunately, it does the same for you. Whether you're making the real thing or rehydrating potato flakes, use evaporated skim milk instead. "It's thicker, so you get the creaminess but not the fat," says Sass. You also get three times the calcium per cup (742 mg). Cans of it hide in that most alien of grocery store aisles: the baking section.

OUR FINAL ANSWERS

The Harder They Fall

Why are some beer bellies hard and some soft? And what's the difference?

—R.M., Boyertown, Pennsylvania

Hard is awesome when it comes to abs, but it's a killer when it comes to beer guts. "Having a hard belly is like having a ticking time bomb in your body," says Jean-Pierre Despres, Ph.D., professor of human nutrition at Laval University in Quebec City. "It increases your chances of heart disease and diabetes, and it's worse than smoking or having high cholesterol." A hard belly is caused by a high accumulation of visceral fat (located in the spaces between organs in your abdominal cavity); it's packed in tightly, so there's no jiggle room. A soft belly is caused by subcutaneous fat (located close to the skin's surface), so it has room to roll. The good news: Losing just 5 to 10 percent of your body weight will strip 25 to 40 percent of your visceral fat.

Quick Fix

I'm 6 feet tall, 230 pounds. I want to get down to 200 in 2 months for a class reunion. Can it be done?

—A.Q., Berkeley, California

Okay, Big Boy, we hope there's someone special coming to the reunion, because you'll need the motivation; your timeline is ambitious. Dropping 16 to 24 of those 30 pounds is actually doable, depending on your activity level. Keep at least 2,200 calories in your diet each day so you don't fall below your basal metabolic rate and send your body into starvation mode, says Heidi Skolnik, M.S., C.D.N., nutritionist for the New York Giants. This is still very low for you—2,500 calories or more, depending on your workouts, is more realistic.

Eat 3 to 5 ounces of protein with every meal. Each day, have at least three servings of dairy, four pieces of fruit, and three servings of vegetables, and limit (but don't eliminate) the starch group. Eat fish at least twice a week. No

AVERAGE WAIST SIZE, IN INCHES, OF AN AMERICAN MAN IN 1988: 37.5

AVERAGE WAIST SIZE OF AN AMERICAN MAN TODAY: 38.8

desserts, booze only occasionally—your party is in 2 months. As for exercise, alternate between intense interval workouts and longer cardio sessions. Every opportunity you get, walk around—and snack smart. The goal is to keep your metabolism burning strong.

Read the Label

What are the most important things on food nutrition labels?

—Y.E., Tampa, Florida

Other than your eyes? Key information is meaningless if you don't read it. A 5-second glance in the supermarket aisle won't hold you up, and it can help slim you down. Check out these three numbers.

1. Serving size is the most deceptive number on a label. The concept was first developed to help diabetics manage their diets, says Audrey Cross, Ph.D., associate professor of nutrition at Columbia University. Snack servings are notoriously small, giving the illusion of fewer calories. Measure a serving onto a dish first and eat it from there.

2. Calories are the forgotten number in the low-carbohydrate frenzy. "Calories always rule. You can't ignore them, regardless of what kind of diet you're on," says Roberta Anding, M.S., R.D., dietitian for the Houston Texans and a spokeswoman for the American Dietetic Association. Also, products that say they're low-cal may simply have a smaller serving size, which means more calories in the long run.

3. Saturated fats may be number three here, but they're the first thing Anding has the football players in her care look at. "You can be fast and lean and still have bad cholesterol," she says. Message to fit men: Don't let your dietary guard down just because you can. "Healthy" men get heart disease, too.

Booze Clues

On the Atkins diet, I'm allowed to drink wine with dinner. But isn't alcohol a major carb?

—L.N., Albuquerque, New Mexico

Wine has 2 to 3 grams (g) of carbohydrates a glass, which leaves plenty of room for the 25 to 50 g permitted per day by Dr. Atkins, may he rest in peace. This doesn't mean, however, that you can booze it up and still stick to a low-carb diet or any weight-loss plan. Alcohol isn't your typical carbohydrate—it's actually a separate nutrient that packs almost twice as many calories per gram (7) as regular sugars or starches (4). One more reason to let only one foot slip off the wagon: Alcohol stops your body from using fat for fuel; you have to burn through all of it before you get back to breaking down fat. Better to relax at the end of the day with a nice long run and a big bottle of water.

Drink to Your Health

I hate water. What else can I chug that's not going to kill me?

—A.J., Lexington, Kentucky

Tea. Iced, green, low-cal, and decaffeinated, of course. Studies have shown that people who drink tea lower their risk of cancer, osteoporosis, and heart disease. Stash some AriZona diet green tea in your fridge and pour early and often. It beats plain water by a mile. For an added boost of cancer-fighting substances, try a mixture of black and green teas that's been infused with a broccoli extract (you can't taste the broccoli). Order the tea at brassicatea.com for $5.

Go Wild

You keep telling me to eat salmon. Does it matter if it's farmed or wild? Canned or fresh?

—W.G., Asheville, North Carolina

If you're going to eat salmon more than once a week, buy the wild, fresh variety. A new study has found that, on average, farmed salmon has 16 times more PCBs (toxic compounds) than wild salmon contains. (The bad stuff is concentrated in the fish pellets salmon farmers feed their captives.) So if you did Atkins by eating farmed salmon five times a week, these industrial pollutants might just encourage a bout of cancer or nervous-system damage. It's unlikely, but why risk it, right? So check the source before you buy. Of course, the reason you're probably after the pink flesh is the omega-3 fatty acids, which help your brain, blood, and heart. Your best omega-3 booster is, once again, wild Atlantic salmon, with 2.2 grams (g) per 3.5-ounce serving (you need about 4 g a week) and no toxic chaser. Canned pink salmon (which generally contains wild fish) is the next-best option, with 1.7 grams of omega-3s per 3.5-ounce serving. The fresh, farmed stuff rings up slightly more omega-3s per serving than wild salmon, which makes it a pretty good source—as long as you don't fish in that pool too often. So how do you know if the salmon is wild? You'll have to ask—labels don't always say. Just remember, "fresh" doesn't mean "wild."

A Cut above the Rest

What's the healthiest cut of beef?

—J.F., St. Louis

Round. This cut from the rear end of the cow has the least fat and the most protein, according to the USDA. A more active part of the body produces more muscle, which provides naturally leaner cuts of beef, says Sara Goodwin, of the National Cattlemen's Beef Association. Look for a cut with the word "round" in its name. The second-best choice is loin.

Don't Pass the Vegetables

If vegetarians can eat a balanced diet without meat, can I eat a balanced diet without vegetables?

—D.A., Calverton, New York

Nice try, but the nutrients in vegetables aren't available in dinner with hooves or in pill form. And a new Yale study suggests that folks who avoid vegetables have an increased risk of colon cancer. Researchers found that men who shunned vegetables because of their bitter taste were also the most likely to

PERCENTAGE OF MEN WHO DON'T EAT THE SUGGESTED 9 FRUITS AND VEGETABLES EVERY DAY: 96

have colon polyps—a precursor to cancer. So if you really hate vegetables, learn to hide 'em. Try pureeing your vegetables and adding them to marinara sauce, soup, chili, stew, or guacamole, advises David Grotto, R.D., spokesman for the American Dietetic Association. The more you chop and puree vegetables, the more invisible they become, and the easier it is for your body to absorb their nutrients. And if you're willing to choke down just one, make it broccoli. Two cups has more vitamin C than an orange and as much calcium as a glass of milk, and this veggie is one of the best sources of vitamin A, Grotto says. Broccoli is also high in fiber and isothiocyanates, which stimulate the body's production of cancer fighters. Sautéed in garlic and olive oil and doused with hot sauce, broccoli is a whole different animal.

Get Steamed

What's the best way to cook vegetables?

—R.T., Boise, Idaho

Steam them. A recent study published in the *Journal of the Science of Food and Agriculture* found that microwaved broccoli lost an average of 86 percent of three major antioxidants, compared with only 6 percent when steamed.

The Musical Fruit

What gives you gas after you eat beans?

—M.G., Spokane, Washington

Oligosaccharides. Beans are loaded with these sugars, but you lack the enzyme to digest them. So your body pushes them into your lower intestine, where microorganisms are waiting for dinner. The by-product of their feast: gas. And you know what happens next. Limit eruptions by adding beans to your diet slowly, not all at once. Your body will tolerate them better. Beano is another option.

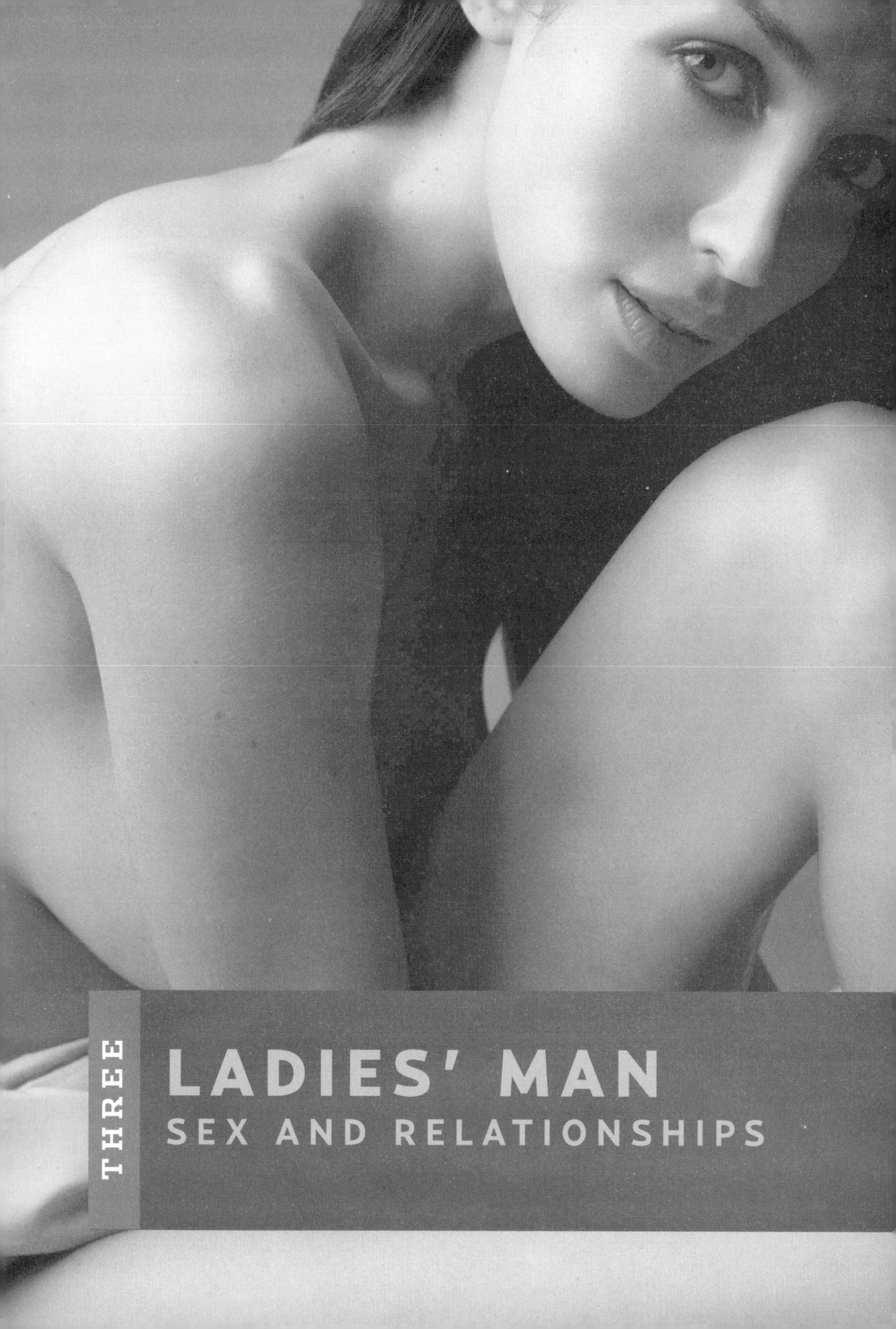

THREE

LADIES' MAN

SEX AND RELATIONSHIPS

MUST READS

Getting to Yes

A redhead, a brunette, and a blonde walk into a bar. Is this a joke, or will one of them leave with you? Here are 39 strategies she wishes you'd use in the dating and mating game

By Lisa Jones

You pick me up at 8:00, and it's game on. I want you to win. But I fear failure. Yours. Mine. Ours.

In the court of dating and mating, women are judge and jury, but the testimony we hear—mostly from our hearts, but also from our Greek chorus of girlfriends—will all take place out of your earshot. The rules are unwritten (until now), but they are set in stone. Give us a really good reason, however, and we'll toss the tablets aside, along with most of our clothing and inhibitions. That's because we want you, the right guy, to make the decision easy for us: not guilty by reason of insanity (i.e., crazy in love).

We hear every message you send—intentional or not. So your attitude is nearly everything. We want you to show a certain degree of eagerness, but not desperation. We want you to believe in yourself and demonstrate why we should believe in you, too. We want you to be spontaneous, but also a man we can count on.

Sound like a lot to ask?

It should be, because this is the process whereby we'll choose a mate for life. Yes, the burden of proof is on you, but we're looking for the case of a lifetime.

Ready to go? Here's how to clear all objections, from the best counselors I know: the single, the available, the hotties who've been waiting for you to come along.

So, see you at 8:00?

THE FLIRTATION

Watch the signals. I've already sent you the Zoolander eye lock, the eyebrow raise, and/or at least two smiles (full, open-lipped, teeth smiles). Come over here and talk to me already. Caveat: There's a small chance I just think you're funny looking, but go ahead, have some balls. I'm worth it.

Convince me (quickly). Once you have the green light, it doesn't matter what you say first. You now have 5 minutes to convince me to keep talking. Make the most of it.

Give me a reason. If you want my number, say something simple and direct. "You're fun. Can I give you a call?" works. Pound the number into your cell phone, or borrow a pen from the bartender. (It's your job; you're the asker.)

Ask me, don't "e" me. Don't be a wuss. If you want to see me, pick up the phone. E-mails can wait for later.

Obey the 2-day rule. If you call within 24 hours, you'll seem desperate. If you wait 3 days, I'll be annoyed that you purposely waited 3 days. So call on day 2.

One of two things will happen:

I'll pick up. You say, "Hey, Lisa, this is Will—the guy you danced to 'Blue Monday' with on Saturday night. How was the rest of your weekend? I want to see you again. Are you available on Wednesday? There's a new tiki bar/restaurant/museum exhibit I've been meaning to check out."

You'll get my voice mail. Identify yourself and your intentions. Then make sure to say these crucial words: "Sorry I missed you. Give me a call back.

SEVEN IMMUTABLE LAWS OF FIRST-DATE ETIQUETTE

1. Help me with my coat.

2. Turn off your cell phone. If you've forgotten to turn off your phone and it rings, turn it off immediately without checking who's calling. Apologize.

3. Always take the seat facing the wall. The woman faces the room. This automatically prevents you from eyeing other women when I'm telling you about my job/childhood/fear of drinking soapy water.

4. Ignore my décolletage. Even if I'm wearing a shirt so sheer it seems constructed of gauze, do not steal furtive glances at my breasts. I will catch you and respect you less for it.

5. Tell me what you're thinking about ordering as you're looking at the menu. (I'm waiting to see if you're going to order an appetizer.) Ask for my opinion when choosing wine, but don't ask me to select the specific bottle. (I'm assuming you're going to pay, but I don't know yet what you want to spend.)

6. Offer me a taste of something.

7. Pay swiftly, without consulting me. And never ask me what you should leave for a tip; it appears you're trying to show me how much you just spent on me.

Otherwise, I'll try you again, and we can make plans." This allows you to call back without wondering whether I got your message.

Remember, a man plans ahead. If you want to see me this weekend, call me by Thursday, please. If you want to see me naked tonight, call me before you're drunk at 1:00 A.M.

Don't ask me to "hang out." When you ask me to "hang out" and it's just the two of us and you don't have a girlfriend (or boyfriend), I assume it's a date. To avoid confusion, say, "I'd like to take you out" instead of, "Wanna hang out?"

Know when to quit. If you call me twice and get no callback, game over. Don't keep calling, e-mailing, or sending flowers. In Meg Ryan movies or when Keanu Reeves performs them, these gestures say "bold romantic." In reality, when you do them, they say "stalker."

THE DATE

Observe the 4:00 P.M. deadline. As the big date approaches, women worry that they'll be stood up. This is why there's a 4:00 P.M. deadline. If you call at 4:20 to confirm the 8:00 P.M. date, I'll have already made other plans just to protect myself from the letdown. Call between noon and 4:00, or risk being set adrift like a hard-luck astronaut.

Choose the location well. If we live in a city, the first date should be closer to my place than to yours—so you can walk me home. You should reach the meeting place on time or a little early. If you're driving to my place, pick me up 5 minutes late. There may be a stray hair that needs taming. And observe proper car etiquette. Always open the door for me, whether or not your car has power locks. Pressing a button does not a gentleman make.

Money matters. Spending too much on a date makes me think you're trying to buy my affection. Or worse. I'd rather see evidence of your personal interest than your interest-bearing accounts. Special note: If you're spending more than $200 on a woman who isn't sleeping with you, you're a sucker. And she sucks.

Pay attention. Girls spend a lot of time getting glam. They also spend a lot of time wondering if guys notice. Respond to my efforts.

But chill with the compliments. Give me a couple of sincere snaps—but make sure they're thoughtful. If you say you like my smile or my eyes, I've heard it before. Say, "Look at that dimple," or, "Wow, you have great eyelashes." Now you have my attention. Compliment my intelligence, sassiness, or unfaltering talent for ordering the best guac. Now you might get some ass.

Introduce me. If you stop and talk to absolutely anyone, introduce me within 30 seconds without using the words "my friend." Personal details are required. By date six, I should have met all your important friends.

LINGERIE SEMIOTICS

The only time I wear thigh-high stockings is when I'm expecting a man to see them. Other sure ways to interpret my underthings:

Thong or no panties. I was trying to avoid panty lines, but sex is on my mind, too.
Cotton briefs. I had no intention of getting naked with you tonight.
Nude-colored panties. I'm not trying to impress you.
Black, red, pink, leopard print, or lace. I want you.
Sheer bra. I wore this to show nipples, of course. It's a test of your willpower.

Don't go all Donald on me. Unless a woman is a hopeless climber, you won't impress her with what you own (that is, if you own anything). Instead, let me discover what's valuable about you, not what you've bought.

Notice what I drink. Ask me if I'd like a refill when I leave an empty glass behind and head for the ladies' room. This makes you attentive and thoughtful. This makes me happy and socially lubricated.

Walk me to my door. It's a scary world, and I want you to protect me. If you're welcome inside my apartment, I will invite you. Do not ask to use my bathroom.

Kiss me. If the date has gone well, lips must come into play. Even if it's just a peck. It gives me more peace of mind than you can imagine. Don't be discouraged if I hesitate to kiss you in return. I might be shy or nervous because I really like you. Or maybe you have bad breath. It doesn't mean I don't, or won't, want you.

Recognize the kiss-off. Game over if I don't kiss you on a second date. Take the hint.

NAKED DATING

Watch the telltale signs. I'm crushing on you if I touch you for any reason. Other signs: I lean forward when you're talking or ask you endless questions. The only way to shut me up is to undress me.

Extend an invitation. Make it very clear you want me to spend the night. "Are you staying over?" is not an invite. "Will you spend the night? I can't wait to wake up with you" is. Offer me a T-shirt, boxer shorts, a toothbrush.

Know the ropes of first-time sex. It's usually a hi-nice-to-meet-you sort of fusion. More groping than soul melding. I'm not overly concerned about whether I'll have an orgasm, and you shouldn't be, either.

Heed the rules of FTD. Flowers on or after the first few dates: too much too soon, and reeking of desperation. Flowers anytime after we've had sex: welcome, romantic, and thoughtful.

. . . And the rules of STD. If you have herpes or any other STD, you must tell me way before pants are removed.

Show, don't tell. If I'm ready for sex, I'll make sure you know it. And nix the safe-sex conversation. Take out a condom. We know what to do.

Remember, this ain't a peep show. Don't ask me to "show you" how I get off. Early on, women aren't comfortable touching themselves for your entertainment. I'll reconsider after four or more sex episodes, or four or more cocktails.

Avoid the label. Being a "selfish lover" is the worst rap a man can get. Avoid it by going down eagerly and often. Go down on me before I go down on you.

Pay attention, part 2. Taking care of your body is sexy. Being obsessed with mine is sexier.

Obey the 2-day rule, part 2. Call me within 48 hours of a date to say you had a good time and to ask me out again. XXX-ception: Call me within 24 hours of any date involving sex or south-of-the-border touching. Subrule: If you don't call when you say you will, you immediately become unreliable.

Know when to shut up. Game over if you say another woman's name for any reason while in bed with me.

Seven Signs She's Good in Bed

Subtle (and not so subtle) ways to tell if a woman will let it all hang out

By Chris Connolly

It's an enigma as enduring as Mona Lisa's small, knowing smile: Sometimes meek women turn wild in bed; sometimes they just lie there, waiting to inherit the earth. Sometimes the chestnut filly with the riding crop turns out to be all packaging; sometimes she's as thrilling as the signs indicated she'd be.

It made me wonder: Is it possible to reliably predict what a woman is like in bed? The love scientists say yes—sort of.

"It's very hard to gauge," explains Helen Fisher, Ph.D., an anthropologist at Rutgers University and author of *Why We Love,* a new book about the nature and chemistry of romantic love. A woman's high heels, short skirt, and follow-me walk mean little. "Those are signs of intention. But they are not signs that this person is actually good in bed and is compatible with you."

So, besides that old cliché about how she dances, what signs can a man go by? Start with these.

SHE SUGGESTS THAI FOR DINNER

Beware the "I-don't-know, what-do-you-want-to-do?" camp of passive babes. A woman who knows and says what she wants, even when answering a mundane question, is more likely to be assertive in bed. Good lovers take responsibility for their pleasure. They remove a lot of the guesswork.

"Human tastes in bed are just as varied as tastes in food," Fisher says. "A person may like Japanese food but hate pizza. Some women want their nipples chewed on; others need you to be more delicate." Today's women aren't shy. "In the past, women didn't get to sleep with enough men to know what they liked," Fisher says. "But now, women are becoming more experienced and more demanding."

SHE EATS IT UP

Take note of how she handles her food. "Watch how she uses her fork. Does she enjoy things? Is she sensuous? Is she poky and grabby?" says Candida Royalle, a producer of femme-friendly adult films and a veteran adult-film star. "If someone eats slowly, it's likely that they like to make love for a long time. I'm one of the slowest eaters I know."

SHE SCREAMS . . . FOR COFFEE ICE CREAM

You may find the perfect lover by comparing tastes in ice cream, says Alan Hirsch, M.D., a neurologist and director of the Smell and Taste Treatment and Research Foundation in Chicago. Researchers call this "ice-cream hedonics." Dr. Hirsch conducted a study of 720 people, ages 24 to 59, in which he correlated personality tests, their favorite ice-cream flavors, their partners' favorite ice creams, and relationship status. Coffee-ice-cream lovers—found to be dramatic, seductive, flirtatious—are most romantically compatible with strawberry fans. Vanilla gals (emotionally expressive and fond of PDA) melt best with rocky-road guys. And mint-chocolate-chip fans are meant for each other.

SHE TALKS LIKE YOU

There's a scene in *Broadcast News* in which William Hurt tells Holly Hunter that listening to her talk in his earpiece while he was on the air was "like great sex!" See if you get a similar buzz from your potential bedmate. "The first thing to look for is mirroring of verbal behavior and pace," explains Michael Cunningham, Ph.D., professor of social psychology at the University of Louisville. "That is, if her pace and her nonverbal behavior match yours, her sexual behavior, which is also nonverbal, will also likely match. If one person seems really slow-moving and the other person seems fidgety, they're going to have different sexual paces.

"If somebody says something and the other person goes on to another subject," he says, "they're not tuning in very well. They probably won't tune in during sex, either."

SHE KNOWS WHO SID VICIOUS IS

"Young women often aren't relaxed enough to have an orgasm," Fisher says. Older women know what they like and will tell you. "They realize that if they have frequent orgasms, it's better for the man in the long run."

At menopause, "levels of estrogen recede, unmasking the power of testosterone," Fisher says. "This allows women to be more assertive and demanding, and many of them become more interested in sex." Sure, Ms. Keaton, we'd love to see your golden globes!

SHE GIVES GOOD LIP

"The way you kiss says a lot about how you make love," says Ava Cadell, Ph.D., an L.A.-based sexologist and author. "I call kissing 'facial intercourse.' It's not just using the lips; it's using the entire body. If she uses her hands on you and presses her breasts into you and moans and groans, she's going to be a great lover. The best female lovers also create sexual anticipation. They start with baby kisses, and then maybe lick your top lip and suck your bottom lip, and as they're doing that, they play with your hair, or put your hands on them. It's sort of like a dance." Speaking of dance . . .

OKAY, FINE: SHE'S A GOOD DANCER

As I was researching this article, every single friend I asked suggested looking for a good dancer. I was reluctant to include this. I'm married to a dancer, and I hate the implied nudge I get when a guy finds out what my wife does. Second, I dreaded asking a respected anthropologist, "So, if a chick is a good dancer, will she be, like, a dynamo in the sack?"

Fisher didn't flinch. "There is a certain amount of dance to copulation. And dancing is energetic, which suggests someone who's in good shape," she said. "But I think what's really going on is that dancing indicates someone who's social and self-confident."

I'm so relieved. All those guys fantasizing about my wife are really thinking, Wow. Check out the self-confidence on her!

Checkout Points

A complete workout for the body parts women notice most

By Lauren Russell

You know that women have a thing for abs. We peek at them when you reach up high for something, we look right at them when you peel off your shirt at the beach, we feel them when you hug us. And we love to run our hands over them.

But you knew this already. (Well, maybe not the reach-and-peek part.) It's why you did crunches today. But there's more to lust than abs.

You sweat to build a body that'll make women sweat you. The mystery—to us—is why you focus on working the muscles that impress guys. "Men want big biceps because they can see their big biceps and because other men can see their big biceps," says Pega Ren, Ed.D., who's a woman and a clinical sexologist in Vancouver, British Columbia. "People get fit not only to attract others sexually but also to stand tall among our peers."

That's fine, but don't forget us. When you walk past a woman, she's checking out her favorite body parts. Biceps are fine, but they're pretty far down our list of favorites. Let us tell you what those favorites are, why we love them, and the exercises you need to do to build them.

A BROAD BACK

Why she likes it: A wide back is essential for a V-shaped torso, and women's attraction to it is ancestral. "When it was important that our mates protect us from woolly mammoths on the plains, we looked for a gene pool that could provide us with protection," says Ren. A broad back promises survival. "It's a domination and protection thing," says Kyra, 26. "Like he's going to take care of you."

To build it: You need to stretch the muscles to the maximum to develop a big back. "A maximum stretch means working the muscle in a full range of motion," says Carter Hays, C.S.C.S., a performance-enhancement specialist in Houston. The straight-arm alternating pullover develops the muscles best.

STRAIGHT-ARM ALTERNATING PULLOVER

Lie faceup on a bench with your right leg straight, the thigh flat on the bench. Keep your left foot on the floor. Hold a dumbbell in your right hand above your thigh, palm facing in. Keeping your arm straight, lift it up and back so it makes a 180-degree arc. Pause, then return to the starting position. Switch legs and hands after each set. Do three sets of 12 repetitions with each arm.

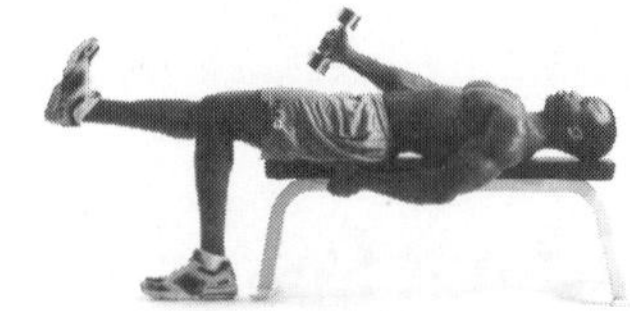

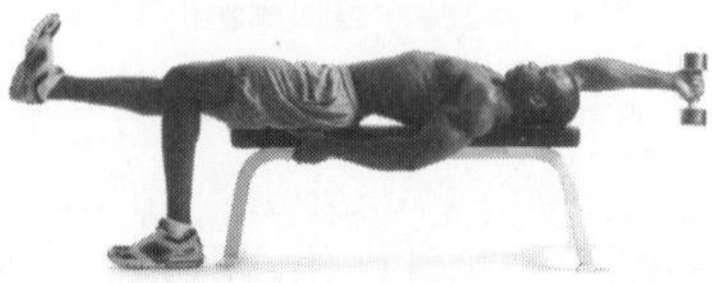

SCULPTED SHOULDERS

Why she likes them: "The shoulder muscles are really the muscles of love and war," says Nancy Etcoff, Ph.D., a psychologist and author of *Survival of the Prettiest: The Science of Beauty*. They also make the whole look when combined with a broad back. "Strong shoulders literally sweep women off their feet," says Laura, 24. "That's where we can wrap our arms around and snuggle up."

To build them: "Strong lateral deltoids add width to your shoulders," says Mike Gough, C.S.C.S., owner of athleticedgesports.com. Try the Swiss-ball leaning lateral raise. "Because of the angle of your torso when leaning against the ball," he says, "the weight has to travel through a greater range of motion."

SWISS-BALL LEANING LATERAL RAISE

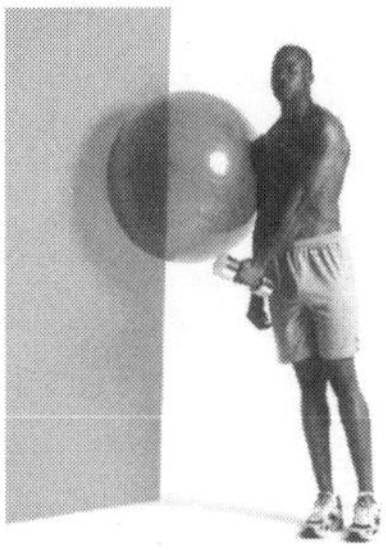

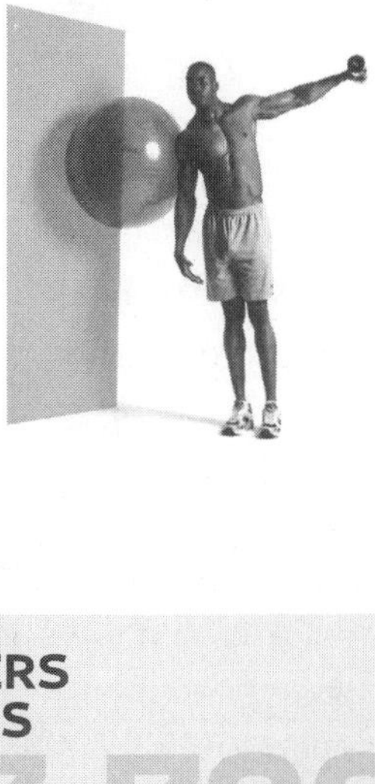

Lean your right shoulder against a Swiss ball that's placed against a wall. Keeping your body straight, place your feet less than shoulder-width apart and far enough from the wall so that your body is at a 30-degree angle from the floor. Hold a dumbbell in your left hand, and let the hand hang down below your right leg, palm facing the wall. Lift your arm up and out to your left until it forms a straight line with your shoulders. Pause, then slowly lower the weight. Do three sets of 12 repetitions with each arm.

THE NUMBER OF *COSMOPOLITAN* READERS WHO SAID THAT STRONG BACK MUSCLES ON A MAN MAKE THEM MELT: 233,700

THE NUMBER WHO SAID SO ABOUT STRONG SHOULDERS: 506,400

NICE BUTT

Why she likes it: It's something to hold on to. "During sex she can reach around, grab it, and literally pull you toward her," says Timothy Perper, Ph.D., a biologist and author of *Sex Signals: The Biology of Love*. It's a subconscious thing, he theorizes, but Jane, 36, says she's fully conscious: "A great butt is one that looks like you can grab on and maneuver. That's what it's there for."

To build it: The one-legged squat isolates the smaller gluteal muscles better than other squats. "You work the gluteus minimus and the tiny muscles that stabilize the hip joint," says Frederick Carl Hatfield, Ph.D., who holds the International Powerlifting Federation record for his (two-legged) squat of 1,014 pounds.

ONE-LEGGED SQUAT

Stand on one leg with the other leg out in front of your body so your heel is just off the floor. Extend your arms out to your sides for balance or hold on to a doorway. Bend the supporting leg to lower yourself as far as you can. Pause, then return to the starting position, and finish the set with that leg before repeating with the other. As this gets easier, try holding a 5- or 10-pound dumbbell in each hand while you squat. Do three sets of 10 repetitions on each leg.

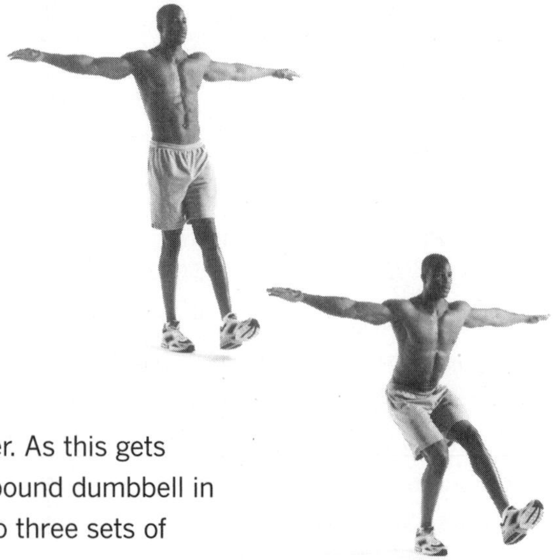

ROCK-HARD CALVES

Why she likes them: "Women want an overall sense of strength and fitness," says Etcoff. "If a man looks as if he can lift something but can't run, it looks disproportionate." Dawn, 25, says, "They don't have to be enormous, but muscular calves are a very masculine trait—and that's sexy."

To build them: Train your anterior tibialis—the muscle opposite the calf—as well as your calves. "Most people are unaware that the calves have an opposite muscle group," says Scott Rankin, C.S.C.S., a strength coach in Toronto. Train it and you'll be able to lift more weight during calf exercises and other lower-body moves.

TIBIALIS CURL

Sit on a bench with your feet together and flat on the floor. Place a light dumbbell across your toes. Lift your toes off the floor as high as possible without raising your heels, then return to the starting position. Do three sets of 10 to 15 repetitions whenever you work your calves.

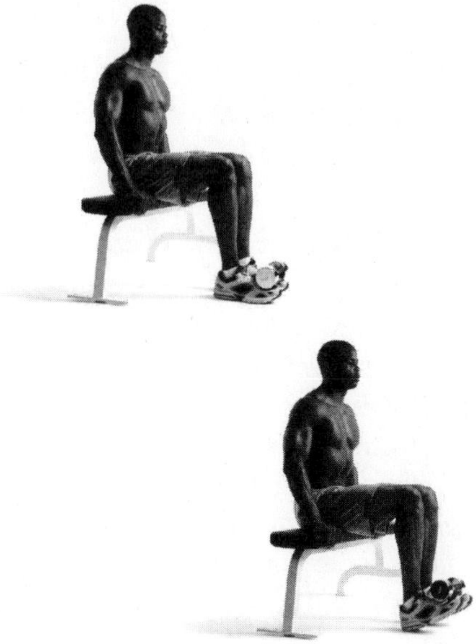

CALF RAISE

Balance on one foot on a step and hold a dumbbell in the hand opposite the leg on the step. Keeping the knee bent, rise onto the ball of your foot, then ease back down. Do three sets of calf raises. Work up to 25 repetitions per set.

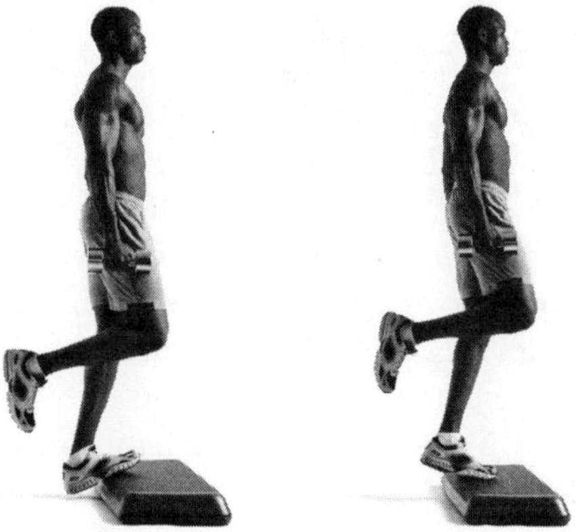

NEED TO KNOW

Take Her to the Movies

The adrenaline produced by scary movies can stimulate sexual arousal because of a phenomenon called spillover, says social psychologist David Myers, Ph.D., in his textbook *Psychology, 7th ed.* "The arousal that lingers after an intense argument or a frightening experience may intensify sexual passion," writes Myers. So your date's excitement doesn't disappear when the movie ends—make a romantic overture and let her excitement spill over to something else.

Likewise, a couple of minutes of an erotic video, with or without sound, is all it takes to sexually arouse a heterosexual woman in her 20s or 30s, according to a recent report in *Fertility & Sterility* magazine. Researchers monitored the vaginal bloodflow, breathing rate, blood pressure, and pulse of 20 women as they viewed erotic and nonerotic tapes, and the women reported their levels of arousal. Audio neither increased nor decreased the effects.

Love Shack

Shacking up makes men happy, according to the British Household Panel Survey. Ten years of data from 10,000 people under age 65 show that men enjoy better mental health when living with a lover than when married or single. Women are happiest when married. It may be because men "benefit from the shared resources without the commitment associated with marriage," says study author Michaela Benzeval, M.D., of Queen Mary College at the University of London.

But while you may be happy now, you might want to rethink cohabitating if you see wedding bells in your future. Shacking up before marriage means a rockier relationship after marriage. According to the *Journal of Marriage and Family,* a half-assed approach to commitment leads to a half-assed approach to solving relationship problems and being a supportive partner—issues that may worsen after a stroll down the aisle.

Lovers' Quarrel

Do what you can to keep the peace. Miami University researchers say heated arguments can cause severe, long-lasting spikes in blood pressure. Over time, these changes could be enough to lead to heart disease, the researchers warn.

PERCENTAGE BY WHICH HAVING AN UNHAPPY MARRIAGE INCREASES YOUR CHANCES OF GETTING SICK: 35

NUMBER OF YEARS BY WHICH AN UNHAPPY MARRIAGE SHORTENS YOUR LIFE EXPECTANCY: 4

Love Heals All Wounds

According to an Ohio State University study, happily married people heal more quickly. Researchers used a tiny vacuum to create blisters on the inner arms of a group of married volunteers, then measured how quickly the blisters started to heal. They found that individuals with low levels of the stress hormone cortisol began healing sooner than those with more cortisol. And those with lower cortisol levels also turned out to be the couples reporting the happiest marriages.

Start the Day Off Right

What's the best time of the day to have sex? Dawn. Okay, okay, any time is good. But technically, early morning is best. Key male and female hormones peak between 5:00 and 9:00 A.M. (hence that mysterious Norwegian wood you wake up with every morning). The hormone supply is a powerful sex stimulant, which will maximize performance and pleasure for both partners. Early morning is also the best time to conceive a child, because that's when your testosterone levels are at their highest. This gives a fertility boost to men with slow-moving sperm or low sperm counts.

Take Your Time

If you rush things when, uh, taking matters in your own hands, you may be setting yourself up for sexual dysfunction. "Every time you masturbate and reach orgasm within 1 to 2 minutes, that timetable becomes more deeply reinforced in your brain," says Sheldon O. Burman, M.D., medical director of the Male Sexual Dysfunction Institute in Chicago. Then when you do have a partner, you're likely to stick to the 2-minute schedule—which eventually could make you a solo act again.

Last Longer

You know what Viagra does. And maybe you know that antidepressants show promise in treating premature ejaculation (PE). Researchers at Tel Aviv University in Israel combined both and reported impressive results in treating men with PE. The men were given paroxetine (Paxil) 7 hours before sex and sildenafil (Viagra) 1 hour before. The men reported lasting an average of about five times longer than usual. And 56 of 58 men who took the combo reported satisfaction, according to the journal *Urology*. Michael O'Leary, M.D., director of the men's clinic at Brigham and Women's Hospital, Boston, adds that the combination has helped some of his patients. Be aware that antidepressants can have serious side effects, but if you're interested, consult a sex specialist or urologist.

Worth the Wait

A combination of injections and implants that serve as male birth control is being researched but is years away from market. The treatment uses the hormone progestin to stop sperm production. But this reduces testosterone levels and may cause lethargy and sexual dysfunction, so testosterone implants are required. When the treatment was studied with 55 couples, none of the women got pregnant, and the only side effect the men reported was increased sexual desire. Sounds like a win-win, but you'll have to wait.

A Less Painful Way to Prevent Pregnancy

The FDA has approved a tiny clamp that makes vasectomies less painful and potentially easier to reverse. The device, called a Vasclip, works by clamping the vas deferens, blocking the flow of sperm from the testicles. Since the Vasclip method doesn't involve cutting or cauterizing the vas, doctors believe the procedure may be much easier to reverse, although full-fledged studies have yet to be completed. In early trials, the procedure was up to 50 percent less painful than a traditional vasectomy. "It's also fast, taking less than 10 minutes in most cases," says researcher David Kirby, M.D.

HIV Results in a Hurry

The FDA has approved a test that can check blood samples for HIV antibodies in as little as 3 minutes. Although you'll still need to visit a doctor, you won't have to wait days to find out everything's okay. The Reveal Rapid HIV-1 Antibody test should already be available at most large hospitals.

FAST FIXES

She's fire and brimstone. You're a deer in the headlights. You've tried pretending to be invisible, but she sees right through you. Before you brush off her verbal assault, remember what happened to former Cleveland Indians pitcher, Chuck Finley, back in 2002: His wife's verbal abuse turned physical when she hit him, scratched his face, kicked him with her high-heel boots, and threw a telephone at his car windshield. She was arrested and thrown in the slammer.

It may stand conventional wisdom on its head, but 1.5 million men are physically assaulted by their partners every year, according to the Centers for Disease Control and Prevention. Next time your little honeybee turns mad as a hornet, here's how to stop the buzzing before her fire turns to fight.

1. Lower your thermostat. Whatever you do, don't get angry. Surprisingly enough, she won't consider it righteous; she'll just get more pissed off, and a little self-righteous besides. If you feel yourself heating up, just remember that "she can't make you angry," says Paul Hauck, Ph.D., an Illinois psychologist and author of *How to Cope with People Who Drive You Crazy* and *Overcoming Frustration and Anger*. "And you didn't make her feel angry. She did. You may be responsible for her problem, but not her emotional reaction."

2. Don't feed her data. "A man generally tries to win an argument by coming up with facts that are totally meaningless to her," says Michael Staver, the author of *21 Ways to Defuse Anger and Calm People Down*. "She filters that as being disrespectful and not listening, which ticks her off all the more."

3. Own up . . . maturely. "If you're wrong, just admit it," says Staver. "But don't do it in a condescending way."

4. Tune in. "If she has a big problem," says Hauck, "you'd better listen." And don't wait till swords are drawn. Like an orgasm, anger follows a bell curve—at the top you're completely out of your mind. So if you're seeing signs of frustration (a sigh or roll of the eyes), you'd better start listening quick, for the apex is near and things are about to go downhill fast.

5. Take a step back. "You don't have to agree," says Staver, "but acknowledge her perceptions as real. It shows that you respect her." Often, her anger is triggered because she believes something's (1) unfair, (2) out of her control, or (3) a personal attack. Address these concerns.

6. Assert your eyes. If you can't make eye contact, it means you're becoming angry. But if you can, it shows you're listening. Psychologists have seen a classic pattern in marital fights: The wife gets mad, the husband shuts down, the wife goes nuts. You shut down because you want to avoid a battle, but she thinks you're avoiding (here comes that dreaded word) intimacy.

7. Get engaged. Ask questions. "It shows you're listening, and it implies you want to listen to her more," says Staver.

8. Hit the road—together. Taking a walk may sound dumb, but it's actually a neat trick. Physically, you just got her to move with you rather than against you. "Taking a walk is calming," says Susan Heitler, a Denver clinical psychologist and author of *The Power of Two*. If the argument reaches crisis mode, however, remove yourself from the situation until it's clear the ranting is over.

9. Use magic phrases. Heitler suggests three: Yes, I agree. You're right. I'm sorry. Nothing disarms an attacker faster than taking her side. So find something, anything, to agree on. We're not suggesting you cave in, but find some small plot of common ground.

10. Use anger as a meter. Heitler compares anger to a Geiger counter—it can alert you to a problem. "What it's not good for," she quickly adds, "is solving a problem."

11. Set limits. "You get the behavior you tolerate," says Hauck. If her rage is a little too melodramatic, a little too frequent, a little too abusive, you want to give her exactly two chances to change, he says.

If you see a pattern of blame, criticism, and complaining, then face it: Cupcake is emotionally unstable, and you may have real trouble on your hands. Don't start sinking into denial. "The problem is, the man often doesn't take the problem seriously," says Martin S. Fiebert, Ph.D., psychologist at California State University at Long Beach. "He doesn't realize he's in an abusive relationship—and that it will escalate."

Five years ago, Fiebert surveyed 978 Southern California college women and found that 29 percent admitted to initiating aggression against the men in their lives in the previous 12 months. Asked why, a majority replied, "I knew I could get away with it." If you're in such a relationship, and your girlfriend habitually handles her frustrations in a physical way, the great danger is that you will get sucked in and, sooner or later, respond in kind.

That's no way to live. If your love life ever turns so hateful, take this advice:

12. Get out of the kitchen. In cases of serious assault, one study found that roughly 80 percent of women attack with a weapon to compensate for their smaller size. If a fight starts in the kitchen, where there are plenty of weapons within arm's reach, don't let it end there. But don't move it to the bedroom. The night Finley's wife was arrested, he searched under their bed and found several knives.

13. Hit the road—alone. "Tell her, 'This needs to stop. If it doesn't stop,

I'm leaving,'" says Philip W. Cook, author of *Abused Men*. "If you stay and find yourself apologizing for 'provoking' her assaults, you're in a controlling and abusive relationship."

14. Swallow your misplaced pride. Call the police. Get medical attention. Check out the Internet site safe4all.org.

15. Stop hitting the bars. Most violence between couples, married or not, is "bidirectional," as the psychologists say. It takes two to tango—and it usually involves too much tequila. Studies have shown that half the women and two-thirds of the men arrested for domestic violence are heavy drinkers.

Drug use can have the same ill effect. At least, that appears to have been the case with Finley's wife. Not long after her arrest, she checked into rehab, agreed to a plea bargain, and was ordered to stop visiting her posse of doctors for multiple prescriptions to medications. Oh, and she was ordered to avoid contact with Finley. Those boots of hers were made for walking—not kicking.

OUR FINAL ANSWERS

Pills for Thrills

Is it okay to take Viagra, Levitra, or Cialis for recreational use? I'm healthy—how risky can it be?

—R.H., Milwaukee

None of these is cleared for nonmedical use. How risky? For one, you could waste money on a look-alike pill if your supply doesn't come from a reputable pharmacy. Or you could have a heart attack and die—it has happened to men taking Viagra, although underlying heart disease and not the medicine might have been the cause. But these three drugs have been prescribed to diabetics (who have a high incidence of heart disease) with little problem. Talk to your doctor and make sure you're at low risk of heart problems. And never take any of these with nitrates (nitroglycerin, or amyl or butyl nitrate). That combo can kill.

Marathon Sex

Is it possible for a man to have too much sex? How about a woman?

—L.G., Pittsburgh

Big plans tonight, L.G.? It's difficult for a man to have too much sex, assuming you have a partner or partners who will let you try. Women, on the other hand, can suffer from the aptly named honeymoon cystitis. "With repeated sexual intercourse, the urethra can become bruised, and the woman can develop what feels like a urinary-tract infection. But it's really bruising from too much sex," says Mark Elliot, Ph.D., director of the Institute for Psychological and Sexual Health in Columbus, Ohio. The condition usually goes away after a few days of abstinence. And in the do-we-need-more-pressure department: Repeated failure to bring a woman to orgasm can cause a female version of blue balls that can lead to infection. "Every time she has sex without an orgasm, the blood flows away [from her sex organs] less and less," says Elliot. Two weeks of sex without orgasm can lead to a buildup of blood, which can lead to constant lubrication, which creates a breeding ground for yeast. To recap: more orgasms, better vaginal health, more sex, world peace. Simple, right?

PERCENTAGE OF AOL TRAVEL USERS—MEN AND WOMEN—WHO SAY THEY LOOK TO MEET SOMEONE RELATIONSHIP-WORTHY WHILE ON VACATION: 43

Of Mice and Men

I'm happy with my wife, but I still get tempted by other women. Why?

—Z.K., Pasadena, California

Your feelings are likely linked to the hormone vasopressin, explains psychiatrist and brain-imaging specialist Daniel Amen, M.D. In studies of male voles (little rodents), those with one brain level of vasopressin were monogamous, while those with a different level played the field, literally. Same with men. Unlike rodents, however, you have a strong judgment center, or prefrontal cortex (PFC), which controls impulses. And it takes up to 30 percent of the human brain, compared with 1 percent of a vole brain. So which are you, a man or a mouse? Use your PFC to focus on keeping your family intact.

Make Your Approach

Where do women feel most comfortable being approached by a man they don't know?

—M.M., Plainfield, New Jersey

We asked 800 women who don't know us—comely visitors to the Web's cosmopolitan.com—where they'd be most receptive to our advances, and yours. Straight from the mouths of babes, here are the facts.

- 61% of respondents say they'd feel most comfortable being approached at a friend's party, and 65% say that's where a serious relationship would most likely spring up.
- 51% say that if a one-night stand occurred, it would probably be with a guy they met at a bar or club.
- 48% think the best opening line is a "straight-up introduction."
- 51% say you'll have a better chance if you approach a woman when she's "talking with one or two friends."
- 66% think you don't have to wait for eye contact before approaching.

Need to know key places to avoid? The grocery store, the street, and public transportation consistently ranked at the bottom of the respondents' comfort scales.

Go It Alone

What's a better idea: bringing a date—any date—or going solo to my high-school reunion?

—J.J., Louisville

We know you want to look good, but explaining all night to your old classmates who your date is will be annoying. And obvious. Fact is, this party is primed with available women who no longer think you're a doof. Wouldn't you rather talk to them than a random date? The reunion rule: Wives and committed girlfriends go along. Having anyone else in tow will just keep you from seeing the real possibilities.

Thought Control

In order to enjoy sex with my fiancée, I often have to fantasize about other women. Is my sex life doomed?

—R.D., St. Louis

No, but it needs work. The problem isn't the Victoria's Secret models that slink into your head during sex—they're expected. The problem is that you allow them to stay. You are in control of your thoughts and can train your mind to be helpful instead of disruptive. Focus on arousing her for a change. Frankly, you're being self-centered, and if you make her moan loud enough, you won't be able to think about other women.

The Right Touch

My girlfriend complains that I have rough hands. What can I do?

—C.B., Richmond, Texas

You may not give much thought to your mitts, but women notice because your hands are an important tool to them. Think about wearing a Speedo made of sandpaper. The thought is enough to lift your voice a couple of octaves, right? If you want your woman to let you touch her smooth, soft body—or even hold her hand—grab your girl's nail file or pumice stone and rub those

PERCENTAGE OF MEN WHO THINK ABOUT A FORMER LOVER EVERY DAY: 17

scaly spots smooth. Try lathering with pumice-infused Lava soap or using a thick body moisturizer to polish your rough edges smooth. The final touch: Give her an oil massage—it's great for her back and terrific for your calluses.

The Ex Files

So I went out with this girl for 8 months, and then I broke up with her. Now I realize I made a mistake, and I want her back. She won't talk to me. Any advice?

—B.H., Middlebury, Vermont

Forget calling her or trying to see her. What you need to do is write her a note. Not an e-mail, a handwritten note. Remind her of your first date and what she was wearing or some other stuff that shows you remember something about her she'd never suspect you would. Don't beg, don't whine, don't grovel. Remind her that you are a man with a memory—and maybe some of her fond memories of you will come to your rescue.

Don't Let Your Friends Down

My girlfriend hounds me about my friends and doesn't like it when I go out after work. She even told one of my friends I was busy—before I got to the phone. She's great, but this makes me uncomfortable.

—T.S. Jackson, Mississippi

You get in a relationship, sure, you give up certain rights, like the right to wear underwear with holes in them or to eat frozen dinners every night. But you never, ever give up the right to friends, beer, sports, and whatever else makes you a man. Your girlfriend crossed the line, a double-yellow one at that. She needs a warning: You're into her, but you're into other things, too. She crosses the line again, and you have no choice but to write her a ticket—right out of your life.

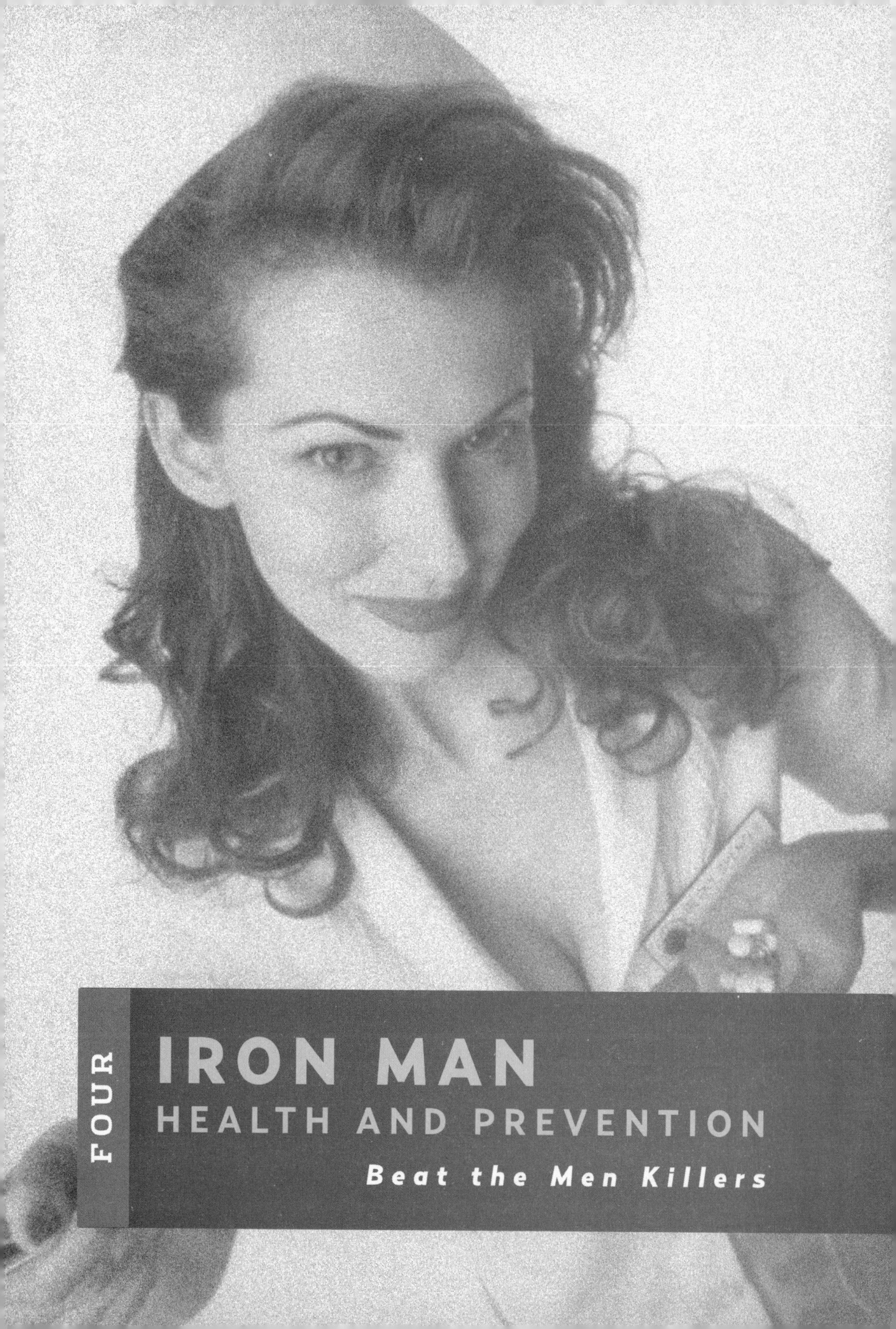

FOUR

IRON MAN

HEALTH AND PREVENTION

Beat the Men Killers

MUST READS

All in the Family

Is disease in your genes? Determine your odds—then lower them

By Matt Marion

The cookies-and-milk memories I have of my grandmother are inevitably interrupted by thoughts of her colon. That was where a polyp sprouted and later turned into the tumor that killed her at the age of 81.

Within months of Flo's death, I was lying facedown on an examination table as a doctor searched for any polyps in the making. (I was clean.) My fear was that I was about to come into an inheritance of colon cancer. The reality is that Flo's kid, my father, is the one who should have been getting a look-see in his large intestine. (He finally had the exam—and he was clean, too.)

What about you? Do you know if your closest relations are putting you at risk of a deadly disease? Now you will. Just enter the medical history of your parents, siblings, grandparents, aunts, and uncles into the Family Risk Calculator, then sit back and watch as it diagnoses your DNA.

DISEASES THAT DISCRIMINATE: THE ADDED GENETIC RISKS FOR AFRICAN-AMERICAN MEN

Certain illnesses play the race cards—they affect black men more often than they do white men. Unfair? Absolutely. But with the following strategies, you can make these conditions color-blind.

Type-2 Diabetes

Odds of getting it: 1 in 15 for black men; 1 in 23 for white men

Improve your odds: Drink milk. Harvard researchers found that a daily dairy fix may reduce the risk of early-stage diabetes by up to 72 percent. One problem: "Sixty percent [of black men] are lactose-intolerant," says Edward S. Cooper, M.D., professor emeritus of medicine at the University of Pennsylvania. If that's you, pop some Lactaid before you pour a glass.

Prostate Cancer

Odds of getting it: 1 in 5 for black men; 1 in 6 for white men

Improve your odds: Make a muscle. Research has shown a link between

(continued on page 122)

THE FAMILY RISK CALCULATOR

Find out if your genes add up to illness

The average man's odds*	If a sibling had the disease, your risk is . . .	If a parent had the disease, your risk is . . .	If two or more relatives had the disease, your risk is . . .
HEART DISEASE			
36%	48% (either sibling)	50% (either parent)	>50%
TYPE-2 DIABETES			
14.8%	24.2% (either sibling); 76% (twin)	22% (either parent)	41%
ALZHEIMER'S DISEASE			
6.3%	37% (either sibling)	37% (either parent)	54%
PROSTATE CANCER			
6%	26% (brother)	13% (father)	30%
COLORECTAL CANCER			
4%	9% (either sibling)	9% (either parent)	16%
STROKE			
2%	4.8% (either sibling)	4.9% (father); 3.9% (mother); 19% (mother died of one)	>5%
TESTICULAR CANCER			
0.35%	2.2% (brother); 14% (twin brother)	1.75% (father)	Unknown

* These numbers are by nature imprecise but can function as a general indicator of your genetic risk. The data were taken from research that studied people with a family history of these diseases and how frequently they developed them, compared with those who had no family history. Other factors such as age, smoking, inactivity, and diet were not considered when calculating these numbers, so your overall risk may be higher or lower.

How and when to get tested

No affected relatives: Have your blood pressure, triglycerides, and HDL and LDL cholesterol checked every 5 years, beginning at age 20. Also, consider having your levels of C-reactive protein (CRP) measured. **One affected relative:** Have the above checked annually. **Two or more affected relatives:** Have all of the above checked annually, beginning now.

No affected relatives: No testing needed. If your body-mass index is 27 or higher, see "One affected relative." **One affected relative:** Have your blood sugar tested every 3 years, beginning at age 45. **Two or more affected relatives:** Get tested now. If your blood sugar is between 70 and 110 milligrams per deciliter, no further testing is needed for 10 years, or until age 45.

No affected relatives: No testing needed. **One or more affected relatives diagnosed prior to age 60:** Go for memory tests every year, beginning at age 50.

No affected relatives: At age 50, begin getting annual PSA (prostate-specific antigen) tests and digital rectal exams. **One affected relative:** Begin at age 45. **Two or more affected relatives:** Begin at age 40. If your PSA is below 1.0, no further testing is needed until age 45.

No affected relatives: Go for a colonoscopy every 10 years, beginning at age 50. **One affected relative:** Begin at age 40. **Two or more affected relatives (or one diagnosed before age 60):** Go for a colonoscopy every 3 to 5 years, beginning at age 40.

See Heart Disease, above.

All men, regardless of family history: Perform a monthly self-exam. While taking a warm shower, gently roll each testicle between your index finger, middle finger, and thumb, feeling for any unusual lumps.

high insulin levels and prostate cancer (excess insulin stimulates a key growth hormone). But Finnish researchers found that men who lifted weights three times a week improved their insulin sensitivity by 23 percent, thereby lowering their overall insulin level.

High Blood Pressure

Odds of getting it: 1 in 3 for black men; 1 in 4 for white men

Improve your odds: Take a daily magnesium supplement. African-Americans are much more likely than Caucasians to be deficient in magnesium, a mineral that may help lower systolic blood pressure (the top number) by as much as 5 points and diastolic pressure by 3 points. Take 250 milligrams twice a day.

Lung Cancer

Odds of getting it: 1 in 12 for black men; 1 in 13 for white men

Improve your odds: Quit smoking and eat an apple a day. A study published in the *American Journal of Clinical Nutrition* shows that just half an apple a day can reduce the risk of lung cancer by 60 percent. *Note:* Red Delicious and Granny Smith apples contain the most disease-fighting compounds.

KEEP IT FROM THE KIDS: CHOLESTEROL SCREENING CAN HEAD OFF INHERITED HEART TROUBLE

It seems obvious that if a lifetime of lousy food and little exercise is what causes clogged arteries, then kids must have pretty clean pipes. But many don't, mainly because of genetic factors. That's why, since 1998, the American Academy of Pediatrics (AAP) has recommended that certain at-risk children between the ages of 2 and 10 have their cholesterol checked every 5 years. Your kid qualifies if heart disease runs in the family or if you or your wife has a total cholesterol of 240 or higher.

Still, some doctors don't think the AAP's guidelines go far enough. "I personally feel that every American child should have his or her cholesterol checked around age 10," says Peter Kwiterovich, M.D., professor of pediatrics and director of the lipid-research program at Johns Hopkins University school of medicine. "Ten is a good age because you get them before their cholesterol levels fluctuate during adolescence."

Whether you just want to play it safe or you have the poster child for family risk factors, the blood work is the same: If total cholesterol is 200 or higher, follow up with a fasting test of HDL and LDL cholesterol. If the LDL score is 130 or higher, cut out the Happy Meals and discuss additional dietary changes with your pediatrician.

The Total Cholesterol Picture

Every man carries deadly forms of cholesterol in his blood, and they can increase his heart-disease risk by up to 300 percent. The really scary part: A standard cholesterol test won't tell you if you have them

By Robert Superko, M.D.

Back when researchers first discovered the correlation between cholesterol levels and heart disease, many of us thought we'd discovered the root cause of coronary heart problems. We thought that doctors were finally in a position to intervene and save patients from a pernicious and deadly disease. Those on the front line felt on top of the world—or at least on top of the summit they had been scaling for so many years.

IT'S IN YOUR BLOOD

A new generation of blood tests can screen for an array of heart-attack predictors. Here are 10 new measures of a healthy man.

Apolipoprotein B (apo B). The most accurate indicator of the number of LDLs—not just the amount of cholesterol—in your blood. This alerts your doctor to the presence of small LDLs.

Apolipoprotein E4 (apo E4). A real indicator of heart-attack risk. Apo E4 test results tell how well you'll respond to dietary changes.

Chlamydia pneumoniae. A bacterium that can have serious consequences for your heart.

C-reactive protein (hs-CRP). A telling sign of arterial inflammation—and *twice* as likely as LDL to predict heart attack.

Fibrinogen. A substance that promotes blood clots, a contributing factor in many heart attacks.

HDL2b. The subclass of high-density lipoprotein that offers the greatest level of protection for your heart. You can't have too much!

Homocysteine. A natural and harmless amino acid by-product, produced and eliminated by the body—unless you've inherited an inability to metabolize it. In that case, levels can become too high, putting you at serious risk of heart disease.

Insulin. A hormone that, in elevated levels, has been linked to heart disease. When excessive insulin is detected in combination with some of the other markers, it can mean real trouble.

Lipoprotein (a) [Lp(a)]. A protein that, in high levels, increases your risk of heart attack by 300 percent, even if everything else is normal.

Small LDL. A small, dense, and very dangerous form of low-density lipoprotein. People with a predominance of these small LDLs are called LDL pattern B and carry a much higher risk of heart disease and heart attack.

The researchers were wrong. How do I know? Because I was one of them. In fact, I participated in one of the original studies to determine the effects of lowering cholesterol on heart-disease risk. Over the course of the study, we met with patients periodically to review their progress. Since that study included only male participants, I was surprised one afternoon to see a woman waiting for me. Her question was simple: "My husband's cholesterol numbers were perfect, and you told him that based on those numbers, he was at low risk of heart disease. So why did he drop dead suddenly of a massive heart attack?"

As you can imagine, I was devastated, but at the time I didn't have an answer to give her. Almost 20 years have passed since that day, and I now believe that I can finally offer her—and the many others who have lost husbands and wives, fathers and mothers, sons and daughters to an unexpected heart attack—an answer to that question.

THE TIP OF THE ICEBERG

It's certainly true that the correlation between heart disease and cholesterol was a discovery of critical importance, and the standard cholesterol blood test—total cholesterol, LDL, HDL, and triglycerides—became (and remains) routine at every physical. Our mistake was in thinking that it gave us all we needed in a blood test for heart disease.

The sheer, horrifying frequency of "surprise" heart attacks was the tip-off that the cholesterol breakthrough was a false summit. For anyone not yet convinced, here's an ice-cold wake-up call: If we use the total-cholesterol test as our sole predictor of heart-disease risk, we miss 8 out of 10 cases. That's a shocking percentage, and it means that—contrary to what you've heard and read—normal cholesterol results aren't necessarily reliable measures of your risk.

The good news is we now have the ability to go beyond basic cholesterol and screen for a far broader spectrum of risk factors that show up in your blood. While there are a number of these "metabolic markers" (see "It's in Your Blood" on page 123), one of the most important—and deadly—is an especially small, dense form of LDL. If you have it—and one study indicates that 50 percent of men with heart disease do have it—you're three times more likely to have coronary artery disease, even if everything else (such as your body weight and your standard-cholesterol-test results) is perfect. And that risk doubles to six times if you have a lot of these LDL particles.

Scary? Yes. But fortunately, we know that small LDL responds remarkably well to lifestyle changes such as diet and exercise. This means that many of those stealth heart attacks are preventable. Maybe even yours.

SIZE MATTERS

If the LDL in your blood consists of predominantly small, dense LDL particles, we say that you're LDL pattern B. (People whose LDL is predominantly large are called LDL pattern A.) Why is this tiny lipoprotein such a big deal? First of all, the size of these particles makes it easier for them to weasel their way into the artery walls, where they cause all kinds of damage. And the presence of small LDL also implies the presence of a truly nasty metabolic stew.

HOW TO GET TESTED

Screening for small LDL—as well as other newly identified risk factors—isn't standard in most physicals. Here's a primer addressing basic questions about how you can learn your real heart-disease risk.

Will my doctor know about these new tests? There's so much new science being reported these days that it's almost impossible to keep up, so your doctor may very well not yet be familiar with these tests. But there's nothing wrong with taking information to him. Just remember, tone is everything. If you give your doctor this information in a way that implies you've caught him napping on the job or trying to deny you the best possible care, he's going to get defensive. So take some documentation when you go (this article should do nicely). Ask him what he thinks of testing for small LDL and the other metabolic markers, and whether or not he thinks you're a good candidate.

What if he says I don't need the tests? If you want to have the tests anyway, you're within your rights to explain your feelings and ask that your doctor arrange to have them done. Or you could ask him to put you in touch with a cardiologist who'll do the testing for you. Obtaining a second opinion is a time-honored tradition in medicine and one you should exercise when you have doubts.

How do I find a doctor to do the tests? If you or your physician needs to find a doctor who specializes in lipid metabolism, which involves the advanced metabolic markers, Berkeley HeartLab will provide you with the names of doctors in your area. Its toll-free hotline is (866) 871-4408.

How much do the tests cost? A battery of tests can cost as little as $200. If your physician is suspicious that other problems may be present, additional tests may bring the cost up to $600, which is not insignificant, but it might turn out to be the best investment you ever made.

Who's paying, me or my insurance company? The only way to tell if you're covered for these tests is for you or your doctor's office to call your carrier directly. In most cases, it's the difference between primary and secondary care. If you have no evidence of coronary heart disease and no evidence of other medical problems such as diabetes, high blood pressure, or high blood fats, these tests count as primary, or preventive, care because there's "nothing wrong with you." As you probably know, preventive care is largely in the hands of the patient in this country. If you or your doctor think you're at risk because of your family history, you may decide to go ahead and pay for the testing yourself.

If you already have coronary heart disease or a heart-disease-related diagnosis, you have a much better chance of being covered. All you need is an appropriate diagnosis of coronary heart disease or a heart-disease-related problem such as high blood pressure, hyperlipidemia, or diabetes.

The stew includes rapid progression of partially blocked arteries; arteries that are more prone to sudden spasm; an increased number of blood fats after a meal; lousy removal of cholesterol from the blood supply; platelet stickiness that increases the likelihood of a heart attack caused by a blood clot; insulin resistance; plaque instability; and more.

You may not have all of these things if you have small LDL, but all of them are associated with it. People with small LDL are also more likely to have low HDL, or "good" cholesterol, which means that cholesterol isn't taken out of blood vessels as well or as fast as it might be. Low HDL is also associated with an increased risk of cardiovascular disease.

So these are some of the very good reasons why we worry so much about catching and treating small LDL.

There's another danger to being LDL pattern B: If you have small LDL and have heart disease, the disease will get worse twice as fast as it will in someone who doesn't have small LDL. But if you treat it, you can seriously retard the further development of the blockages and, in many cases, stop the progression of the disease more easily than a person without these small particles could. In fact, in a small percentage of cases, you can actually cause the disease to regress. In other words, LDL-pattern-B patients have the most rapidly progressive disease, but they are also the patients who respond best to treatment.

Still not convinced you should be tested for small LDL? Consider this: People with small LDL may also have elevated levels of the metabolic marker apo B, the combination of which may increase the risk of coronary artery disease by six times. Worse, the presence of small LDL, elevated apo B, and high insulin ratchets your risk up to an alarming 20 times normal.

Here's some good news: Although the size of your LDL particles is genetically linked, your risk can be modified through treatment.

In fact, we can actually convert you from a high-risk LDL pattern B to a low-risk LDL pattern A. And the treatment isn't complicated or expensive. Weight control, a diet relatively low in saturated fat and simple sugars, and an adequate amount of exercise will often do the trick. So if you have this risk factor, don't despair. Just get busy.

Excerpted from *Before the Heart Attacks*, by H. Robert Superko, M.D. © 2003 Rodale, Inc. For more information, go to menshealth.com.

EACH YEAR, THE NUMBER OF MEN WHOSE FIRST SYMPTOM OF HEART DISEASE IS DEATH: 80,000

Pressure: Treated

New, tougher guidelines on blood pressure have suddenly dumped millions of men in hypertension purgatory. Are you one of them?

By Jim Gorman

My friend Porter's blood-pressure numbers are high. Scary high. He just clocked in with a BP of 168 over 137. I gave him a pep talk, told him to visit his doctor, pronto, then hung up the phone with smug assurance. Glad I'm not you, bro.

Turns out ol' Porter and I have more in common than I knew. The National Heart, Lung, and Blood Institute (NHLBI) recently got tough with its revised blood-pressure guidelines. Numbers previously considered "normal"—a blood pressure of between 120 and 139 systolic (the pressure in the arteries as your heart pumps) or 80 and 89 diastolic (between heartbeats)—now qualify as "prehypertension." My own blood pressure is 122 over 84. This makes me one of nearly 23 million men who used to be in the safe zone but now face a major health challenge.

WAKE-UP CALL

If your snoring shakes the ceiling joists, you may have obstructive sleep apnea, a condition that affects 10 percent of men and is one of the root causes of elevated blood pressure. Obstructive sleep apnea occurs when a person's throat muscles relax to the point that they actually block the upper airway, resulting in an evening of oxygen deprivation. This shortage of O_2 leads to constricted blood vessels, which in turn leads to elevated blood pressure. A mild case of obstructive sleep apnea, in which breathing stops for longer than 10 seconds up to five times an hour, increases the risk of developing hypertension by 40 percent. A bad case of apnea triples the risk.

To find out if you're suffocating yourself, ask your doctor for a referral to a sleep lab. (The American Academy of Sleep Medicine has a searchable list of accredited labs at www.aasmnet.org.) If the diagnosis is dire, you'll probably be prescribed a CPAP machine, a masklike contraption that blows air into your throat to keep it open. Think you'd prefer a remedy that goes in your mouth rather than over it? Ask about the antidepressant mirtazapine. While it's not specifically FDA approved to treat sleep apnea, researchers at the University of Illinois found that apnea sufferers who took mirtazapine an hour before bedtime had 50 percent fewer incidents of suspended breathing than those taking a placebo. (The drug may stimulate the muscles in the throat to contract.) "There probably are a million patients who know they have sleep apnea and don't have an effective treatment that they can tolerate," says David Carley, Ph.D., the lead study author. "This is an alternative that would work for that huge group."

"Prehypertension," like "precancerous," definitely grabs your attention, which is the whole point behind the new, steeper grading curve on blood pressure. Public-health officials are alarmed that millions of Americans aren't doing enough to control their high blood pressure—before or after a diagnosis of hypertension. "The old guidelines conveyed a sense of complacency," says Edward Roccella, Ph.D., head of the high-blood-pressure education program at the National Institutes of Health (NIH). "We now know that if you live to 55 as 'normal,' or now 'prehypertensive,' there's a 90 percent chance that you will develop hypertension in your lifetime."

A certain level of pressure within your arteries is essential to continued daily living. Pressure is what propels blood through your body's 60,000 miles of blood vessels. Without pressurization, blood couldn't overcome gravity to reach your brain. Then you'd know how Jessica Simpson feels.

To generate blood pressure, the human body relies on the heart as well as muscle fibers lining the arteries. When necessary, the brain increases blood pressure either by signaling the heart to speed up or pump harder or by directing the arteries to contract. Or some combination of the three. This is exactly what happens in the morning as you hop out of bed. When you stand after being horizontal for so many hours, blood pressure in your head plummets while pressure in your legs shoots up. Without an immediate correction in this imbalance, you'd crumple to the floor midyawn. On cue, arteries in the lower body constrict while the heart dramatically increases output. The instant result: Blood pressure rises, and blood flows to the brain. Now go brush your teeth.

It's an ingenious system, one that's idiotically easy to throw out of whack. Chow on salty foods, and your body will retain more water in order to dilute the excess sodium, increasing overall blood volume. Lard your butt or belly with extra fat, and your heart will have no choice but to work harder to force blood into new tissue. Clog your arteries by eating fatty foods and lazing around, and your heart will pound away to push blood through narrower

NUMBER OF MEN WHO ARE ESTIMATED TO HAVE HIGH BLOOD PRESSURE: 30 MILLION

NUMBER OF MEN WHO HAVE HIGH BLOOD PRESSURE BUT ARE UNAWARE THAT THEY HAVE IT: 10 MILLION

pipes. Consume yourself with stress and worry, and your brain will kick heart and arteries into a perpetual fight-or-flight mode characterized by increased cardiac output. In each case, the net effect is the same: chronically elevated blood pressure.

Unlike your home's water heater, your circulatory system doesn't come equipped with a pressure-relief valve. As a result, thin-walled vessels in the brain can burst under extreme pressure, causing the wholesale slaughter of brain cells that's known as a hemorrhagic stroke. Or hypertension can cause plaque buildup in one of the brain's arteries, eventually cutting off bloodflow. (High blood pressure damages smooth artery walls, creating anchor points for plaque to latch onto.) Kidney failure or heart attack can also follow from dangerous plaque accumulations.

Then there's the plain old wear and tear that high blood pressure causes on your ticker. Over time, the extra work brought on by high blood pressure causes the walls to stiffen and thicken. With thick, rigid walls, the heart becomes a less efficient pump, unable to push out as much blood as it takes in. Blood backs up, the heart gives out, and the coroner scribbles "congestive heart failure" on your chart.

MONITOR YOURSELF

No matter where you have your blood pressure checked, here's how to ensure an accurate reading.

At the doctor's office: Mercury-based gauges are the most accurate, but even they can be off. Ask how often the gauge is recalibrated, or look for a service certificate on the housing, says Jeff Wells of Prestige Medical Corporation, a maker of blood-pressure monitors. Once a year is standard. Medical facilities make you jittery? This stress, called "white-coat hypertension," can drive up your numbers. "Ask your doctor to take several measurements; by the third reading, your blood pressure should have settled down to its usual level," says R. Curtis Ellison, M.D., professor of medicine at Boston University.

At home: Nearly 20 percent of home BP monitors are inaccurate, according to a recent Mayo Clinic study. Two models you can trust: the Omron HEM-711AC ($90) and the Lifesource UA-787V ($110); both have been certified accurate. It's important to cuff your biceps, not your wrist. (BP rises in your extremities.) Big biceps? Spring for a larger cuff to avoid an artificially high measurement. And whichever monitor you choose, bring it to your doctor's office once a year so it can be checked against a mercury gauge.

In a store: Treat the results from an in-store monitor as you would a horoscope. "These machines aren't maintained, so they lose calibration," says Alan Rubin, M.D., an endocrinologist and the author of *High Blood Pressure for Dummies.*

BETTER MEDS THAN DEAD

Sometimes blood pressure won't budge no matter how many lifestyle changes you throw at it. Plan B? If you're still prehypertensive after 6 months of rehabbing your routine, see your doctor about medication. There are literally dozens of drugs that can knock points off your systolic and diastolic bottom line.

Chances are, hypertension hasn't appeared on your radar screen, setting off the same alarms as cancer or heart disease. But it should. "It may well be the number one public-health issue in the United States," says Michael Weber, M.D., past president of the American Society of Hypertension. "Right now, 50 to 60 million Americans have high blood pressure, and that number is going to rise as the population ages and as kids today stay so sedentary."

That said, if you fall into the new prehypertension category, don't panic (and not just because panicking will raise your pressure). Hypertension is not a foregone conclusion, and neither is a lifetime of expensive pressure-lowering drugs. "Many prehypertensives can lower their blood pressures by modifying their lifestyles," says NIH's Roccella. In other words, you need a plan, not a pill. Starting tomorrow, here's what that plan will look like.

7:00 A.M.

Down a can of low-sodium V8. Make that two 5.5-ounce cans. "I've had patients lower their blood pressure just doing that," says Julian Whitaker, M.D., president of the Whitaker Wellness Institute in Newport Beach, California. One reason for the reduction: Eleven ounces of V8 contains nearly 1,240 milligrams (mg) of potassium. In a study published in the *Journal of Human Hypertension*, researchers found that prehypertensive patients who added more potassium to their diets lowered their systolic pressure by 2.5 points and their diastolic by 1.6 points. Potassium helps sweep excess sodium from the circulatory system, causing the blood vessels to dilate. What makes V8 better than a banana (another good source of potassium)? It also contains lycopene and lutein, two phytochemicals that have their own blood-pressure-lowering properties.

10:00 A.M.

Head off office anxiety. Job stress isn't all in your head—it's in your circulatory system, too. "Long-term stressful situations readjust the blood-pressure set point upward," says Rollin McCraty, Ph.D., director of research at the HeartMath Institute in Boulder Creek, California. But McCraty has a fix. Retreat to your office and sit quietly while focusing for 10 seconds on the area around your heart. Breathe deeply and try to replace any negative sensation by reexperiencing a positive, fun feeling or event from your past. (Heck, use someone else's past if you have to.) "Practice doing this 5 to 10 times a day, five times a week, to achieve a drop in blood pressure," says McCraty. According to a 3-month study of 38 computer-company employees, that drop could be as much as 10 points systolic and 6 points diastolic.

12:00 P.M.

Cut out the cold cuts. One slice of ham contains 240 mg sodium, more salt than you'll find on the outside of two pretzel rods. The point: Lose the lunchmeat, and you'll lower your blood pressure. A recent NHLBI study found that prehypertensive people who reduced their daily sodium consumption from 3,300 mg to 1,500 mg knocked nearly 6 points off their systolic BP and close to 3 off their diastolic. If you want to have your hoagie and eat it, too, at least switch to the Boar's Head line of low-sodium meats—ham, turkey, roast beef—and leave the pickle (833 mg sodium) on your plate. Another rule of thumb: If a food comes canned or jarred, it's probably a salt mine. "Many canned and bottled foods contain extra sodium added during processing," says Mary Ellen Camire, Ph.D., a nutrition advisor for *Men's Health*. "Whenever possible, buy fresh or frozen instead."

5:30 P.M.

Ease up at the gym. If your workout style is all about running full tilt or lifting full loads, dial it back a bit. In a recent study published in the *Annals of Internal Medicine*, researchers found that a regular program of moderate exercise reduced blood pressure by an average of 3.8 points systolic and 2.6 diastolic. "I recommend staying in the 70 to 85 percent heart-rate range for the most benefit in lowering blood pressure," says S. Michael Clark, M.D., a specialist in preventive medicine at the Cooper Clinic in Dallas. Fast walking, running at a relatively easy 8:30 pace, and what Dr. Clark calls "endurance

BUTTS AND GUTS

Anything you do to lower your blood pressure will be worthless if you don't address the two biggest risk factors for hypertension: smoking and being overweight. Besides doing a number on your lungs, smoking elevates blood pressure by increasing heart rate and constricting blood vessels. As for that jelly belly, each pound of fat needs servicing by literally miles of new blood vessels, which means the heart must beat harder with each stroke to push blood through that tissue. Drop just 10 pounds, and you'll knock an easy 5 points off your blood pressure and as a result lower your risk of stroke by 42 percent.

lifting"—three sets of 10 to 12 repetitions at 70 percent of maximal effort—will get you into the right heart-rate range. Played out over the course of a week, a BP-lowering workout regimen looks like this: 1 day each of jogging, swimming, and cycling, and 1 or 2 days each of walking and lifting.

7:00 P.M.

Make stir-fry for dinner. And use sesame oil. Indian researchers found that when hypertensive patients used sesame oil in place of the other oils in their diets, their BP readings dropped from an average of 166/101 to 134/85 in just 2 months. The reason? It may be the polyunsaturated fatty acids (sesame oil contains 43 percent; olive oil, 11 percent), as well as the compound sesamin, which inhibits the synthesis and absorption of cholesterol, says Devarajan Sankar, D.O., Ph.D., the lead study author. Try using sesame oil on salads, as a marinade for meats, and even in peanut-butter smoothies. (The nuttiness will complement the sesame flavor.)

9:45 P.M.

Go two rounds and out. Make the second drink of the night your last call for alcohol. In a landmark study published in the *New England Journal of Medicine,* researchers found that one or two drinks a day actually decreased blood pressure slightly. Three drinks or more a day, however, elevated blood pressure by an average of 10 points systolic and 4 diastolic.

How crossing the two-drink threshold turns booze from benign to dastardly is still not fully understood. "Heavy drinkers may impair their kidneys' ability to excrete sodium," says R. Curtis Ellison, M.D., professor of medicine at Boston University. As for the type of alcohol, it really doesn't matter. Heck, order a screwdriver: Orange juice is one of the best sources of blood pressure-lowering potassium.

Cancer-Proof Your Prostate

Eight ways to dodge, detect, and defuse a potential gland mine

By Matt Bean

It's one of those weird anatomical-arboreal coincidences: The human prostate is about the size and shape of a walnut. But what if it really were a walnut? For one thing, you'd never get prostate cancer. Which sounds great, until you realize that you could get "walnut curculio" or "walnut-husk maggot" instead. Better to deal with the devil you know.

And what a devil it is. Last year, 221,000 men were diagnosed with prostate cancer; that's more than lung, colon, and brain cancers combined. And nearly 29,000 men died of it.

These are grim statistics, but there's reason to be optimistic. Make that eight reasons. What follows is the latest, hot-out-of-the-lab research on how you can prevent, detect, and treat the disease. Putting this science into action (read: more sex, more wine) won't confer absolute immunity, but it will make your prostate one tough nut to crack.

PREVENTION

Love thyself. As if masturbation didn't already provide enough of a payoff, a recent Australian study found that DIY sex may also help prevent prostate cancer. The study of 2,338 men showed that the guys who masturbated five or more times a week were 34 percent less likely to develop prostate cancer by age 70 than those who handled matters less often. "Seminal fluid contains substances that are carcinogenic," says Graham Giles, Ph.D., the lead study author. "Regular ejaculation may help flush them out."

And in case you're wondering, no, masturbating more than once a day won't offer more protection, and yes, straight-up sex works, too. But before you have unprotected nookie with your partner, be sure she's been tested for cytomegalo-virus, a type of herpes recently found in cancerous prostate tissue.

Be happy you're going bald. Turns out the hair-loss drug Propecia has one impressive side effect. In a National Cancer Institute (NCI) study of 18,882 men, researchers found that the men who took 5 milligrams (mg) of Propecia, a.k.a. finasteride, every day for 7 years had a 25 percent lower risk of prostate cancer than those taking a placebo. Finasteride blocks production of dihydrotestosterone, a hormone that triggers hair loss and prostate growth. "It's the first study to prove that prostate cancer is preventable," says Peter Greenwald, M.D., the NCI's director of cancer prevention.

One caution: Men on finasteride had a slightly greater chance of being diagnosed with a more aggressive form of the disease than did the placebo takers. More research on the drug is needed, but if you're concerned about prostate cancer, discuss these findings with your doctor.

Wine and dine. There's a good reason Western European men have lower prostate-cancer rates than we do. And it has nothing to do with Speedo thongs. New research suggests that certain staples of the Mediterranean diet have prostate-cancer-fighting properties. For starters, a recent study published in the *Journal of the National Cancer Institute* shows that men who eat more than 10 grams of garlic or scallions (about three cloves of garlic or 2 tablespoons of scallions) daily have a 50 percent lower risk of prostate cancer than those who eat less than 2 grams. (Give credit to organosulfur compounds, which are common to both vegetables.)

Then there's red wine; red grapes are flush with resveratrol, an antioxidant found in some plants that may help inhibit the growth of prostate cancer, according to a report from the M.D. Anderson Cancer Center at the University of Texas. A glass or two of red wine daily should suffice. "If you drink too much," says Catherine O'Brian, Ph.D., the lead study author, "you can neutralize the beneficial effects."

DETECTION

Lower the bar. Here's a PSA (public service announcement) regarding your PSA (prostate-specific antigen): Using a score of 4.1 or greater as the alarm for prostate cancer could prove fatal. A recent study of 6,691 men, published in the *New England Journal of Medicine (NEJM)*, showed that this traditional threshold for ordering a follow-up biopsy may be missing 82 percent of prostate-cancer diagnoses in men under 60. "The threshold of 4.1 that's being used has never been rigorously studied," says Karen M. Kuntz, Sc.D., one of the study's authors. And while critics say a lower threshold will lead to unnecessary biopsies, Rinaa Punglia, M.D., another of the study authors, believes that the broader standard could be worth it. "It's a trade-off," she admits. "But it could save lives."

So how low should you go? Dr. Punglia recommends that when you have your PSA level checked (annually beginning at age 50—or 45 if you have a family history or are African-American), you observe a threshold of 2.6, especially if you're under age 60; according to the *NEJM* study, following this guideline doubled the cancer-detection rate, from 18 percent to 36 percent.

Calculate your risk. Let's say your PSA is 2.6. You still may not need a biopsy. Instead, ask your doctor to use a nomogram. This needle-free analysis turns a patient's age, PSA density (PSA divided by the volume of the prostate), digital-rectal-exam result, and transrectal-ultrasound result into a score that helps determine whether a biopsy is really warranted. "We can say whether or not, for your prostate, that's a high PSA," says Mark Garzotto, M.D., director of urologic oncology at the Portland VA Medical Center. In a study of 1,200 men, Dr. Garzotto found that if a nomogram had been used in every case, it would have spared 24 percent of the men from unnecessary biopsies. If your doctor can't crunch the numbers, ask for copies of your test results; you can find the same nomogram at menshealth.com and do the math yourself.

TREATMENT

Hit the spice rack. Researchers at the Center for Holistic Urology at Columbia-Presbyterian Medical Center in New York City recently found that a blend of herbs including ginger, oregano, rosemary, and green tea reduced prostate-cancer cell growth by 78 percent in the lab. Sold as Zyflamend, it's thought to inhibit the activity of COX-2, a protein linked to the progression of the disease. You can find retailers of Zyflamend at new-chapter.com. Get your doctor's okay before taking it.

Use CAD (computer-assisted doctor). The radical prostatectomy recently became a lot less radical, thanks to a new robotic version of the procedure. With the da Vinci system, doctors use three-dimensional imaging to

THE CANDY CURE

How a scandal may bring sweet relief to prostate-cancer patients

Four years ago, the hottest herbal supplement for prostate health wasn't saw palmetto but rather PC-SPES (PC for prostate cancer and SPES from the Latin word for *hope*). The study findings were impressive—a 50 percent drop in the PSA levels of three-quarters of the men taking it—and the testimonials even more so. "It was a miracle substance," says Bob Each, 59, who started taking PC-SPES after hormone therapy couldn't completely keep his metastatic prostate cancer in check. "My bone scans lit up like a Christmas tree. I was a dead duck." His cancer is now nearly undetectable.

Then, in 2002, the miracle substance was pulled off the market after it was found to be tainted with prescription medications. One of the medications was diethylstilbestrol (DES), a synthetic estrogen that treats prostate cancer by lowering blood levels of testosterone. It was abandoned in the 1980s because of heart attacks and blood clotting. Many scientists believed that DES, and not an herbal ingredient, was what had made PC-SPES so effective. But a few researchers and hundreds, if not thousands, of patients remain unconvinced.

"The loss of this supplement is unfortunate," says Dan Theodorescu, M.D., Ph.D., chairman of urologic oncology at the University of Virginia. He found that DES by itself left a different "genetic fingerprint" on prostate-cancer cells than did PC-SPES—supporting data that the two work by fundamentally different mechanisms. "Ultimately, we had hoped to find the most active ingredient in PC-SPES and synthesize it."

That ingredient may be *Glycyrrhiza glabra*, or licorice root. Like DES, licorice-root extract has powerful estrogenic effects: In one Italian study, researchers found that men who swallowed 7 grams daily for 8 days experienced a 25 percent reduction in testosterone levels. It may also act as a sort of chemotherapy. A recent Rutgers University laboratory study showed that licorice extract destroyed prostate-cancer cells in much the same way as the chemotherapy drug Taxol. Spurred on by this finding, Rutgers researchers are now conducting a Phase II clinical trial with 30 prostate-cancer patients.

Most health-food stores carry licorice-root extract by the bottle ($8 to $14 for 100 tablets), but don't start taking it to treat prostate cancer without first consulting your doctor. Nor should you write yourself a prescription for Twizzlers three times a day.

direct two nimble robotic hands through a few small slits in the patient's abdomen to remove the cancerous prostate. According to data from the Vattikuti Urology Institute at the Henry Ford Health System in Detroit, 90 percent fewer men became incontinent and 50 percent fewer became impotent with the da Vinci system than with manual gland removal. "It's like playing golf with a titanium driver versus a wooden driver," says chief of urology Mani Menon, M.D. Another plus: Patients spent an average of 1.5 days in the hospital, compared with 2.3 days for open surgery. For a list of da Vinci–equipped hospitals, go to intuitivesurgical.com/patients/maps.

Rehab your erections. Unless you're David Beckham, this one's a no-brainer: Take a nerve graft from your ankle and save your sex life. The cavernous nerves, a.k.a. the boner bugle corps, are often a casualty of prostate removal if cancer has (or might) spread outside the gland. But by replacing the cavernous nerves with the sural nerve that runs along the ankle, as many as 9,000 men a year could recover erectile function, says Peter Scardino, M.D., one of the developers of the procedure and chairman of urology at Memorial Sloan-Kettering Cancer Center in New York City. "If you've got only one [cavernous] nerve left, you're firing on four cylinders, but if I do a graft, it's like you're firing on seven out of eight," he says. And don't worry; a slight numbness in your foot is the only side effect. Talk to your urologist about where to find a surgeon experienced in sural-nerve grafting.

NEED TO KNOW

Super Seven

Imagine a pill that can reduce your risk of heart disease by 80 percent. That's the promise of Polypill, which is actually a cocktail of seven existing heart medications: low-dose aspirin, folic acid, two cholesterol-lowering statins, an ACE inhibitor, a beta-blocker, and a calcium-channel blocker. Researchers at the University of London, where the pill is being developed, say if everyone over 55 started taking Polypill immediately, it would save millions of lives each year. Because Polypill contains mostly low doses of generic drugs, it's cheap and has few serious side effects.

When Seconds Count

A blood test developed by the Cleveland Clinic could prevent thousands of deaths a year by diagnosing heart attacks faster. In lab experiments, the test identified an attack faster than current tests by measuring an enzyme normally found in white blood cells. The enzyme is released when arteries with rupture-prone fatty deposits become inflamed. Doctors are working with drug companies to make the new test available in hospitals.

Keep the Beat

More than one million men suffer from an irregular heartbeat, or atrial fibrillation (AF). But statins can help cure the condition, say Chinese researchers. Two years after receiving electric-shock treatment for AF, 60 percent of patients taking Zocor or Lipitor had no symptoms, compared with 16 percent of those not on statins. Statins reduce inflammation, which can lead to AF, says study author Hung-Fat Tse, M.D. If you have AF, ask your doctor about starting statins prior to electric-shock treatment.

NUMBER OF ADDITIONAL YEARS THE AVERAGE MAN WOULD LIVE IF HEART DISEASE WERE WIPED OUT: 6

Snooze or You Lose

If it takes you 30 minutes or more to fall asleep each night, your risk of dying is twice what it is if you fall asleep immediately, say University of Pittsburgh researchers. That's because sleep problems often disguise serious medical conditions.

Sleep Off Hypertension

The sleep aid melatonin may also reduce high blood pressure (BP), say Dutch researchers. In a 3-week study of 16 men with hypertension, those taking 2.5 milligrams of melatonin an hour before bed saw their systolic blood pressure drop an average of 6 points and their diastolic by 4. Previous studies link disturbed sleep to high blood pressure, so melatonin may help by regulating sleep cycles, says lead author Frank A.J.L. Scheer, Ph.D. Whether you're hypertensive or prehypertensive (120 to 139 systolic, 80 to 89 diastolic), talk to your doctor before taking melatonin for BP.

Bad Air Day

Researchers in Taiwan examining hospital data recently discovered that for every 25 percent increase in air pollution, the incidence of hemorrhagic stroke (a bursting blood vessel) went up by 54 percent. A possible reason: Pollutants cause dangerous fluctuations in heart rate. More research is needed to determine if the same risk factor exists in the States.

Guard against Strokes

Angioplasty is a lifesaver, unless a bit of plaque breaks free from the artery wall during the procedure and goes hurtling toward your brain, triggering a stroke. To keep this from happening, researchers at the Cleveland Clinic have developed a tiny filter capable of catching errant debris released during the procedure. In early trials, the new filters reduced stroke risk during angioplasty by more than 50 percent. Additional trials of the filter, called Angioguard, are currently under way.

New Stroke Treatments on the Way

Scientists at UCLA are testing a tiny metal corkscrewlike device designed to stop strokes. Using the device, doctors are able to latch onto and remove blood clots and immediately restore bloodflow. The device is entering clinical trials.

In addition, studies in Australia indicate that a compound in vampire-bat saliva may be up to 200 times more effective than current medications at breaking down blood clots and could help in treating strokes. The secret to the saliva's effectiveness is a compound called desmoteplase, which helps keep a victim's blood from clotting after a bite. "Desmoteplase is not only more effective at dissolving blood clots than other drugs, it's also much less likely to cause damaging side effects in the brain," says Robert Medcalf, Ph.D., the study author. A man-made version of desmoteplase is currently in development.

High and Unmighty

Finally, an upside to being downsized: Men who are 5'11" or taller have a 20 to 40 percent greater risk of developing prostate cancer after the age of 50 than their shorter peers. Researchers at Boston's Brigham and Women's Hospital made the discovery but haven't yet found the cause of the link. Still, if you're at least 6 feet tall and over 50, this is one more reason to make sure you get a yearly prostate-cancer screening.

Better Prostate-Cancer Tests

Researchers at Northwestern University have developed a new test that's hundreds of times more accurate at detecting changes in levels of prostate-specific antigen (PSA) than are existing methods. To perform the procedure, researchers sandwich strands of DNA between tiny bits of gold called nanoparticles and then analyze proteins from the DNA, looking for signs of cancer. Additional trials on the test are under way.

In related news, a new procedure called Prose may eliminate the need for a painful biopsy in order to confirm the presence of prostate cancer. The noninvasive procedure is straight out of *Star Trek*—doctors use an MRI-like device to scan your pelvis, looking for potentially cancerous tissue. If anything suspicious is spotted, your physician then uses a device called a spectroscope to scan the tissue, checking for chemicals that indicate the tumor's severity. Currently, doctors use Prose after a PSA test and tissue biopsy; but in the future, physicians may be able to bypass the biopsy for a quicker and more accurate cancer diagnosis. Prose testing from GE Medical is available in 20 hospitals nationwide.

Multitasking Medicine

A drug designed to stop the spread of bone cancer may help save the lives of men with other forms of cancer. In a 4-year trial, U.K. researchers found that men taking sodium clodronate had lower PSA levels and were less likely to die of prostate cancer than men not taking the medication.

Get Off Insulin

According to a new study published in the *Annals of Surgery*, gastric bypass surgery may help treat diabetes. Of 191 overweight type-2 diabetics who had the surgery, 83 percent were able to go off their diabetes medication.

Also in the works is a drug made from Gila monster spit, which may help people with diabetes reduce their blood sugar—and lose weight. Since food in the desert is scarce, most Gila monsters eat only a few times a year. So, in order to survive, the lizards have evolved to produce a substance in their saliva that helps their metabolism process infrequent meals. A trial of 105 men and women taking exenatide, the drug version of the magic spittle, showed that nearly half were able to lower their blood sugar to within healthy levels. Even better, those individuals each lost an average of 7.5 pounds. More trials are under way.

No More Needles

For diabetics, checking blood sugar may soon be as simple as slicing an onion. A new study from India reveals that teardrops may be just as effective as blood samples at tracking blood-sugar levels. The discovery will allow researchers to develop a new kind of test strip that could measure blood-sugar levels simply by being placed near the corner of the eye.

Stop the Spread of Melanoma

Doctors at the University of Michigan have developed the first test capable of detecting the spread of melanoma. To perform the new procedure—called sentinel-lymph-node mapping—doctors inject a small amount of radioactive dye into the cancer site. The dye's movement through the body helps clue physicians in to locations to which the cancer may have spread. "The earlier we can find and treat skin cancer that's spread, the better a patient's odds of beating the disease," says Carol Bradford, M.D., the study author.

Genetic Test for Colon Cancer

In the future, a simple blood test may tell you if you're at risk for colon cancer. In a study of 172 men and women, Johns Hopkins University researchers found that people with a family history of colon cancer were nearly five times more likely to have a specific genetic defect in their blood than people with less risk of the disease.

FAST FIXES

We're hardwired to like things fast: fast cars, a fast buck, fast girls. That's why it's little surprise that we die fast, too. Among developed countries, we're pretty far down on the list of men who live the longest. But we can do better. That's where these fast fixes come in. We've put together 14 ways to slow down your demise.

1. Don't weather the storm. Fewer guys would perish at the hands of Mother Nature if they sought shelter when the weather is threatening. A review of data from the National Weather Service found that men are 85 percent more likely to be struck by lightning than are women. Guys are also more likely to be killed in floods, tornadoes, and high winds, the study reports.

2. Survive your next surgery. The old real estate mantra "location, location, location" seems to have a bearing on the outcomes of surgery. A new study conducted at the Moffitt Cancer Center and Research Institute in Florida showed that you're nearly 10 times more likely to die or suffer injury if you have a medical procedure performed in a doctor's office rather than a hospital. The reasons for the increased risk? Underqualified doctors, out-of-date or shoddy facilities, and problems with anesthesia. Currently, more than half of all states have no laws regulating office surgeries. So if you're having any kind of surgery, consider having it done at the hospital rather than in a doctor's office.

3. Eat cranberries for your brain. Don't just eat cranberries at the holidays. According to a new study from the University of Massachusetts, cranberries may help protect your brain during a stroke. In laboratory experiments, researchers found that cranberry extract helped to keep brain cells from dying during simulated stroke conditions. Although researchers are still working to determine the exact dosage of cranberries needed for maximum stroke protection, the amounts tested were roughly the equivalent of consuming half a cup of berries per day.

4. Build iron lungs. Another reason to make sure you get plenty of exercise: Researchers in Finland recently found that exercise can help keep your lungs from aging and losing function. In a 25-year study of 429 men, researchers discovered that individuals performing the most exercise had the strongest, healthiest lungs and were the least likely to die of lung disease. Even getting half an hour of moderate aerobic activity daily should help, says Margit Pelkonen, M.D., the study author.

5. Order a Bloody Mary. Next time you're headed someplace where people will be smoking, pop a vitamin C supplement. Or, if you're going to a smoke-filled bar, make the first drink of the night something containing orange or tomato juice. The reason? Vitamin C may help prevent the damaging effects of secondhand smoke. Researchers at the University of California gave 67 nonsmokers regularly exposed to secondhand smoke either 500 milligrams (mg) of vitamin C or a placebo daily. At the end of the trial, those taking the C had significantly less oxidative damage from the smoke than those popping the placebo.

6. Cut your lung-cancer risk. If you've ever smoked, take note: You may be able to reduce your lung-cancer risk by popping just a couple of pills a day. Start with a good multivitamin containing B_6. Washington State University researchers recently found that many smokers have unusually low levels of B_6, a vitamin that prevents the DNA damage that can cause malignancies. Follow the B_6 with an anti-inflammatory, such as ibuprofen or aspirin. A study published in the journal *Cancer* found that men who take either medication at least three times a week reduce their lung-cancer risk. And if you're trying to kick the habit, opt for maximum-strength patches and gums. New French research shows that men often need larger doses of nicotine replacements so they can give up the habit for good.

7. Make aspirin therapy work. If you're taking a daily aspirin for a heart condition, don't even think about going cold turkey. French researchers recently discovered that heart patients who ceased aspirin therapy were likely to suffer a major coronary event within 1 week, even if their condition seemed stable. Normally, aspirin helps prevent platelets from clogging a person's arteries. Stop taking the drug and "there may be a kind of rebound syndrome; platelets become more and more active," says Emile Ferrari, M.D., the study author. If you'd like to stop, talk to your doctor, who will start you on another medication to prevent the deadly rebound effect.

You also may want to reconsider taking ibuprofen for a headache or sore muscle. In a new study, Harvard researchers found that regular use of drugs called NSAIDs (nonsteroidal anti-inflammatory drugs, including pain medications like ibuprofen) can reduce aspirin's ability to protect the heart. Normally, aspirin reduces heart-attack risk by up to 44 percent in healthy men. However, in a 5-year study of men who took aspirin every other day and painkillers at least 60 days a year, researchers found that the men were as likely to suffer a heart attack as men who didn't take any aspirin.

8. Pop a pre-game pill. Talk about a game going into sudden death. Swiss researchers recently found that men were up to 60 percent more likely to suffer a fatal heart attack during a televised sporting event—in this case, the World Cup—than at other times. "It's the combination of stress, anger, and excitement," says Eugene Katz, M.D., the study author. His advice for at-risk guys: Pop an aspirin before the game, and get up and move around every half hour or so while it's under way; both strategies will help reduce the risk of clot formation.

9. Make yourself a sandwich. Researchers at the University of Virginia Health System found that eating foods rich in magnesium, such as peanut butter and whole-wheat bread, can help protect your heart. The 15-year study of 7,000 men showed that the risk of coronary heart disease nearly doubled in those who were magnesium deficient. "The risk declines significantly with increasing magnesium intake," says Robert Abbott, M.D., the lead researcher. It's believed that too little magnesium may increase the risk of atherosclerosis (hardening of the arteries) and hypertension. Aim for about 420 mg a day; one peanut-butter-and-jelly sandwich on whole-wheat bread will get you a third of the way there.

10. Get two for one. If you have a family history of heart disease and are considering taking an antidepressant, talk to your doctor about Zoloft. According to a new Duke University study, taking an antidepressant such as Zoloft may help reduce your heart-attack risk. "When patients take Zoloft, their blood becomes less sticky and less likely to form heart-stopping clots," says Christopher O'Connor, M.D., the study author. Another reason this is a particularly important finding: An estimated one in four men who've had heart attacks also develop depression.

11. Check your own BP. Researchers in Belgium found that monitoring blood pressure (BP) at home helps reduce medication use. Of 203 hypertensive people, 25 percent of those who cuffed themselves twice a day stopped medication after a year, compared with 10 percent of nonmeasurers. Home monitoring may increase treatment compliance and weed out misdiagnosed patients, since seeing a doctor can cause stress. "Stress increases BP and can give the false impression that the patient is hypertensive," says study author Jan Staessen, M.D., Ph.D. Try the Lifesource Quick Response, $110 (lifesourceonline.com).

12. Cut calories. Two new studies suggest cutting calories could reduce your risk of prostate cancer. A study done in France reports that overweight men are more than twice as likely to develop prostate cancer as men who are carrying fewer pounds. Also, researchers at Johns Hopkins University looked at 440 middle-aged men and found that those with prostate cancer took in the

NUMBER OF POINTS, ON AVERAGE, THAT DRINKING 12 OUNCES OF CONCORD GRAPE JUICE DAILY CAN LOWER YOUR BLOOD PRESSURE: 6

most calories compared with the other men in the study. The findings showed that eating more than 2,600 calories a day was associated with a four times greater risk of developing the disease, regardless of where the calories came from—fat, protein, or carbohydrates. Scientists say more research needs to be done to confirm this connection.

13. Know for sure. A new Harvard study reveals that even the most accurate PSA tests still miss 82 percent of prostate-cancer tumors in men under 60. If your average PSA readings fall between 2.6 and 4.0, the researchers suggest considering a prostate biopsy.

14. Walk away from the reaper. Harvard researchers report that diabetics who take regular, brisk walks are less likely to die of any cause—including heart disease—than men who take slower walks on a less regular basis. In a separate study, doctors found that diabetics who took multivitamins were 73 percent less likely to get sick over the course of a year, compared with diabetics not taking vitamins.

OUR FINAL ANSWERS

Get There Alive

I had read about a journalist who died of a pulmonary embolism while covering the war in Iraq. I travel a lot in cramped business class. Could it happen to me?

—J.M., Huntington Beach, California

Affirmative. In a condition called deep-vein thrombosis (DVT), blood clots form in the deep veins of your legs (the iliac, femoral, popliteal, and tibial veins, which return deoxygenated blood to your heart). If a clot breaks loose and reaches your lungs, it can block a pulmonary artery or one of its branches—this blockage is called an embolism—potentially killing you within hours. "You're putting yourself at risk if you travel in cramped spaces for 10 or more hours in a row, and your risk increases greatly if you are obese, smoke, or don't exercise," says Pierce Scranton, M.D., a spokesman for the American Orthopedic Foot and Ankle Society.

To avoid problems during your flights, follow Dr. Scranton's three key tips:

- Pop an aspirin 1 hour before your flight to inhibit blood clotting.
- Walk to the end of the plane once every hour. Exercise increases your circulation.
- While you're standing in line for the john, do 10 toe raises. Repeat on the hour (which you'll need to do if you're hydrating properly—drinking plenty of water is another clot stopper). This exercise will squeeze the blood out of the veins in your feet—the area that's at the highest risk of developing a clot. Symptoms of DVT may include pain, swelling, discoloration of the affected area, and skin that's unusually warm to the touch.

Shop for a Prostate Doc

My dad has to have his cancerous prostate removed. What's the one thing we can do to ensure a safe procedure?

—G.T., Portland, Maine

Find a surgeon who's cracked more walnut-size objects than your average obese squirrel. "If your father has decided to have radical prostatectomy, make sure the surgery is performed by someone who does a lot of them," says Mark S. Litwin, M.D., professor of urology and public health at UCLA. Dr. Litwin coauthored a recent study published in the *Journal of Clinical Oncology* comparing the numbers of prostatectomies surgeons had performed with their outcomes. His findings: Patients of surgeons who do at least 40 such procedures a year have significantly better results than those whose docs do fewer. Men whose doctors had the most experience with prostatectomy were nearly half as likely to suffer postoperative complications and also had shorter hospital stays. To find Dr. Cutsalot, ask these two questions: (1) "How many radical-prostatectomy surgeries did you do in the last year?" (2) "Do you know what the rates of incontinence and impotence were for your 100 most recent patients?" Says Dr. Litwin, "The surgeon who knows these specific outcomes is one who's interested in his own quality improvement."

Water Down Your Blood Pressure

What is the best way to treat hypertension?

—P.L., Oakwood, Ohio

Piss it away. A new study by researchers at the University of Texas compared the three types of drugs prescribed for hypertension and found that diuretics work best at lowering blood pressure and preventing cardiovascular events. Plus, they're the cheapest—10 cents a day, compared with 78 cents per calcium channel blocker and 30 cents for each ACE inhibitor. "Diuretic" is simply doc-speak for a water pill that acts on the kidneys to make you pee. "They alter your body's distribution of sodium and water into the urine, resulting in changes in total body water and reducing blood pressure," says Barry Davis, M.D., an author of the study.

Missing a Beat

When my heart skips a beat, is there any danger it won't start up again?

—D.M., Aurora, Illinois

There are both benign and dangerous reasons your heart could skip. The harmless one happens when your heart fires off a few extra beats, then pauses to fill up with more blood than normal, resulting in one megastrength heartbeat. According to Richard Stein, M.D., associate chairman of medicine at Beth Israel Medical Center in New York City, this sudden sensation happens to everyone. "Some people notice it coming on when they have a lot of caffeine, alcohol, stress, or sleep deprivation, but it's benign and seems not to have anything to do with how long and well you live," says Dr. Stein.

Things get dangerous when the chambers of your heart beat so fast, they quiver. When it happens in the upper chambers, it's called atrial fibrillation; the blood pools there and can form clots, and there's a risk that a clot could travel to the brain and trigger a stroke. Untreated quivering in the lower chambers, known as ventricular fibrillation (VF), can lead to collapse and sudden death because the ventricles can't pump enough blood to the brain, lungs, and other vital organs. VF affects people who have congenital heart defects or who have already suffered a heart attack. (You know who you are.)

What helps? A dose of fish oil—or more fatty fish (salmon and tuna). According to a large Italian study of patients suffering from fibrillation, daily intake of fish-oil supplements cut the risk of sudden death in half after just 3 months. And just for the record, Dr. Stein insists that your heart does not physically skip a beat when the love of your life walks in the room.

Keep Smoking to Quit

Can Quest cigarettes help me quit?

—P.T., San Diego

If you're one of the rare guys who smoke only because they're nicotine fiends, Quest might indeed help. Here's how: The cigarettes are made from genetically altered tobacco that has less nicotine. Level 1 has 0.6 milligrams (mg) nicotine per cigarette (compared with 1.1 mg in a full-flavor Marlboro), level 2 has 0.3 mg, and level 3 has no more than 0.05 mg. Climbing down the ladder may break your addiction. But will beating cigarettes follow? Not necessarily. Smoking behaviors—feeling more confident, bonding with other smokers—are often harder to give up than nicotine itself, says Thomas Eissenberg, Ph.D., professor of psychology at Virginia Commonwealth University. Still, any tool that might get you off the hook is worth trying.

AVERAGE PERIOD OF TIME A SMOKER NEEDS TO GO WITHOUT LIGHTING UP TO DECREASE HIS RISK OF HEART DISEASE BY 50 PERCENT: 1 YEAR

Better Leave It to the Doctor

Do home cholesterol monitors really work?

—M.S., Seattle

They're a lot like aging Cy Young Award winners—effective but expensive. To win FDA approval, the machines first had to test within 3 percent accuracy compared with traditional lab tests. But that's under ideal testing conditions. Factors like human error and time of day can skew a reading by up to 12 percent. Some tests measure only total cholesterol and give no information about HDL or triglycerides. Many systems ring in at over $100, with test strips sold separately. "From a dollar standpoint, if you're going to do this only once or twice, it's not cost effective," says Michael Rocco, M.D., a cardiologist at the Cleveland Clinic. "Plus, you don't have the value of a doctor interpreting the information and making a recommendation." Our advice: If your doctor wants you to buy one as part of an ongoing cholesterol treatment, pony up. Otherwise, save your money for a gym membership and some salmon.

Killer Smile

My wisdom teeth don't bother me. Is there any reason to have them yanked?

—B.T., Billings, Montana

It's your choice: Keep the useless teeth and boost your heart-disease risk, or pull them and die of something else. "In most people, the mouth doesn't have enough room for wisdom teeth, so they may erupt incorrectly or cause crowding, making them more susceptible to infections," says Edwin Slade, D.M.D., a spokesman for the American Association of Oral and Maxillofacial Surgeons. "And they're very hard to clean, which puts you at an even higher risk." Infections left untreated even for a few months can lead to more serious damage, such as periodontal disease, which increases your chances of heart disease. Chronic infections can cause a cascade of inflammation in your blood vessels, which could lead to a blood clot and the Big One. That's where the tooth wisdom comes in: Smart men call an oral surgeon.

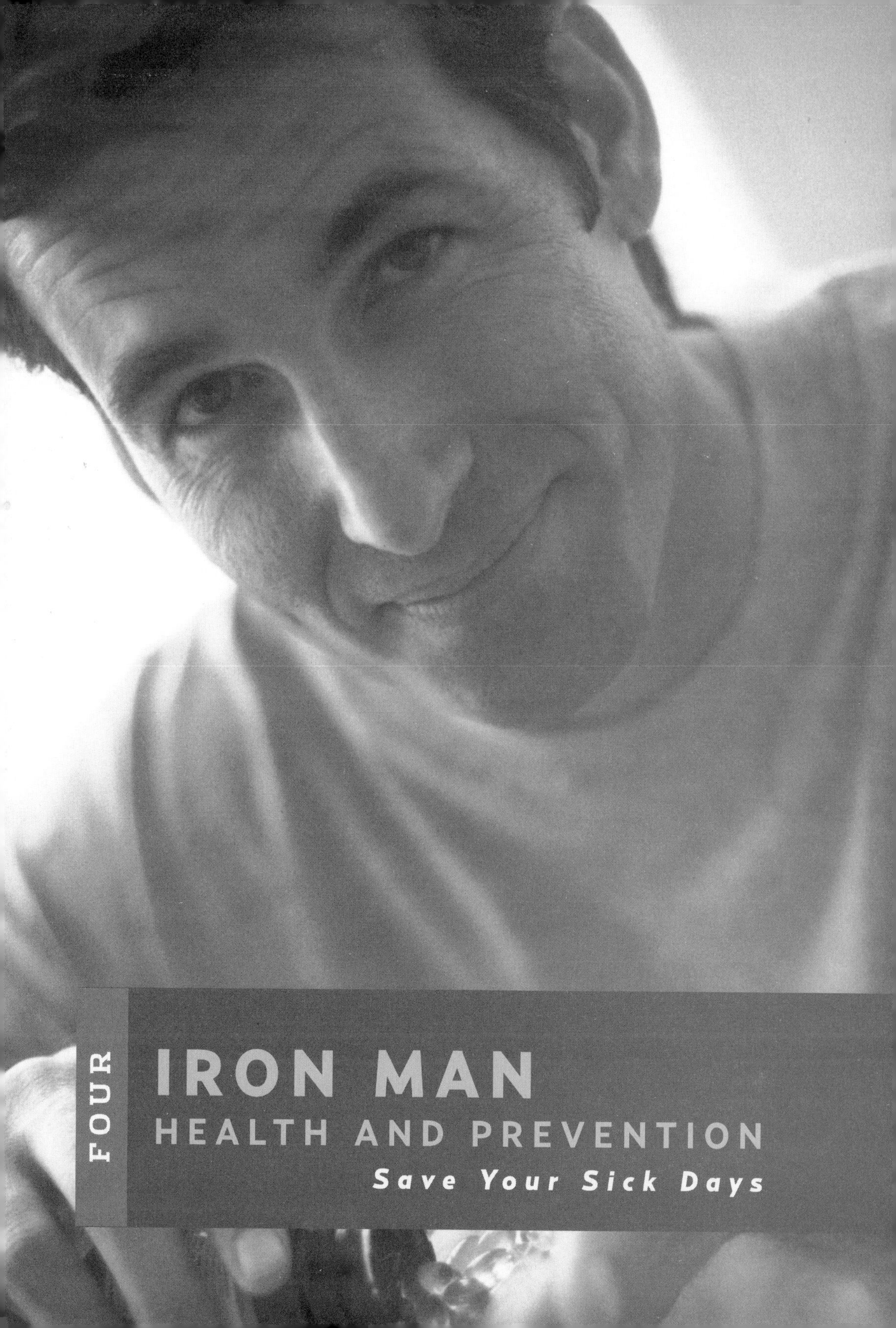

FOUR

IRON MAN

HEALTH AND PREVENTION

Save Your Sick Days

MUST READS

Seven Pains You Should Never Ignore

These common aches could very well be nothing. Or something far, far worse

By Allen St. John

Most of the time, it's good that the little Vince Lombardi sitting on our shoulder tells us to shut up and play through the pain, otherwise we'd never get anything done. On the other hand, there are a few instances in which we can actually talk ourselves out of existence.

That's what happened to NBC reporter David Bloom. While covering the war in Iraq from his specially outfitted armored vehicle, he began to feel pain behind his knee. He reportedly sought out medical advice by satellite phone, decided not to follow the advice—"Go to a doctor"—popped a few aspirin, and kept right on going. Three days later, Bloom died of a pulmonary embolism caused by deep-vein thrombosis. He was 39.

The ache that Bloom blew off is one of seven pains that no man should ever ignore. And no, this isn't negotiable.

SUDDEN GROIN PAIN

Not as severe as a shot to the crotch but pretty close. Sometimes accompanied by swelling.

The condition: Odds are it's something called testicular torsion. Normally, a man's testicles are attached to his body in two ways: by the spermatic cords, which run into the abdomen, and by fleshy anchors near the scrotum. But sometimes, in a relatively common congenital defect, these anchors are missing. This allows one of the spermatic cords to get twisted, which cuts off the flow of blood to the testicle. "If you catch it in 4 to 6 hours, you can usually save the testicle," says Jon Pryor, M.D., a urologist with the University of Minnesota. "But after 12 to 24 hours, you'll probably lose it." Another possible cause of the pain in your pants: an infection of the epididymis, your sperm-storage facility.

The diagnostics: A physical examination, possibly followed by an ultrasound. Antibiotics can stifle an infection. And if your testicles are doing the twist?

A surgeon will straighten the cord, then construct artificial anchors with a few stitches near the scrotum.

SEVERE BACK PAIN

Similar to the kind of agony you'd expect if you'd just tried to clean-and-jerk an armoire. The usual remedies—heat, rest, OTC painkillers—offer no relief.

The condition: "If it's not related to exercise, sudden severe back pain can be the sign of an aneurysm," says Sigfried Kra, M.D., associate professor at the Yale school of medicine. Particularly troubling is the abdominal aneurysm, a dangerous weakening of the aorta just above the kidneys. But don't worry; eventually, the pain subsides—right after your body's main artery bursts. A less threatening possibility: You have a kidney stone. More pain, but you'll only wish you were dead.

The diagnostics: A CT scan using intravenous radiopaque dye does the best job of revealing the size and shape of an aneurysm. Once its dimensions are determined, it'll be treated with blood-pressure medication or surgery to implant a synthetic graft.

PERSISTENT FOOT OR SHIN PAIN

A nagging pain in the top of your foot or the front of your shin that's worse when you exercise but present even at rest. It's impervious to ibuprofen and acetaminophen.

The condition: It's probably a stress fracture. Bones, like all the other tissues in your body, are continually regenerating themselves. "But if you're training so hard that the bone doesn't get a chance to heal itself, a stress fracture can develop," explains Andrew Feldman, M.D., the team physician for the New York Rangers. Eventually, the bone can be permanently weakened.

The diagnostics: Radioactive dye reveals the fracture in the x-ray, and you'll be told to stop all running until the crack heals. Worst case, you'll be in a cast for a few weeks.

SHARP PAIN IN THE ABDOMEN

All the metaphors apply—knife in the gut, bullet in the belly, skewer in the stomach—except this attack is from within.

The condition: Take your pick. Since the area between your ribs and your hips is jam-packed with organs, the pain can be a symptom of either appendicitis, pancreatitis, or an inflamed gallbladder. In all three cases, the cause is the same: Something has blocked up the organ in question, resulting in a potentially fatal infection. Exploding organs can kill a guy. See a doctor before this happens.

The diagnostics: If the pain is in your lower-right abdomen and your white-blood-cell count is up, says Dr. Kra, it's probably appendicitis (out comes the appendix). Pain in your upper abdomen with high white blood cells usually spells an inflamed gallbladder (goodbye, gallbladder). And if it hurts below your breastbone and certain enzymes in the blood are elevated, then pancreatitis is probably the culprit. (The pancreas stays, but a gallstone may be blocking things up. If so, the stone and the gallbladder may have to come out.)

TRANSIENT CHEST PAIN

Not a type of pain that strikes only homeless people, but a heavy ache that comes on suddenly and then goes away just as quickly. Otherwise, you feel fine.

The condition: It could be indigestion. Or it could be a heart attack. "Even if it's very short in duration, it can be a sign of something serious," says John Stamatos, M.D., medical director of North Shore Pain Services in Long Island and author of *Painbuster*. Here's how serious: A blood clot may have lodged in a narrowed section of a coronary artery, completely cutting off the flow of blood to one section of your heart. How much wait-and-see time do you have? Really, none. Fifty percent of deaths from heart attacks occur within 3 to 4 hours of the first symptoms. You're literally living on borrowed time.

The diagnostics: A blood test checks for markers of damaged heart tissue. Treatment: angioplasty or bypass.

THREE HEALTH SCARES YOU CAN IGNORE

We add a dose of perspective to the panic

West Nile virus. While it's true that the West Nile virus killed 284 people in 2002, the chances of it taking a healthy young or middle-aged man are slim. "The healthier one is, the less likely he is to get seriously ill if he's infected," says Stephen Zinner, M.D., professor of medicine at Harvard medical school. In fact, of those bitten by the virus-carrying mosquitoes, no more than 15 percent will develop symptoms, and subsequent death is even more rare. So just do what you've always done: Use bug spray, and then relax.

Mercury in dental fillings. When the American Dental Association (ADA) surveyed adults about whether they believed that dental amalgams (silver-coated fillings) caused illness, nearly half answered "yes." They're wrong. "Mercury vapor can be leaked, but it's minuscule and causes no harm," says Richard Price, D.M.D., a consumer advisor for the ADA. "An amalgam's only downside is that it looks ugly." The FDA and the World Health Organization concur that there is no health risk.

SARS. Toss the surgical mask. "A 35-year-old American male's chances of ever being exposed to this virus in the States are so small that he should worry more about walking across the street," says Stanley Deresinski, M.D., clinical professor of medicine at Stanford University and editor of *Infectious Disease Alert*. But let's say you do somehow get hit by SARS instead of an SUV. As with the West Nile virus, the chances a healthy man will succumb to the virus are low—about 5 percent, Dr. Deresinski says.

LEG PAIN WITH SWELLING

Specifically, one of your calves is killing you. It's swollen and tender to the touch and may even feel warm, as if it's being slow-roasted from the inside out.

The condition: Just sit in one place for 6 or more hours straight and wait for the blood that pools in your lower legs to form a clot (a.k.a. deep-vein thrombosis, or DVT). Next thing you know, that clot will be big enough to block a vein in your calf, producing pain and swelling. Unfortunately, the first thing that you'll probably want to do—rub your leg—is also the worst thing. "It can send a big clot running up to your lung, where it can kill you," warns Dr. Stamatos.

The diagnostics: A venogram, in which dye is injected into the vein and then x-rayed, is the definitive way to diagnose DVT. They'll try to dissolve the clot with drugs or outfit vulnerable veins with filters to stop a clot before it stops you.

PAINFUL URINATION

Relieving yourself has become an exercise in expletives. Also, you could swear (and you do) that your yellow stream has a rusty tint.

The condition: Worst case? Bladder cancer, according to Joseph A. Smith, M.D., chairman of the department of urologic surgery at Vanderbilt University. The pain and the blood in your urine are symptoms of this, the fourth most common cancer in men. Smoking is the biggest risk factor. Catch the disease early, and there's a 90 percent chance of fixing it. Bladder infections share the same symptoms.

The diagnostics: It's a sick joke but true nonetheless: They'll diagnose by process of elimination. Urinalysis first, to rule out bugs, followed by inserting a scope to look inside the bladder. A tumor will be treated with surgery, radiation, or chemotherapy.

Immunity Granted

You already know how to catch a cold. Now learn how to knock one out

By Jamie Beckman

Flip through the *Old Farmer's Almanac* and you'll see how utterly pathetic we've been in our battle against the common cold. Take this strategy employed by American colonists: "[They] pared orange peels, rolled them up inside out, and stuffed them into the nostrils." Using rinds against the rhinovirus sounds brilliant compared with the device patented by Norman Lake in 1977—a modified clothespin. As the *Almanac* tells it, "the FDA told

Lake he could not advertise his device as a cold cure but only as a way of 'keeping foreign material out of the nose.'"

Not exactly our best moments. But this year's cold season is going to be different. Our tactics? Speed and science. We've assembled the latest research on how to arm your immune system so it'll strike at the first tickle in the throat. Or immediately after a suspicious double sneeze. Or right after that vague, blah feeling begins creeping in. In the past we've always allowed the cold virus to establish a beachhead in our bodies before fighting back. This time, the second it lands, we hit and we hit hard.

STRATEGY #1: EAT THE ANTIVIRAL BREAKFAST

Woke up sick and tired? Research shows that the right morning meal can help quash the cold virus. In a recent study from the Netherlands, researchers analyzed the impact that consuming a 1,200-calorie breakfast has on a man's immune system versus eating nothing at all. They found that eating big and eating early increased blood levels of gamma interferon, a natural antiviral agent, by 450 percent. (Going hungry actually caused a 17 percent decrease.) More research is needed to determine if fewer calories will have a similar effect, but in the meantime, shoot for 1,200 every morning until your cold symptoms disappear. Not, however, 1,200 calories of pancake syrup. Instead, hit your quota by eating a bowl of Kellogg's Raisin Bran (with 2 percent milk), a glass of orange juice, and a toasted English muffin with peanut butter and grape jelly, followed by a Stonyfield Farm–brand smoothie.

STRATEGY #2: STRESS OUT YOUR SYSTEM

If you get attacked at the office, strike back with stress. When Ohio State University researchers had 34 men either take a 12-minute memory test or watch a 12-minute video of surgical procedures, they found that the test-takers'

AN OUNCE OF PREVENTION

There are two ways we commonly catch a cold: by unconsciously putting our mitts in our noses or mouths or by sucking in the germs from someone else's sneeze or cough. Compulsive hand washing takes care of the first avenue of infection, but what about the airborne attack? Do the obvious—hold your breath for as long as you can after someone sneezes or coughs near you, recommends Murray Grossan, M.D., an ear, nose, and throat specialist at Cedars-Sinai Hospital in Los Angeles and author of *The Sinus Cure*. "Think of germ-laden air as colored smoke," says Dr. Grossan. "If you hold your nose, the colored smoke won't go in."

levels of SIgA, a key immune-system protein, shot up dramatically. (The SIgA levels of the guys who saw the gore went down.) The moral of the study: Expose yourself to short-term stress, the kind you have some control over, and you'll supercharge your immune system. "Stress response is a normal protec-

WE DOCTOR THE CLASSIC COLD REMEDY

Once a cold takes hold, you need to minimize the symptoms and shorten the duration. Chicken noodle soup does both, and it won't knock you out the way over-the-counter cold medicines can. When researchers at Nebraska Medical Center compared chicken noodle brands, they found that Knorr's was best at short-circuiting those nonstop sniffles. And while Knorr's is powerful right out of the packet, this quick recipe makes it even more potent.

Ingredients

2 c cooked, diced chicken *(Supplies zinc; a University of Michigan study shows that the mineral can reduce the symptoms and duration of a cold.)*

½ c chopped carrots *(Beta-carotene in the carrots helps make immune-system cells better at fighting off infection.)*

2 medium onions, diced, and 3 cloves garlic, minced *(Onions and garlic are potent antivirals. "Compounds in garlic and onions are readily passed to the lungs and respiratory tract, where they can be most effective against cold viruses," says James Duke, Ph.D., author of* The Green Pharmacy.*)*

2 (2.72-ounce) packets Knorr Savory Soups chicken noodle soup mix

1 c enriched egg noodles *(They're a good source of selenium; too little selenium makes it easier for the cold virus to multiply and mutate.)*

1 red bell pepper, chopped *(Peppers are packed with salicylates, the active ingredient in aspirin.)*

2 tsp cayenne pepper *(Supplies more salicylates, and the heat acts as a decongestant.)*

Directions

Pour 8 cups of water into a large pot and bring to a boil. Add the chicken, carrots, onions, and garlic, and boil for half an hour or until the carrots are tender. Add the remaining ingredients and cook for an additional 5 to 10 minutes. Makes eight 1-cup servings.

Per cup: 167 calories, 15 grams (g) protein, 20 g carbohydrates, 1 g fat, 2.5 g fiber, 28 milligrams sodium

tive coping mechanism," says Jos A. Bosch, Ph.D., the study author. "The body prepares itself for potential harm and activates its immune resources."

To use stress as medicine, Bosch suggests taking on a small extra project at work or helping a coworker with a task. "It shouldn't take longer than a day or half a day," he says. "If the stress response is continuous, then the immune system will be suppressed."

Already swamped? Play a video game when you get home; Bosch found that Xbox stress can also boost SIgA levels.

STRATEGY #3: BREW THE COLD-VIRUS KILLER

Swap your 3:00 P.M. coffee for a caffeine-toting cold buster: green tea. When Canadian researchers added green tea to lab samples of the adenovirus (one of the bugs responsible for colds), they found that it stopped the virus from replicating. All the credit goes to EGCG, a chemical compound found in certain kinds of tea, but in the highest concentrations in green tea. Start pumping green tea into your bloodstream at the first sign of a cold, and you should be able to stop the advance of the adenovirus. "It's the difference between staying home for 2 or 3 days and going to work and just sniffling a bit," says Joseph M. Weber, Ph.D., the lead study author and a professor of microbiology at the University of Sherbrooke in Quebec. The best brand to brew? Tetley; it was one of the most effective in Weber's study. Note: To brew the maximum amount of EGCG, boil a mug of water in the microwave, toss in a tea bag, and let it steep for 10 minutes. Sweeten with honey.

STRATEGY #4: RECHARGE YOUR IMMUNE RESPONSE

We love Leno, but call it a night. According to Michael Irwin, M.D., a psychiatrist and sleep researcher at UCLA, if the amount of sleep you're logging decreases by 40 percent or more (for instance, you sleep 4 hours instead of the usual 7), the effectiveness of your immune system will decline by 50 percent. And for the immune system to operate at full strength, you'll need to sleep a straight 8, the amount shown to produce the highest levels of "natural killer cells," which attack viruses. But don't knock yourself out with alcohol, including alcohol-spiked cold medicines like NyQuil. "A single dose of alcohol impairs your sleep," says Dr. Irwin. Instead, wear light clothing—shorts and a T-shirt—during your waking hours at home; Japanese researchers found that this adjusts a person's core body temperature enough to improve sleep quality and boost the immune response.

STRATEGY #5: WORK OUT THE WHITE BLOOD CELLS

It's harder to hit a moving target, and that goes for a cold virus that's throwing punches, too. In a University of Massachusetts study of 547 people, researchers found that the most physically active people had 25 percent fewer upper-respiratory infections over the course of a year than did the couch potatoes. Researchers believe that exercise may strengthen immune function, in part by increasing the body's production of white blood cells. "If you exercise, you should see two benefits: One, you'll have a reduced risk of catching a cold, and two, if you're unlucky enough to get a cold, you should have it for a shorter period of time," says Charles E. Matthews, Ph.D., the lead study author. That said, it is possible to sweat yourself sick. (Marathon runners are at a greater risk of upper-respiratory infections after a race.) So do what Matthews's study subjects did: Aim for 60 to 90 minutes of moderate activity daily, with walking counting just as much as weight training.

Right in the Nose

Allergy-proof your life with our simple five-step plan

By Ted Spiker

Next time you're hit with hay fever, try to remember that things could be worse. You could be Clay Aiken.

The American Idol also-ran is allergic to coffee, chocolate, shellfish, tree nuts, and mushrooms. And mints. Imagine going into anaphylactic shock because you wanted fresh breath.

On the other hand, Aiken *can* easily avoid his triggers, something that, sans a SARS mask, is difficult to do if you're allergic to pollen. Or ragweed. Or her beloved cat.

Inhaling allergens may be inevitable, but suffering isn't. We've developed a five-step plan that's the closest thing you'll find to an "off" switch for your overreacting immune system. Each step provides progressively more powerful medicine, taking you from a simple herbal treatment to cutting-edge science. And at no point will you need to do as Aiken did in his youth: run over the cat.

STEP 1: CONSIDER YOUR OTC OPTIONS

With predicted sales of nearly $400 million in 2004, Claritin is the most popular over-the-counter allergy aid after Kleenex. But Claritin's two main selling points—maximum relief and minimum drowsiness—may be more hype than health benefit. In a study published in *Annals of Allergy, Asthma and Immunology*, researchers found that old-school Benadryl was actually 20 percent more effective in treating the itchiness and sneezing caused by seasonal allergic rhinitis, a.k.a. hay fever, than was Claritin. And in a separate study review, researchers determined that Claritin (as well as its cousins Zyrtec and Allegra) may actually have significant sedative effects, while diphenhydramine, the active ingredient in Benadryl, isn't as sedating as people think.

Bottom line: Try taking the smallest recommended dose of store-brand diphenhydramine: 25 milligrams (mg) every 6 hours. If that doesn't work, then try Claritin or, better yet, the store brand of the stuff (usually labeled "loratadine"). "One drug will work better on some people than on other people," says Richard Lockey, M.D., chief of the allergy division at the University of South Florida. "We're biologically diverse."

STEP 2: GIVE MOTHER NATURE A TASTE OF HER OWN MEDICINE

The herbal supplement butterbur may sound like a turkey, but there's evidence that it really does work. Scottish researchers found that patients with grass and pollen allergies who popped 50 mg of the plant extract twice daily had 13 percent better nasal airflow than those who took a placebo. Another study published in the *British Medical Journal* reported that butterbur treated seasonal allergies nearly as well as the prescription medication Zyrtec. "It's effective against all symptoms of allergic rhinitis, including sneezing, itching, and conjunctivitis," says Andreas Schapowal, M.D., Ph.D., the author of the study.

Butterbur is believed to block leukotriene, a chemical that causes allergic reactions, while at the same time controlling eosinophils, the white blood cells that accumulate when allergic reactions take place, says Dr. Schapowal.

WHEN PEANUTS TURN POISONOUS

Detoxifying the number one food allergy

Today there are more than one million Americans with severe peanut allergies. But it wasn't always "eat a goober, go to the hospital." What changed? The way we process peanuts, according to Sheldon Spector, M.D., clinical professor of medicine at UCLA. "Peanut allergies are more common in the United States, but they eat a hell of a lot of peanuts in China, so the theory is that the way we process them and the way we roast them may bring out the allergen potential."

That's the likely "why" behind the reactions; here's how some of them may be prevented in the future. In a 4-month study published in the *New England Journal of Medicine,* researchers discovered that when an anti-IgE treatment was given to allergy sufferers, their tolerance for peanuts rose from half a peanut to an average of nine. More research is still needed, but in the meantime, Scott Sicherer, M.D., of the Jaffe Food Allergy Institute at the Mount Sinai school of medicine in New York City, recommends being careful when eating in restaurants that serve Chinese, Thai, and other Far Eastern cuisines; the cooks may use the same wok to make more than one dish, allowing peanut oil to leach into your food.

What's more, there's no sedating effect with butterbur. You can buy the supplement ($24 for 60 capsules) at most health-food stores or at iherb.com.

STEP 3: SNORT A LEGAL DRUG

Unless drug companies invent an antihistamine suppository, there are basically two injection-free avenues for allergy meds: down the hatch or up the honker. And while OTC nasal sprays have gotten a bad rap for causing something called "rebound congestion," at least one prescription spray may be worth snorting. When researchers at the Institute for Allergy and Asthma gave allergy sufferers the nasal spray azelastine, Claritin and azelastine, or a placebo spray for 1 week each, they found that the first two groups experienced nearly identical 22 percent improvements in their nasal symptoms. The researchers' conclusion: Azelastine can help, especially those people whom Claritin can't.

"When it comes to nasal symptoms, sprays come out ahead," says Sheldon Spector, M.D., clinical professor of medicine at UCLA and president of the California Society of Allergy and Immunology. If you don't respond to oral antihistamines, talk to your doctor about a prescription for azelastine.

STEP 4: GET THE DROP ON ALLERGIES

They do a lot of things in Europe we'd never think of doing here, like paying to watch soccer. But they may be on to something with their choice of

LET'S CLEAR THE AIR

How to get cheap relief from indoor allergens

Buy the right home air cleaner and you can wipe out invading allergens without breaking your defense budget. Hunter's HEPAtech purifiers are one good choice. Here are some things to consider when looking at other brands.

Filtration. HEPA (high-efficiency particulate air) filters are designed to remove nearly 100 percent of particles as small as 0.3 microns, but most indoor allergens are bigger than that and can be caught with a lower-efficiency (i.e., lower-cost) filter.

Ultraviolet light. It kills mold and germs, but you can also blast their hangouts—leaky pipes and under-sink cabinets, and damp basement crevices—with dish detergent or a bleach-based spray cleaner.

Efficiency. The clean-air delivery rate (CADR) measures how fast a filter makes dirty air clean. Look for one that will filter between three and five room volumes every hour.

Noise. An air cleaner doesn't have to sound like a Harrier jet to keep allergens at bay. Most models offer stealth settings, but test each unit on high speed as well. Watch out for breeze models without fan-powered intakes: Many have ranked poorly in consumer tests.

allergy treatment. "Allergy drops are frequently used in Great Britain and in the majority of European countries," says Russell Roby, M.D., an allergy specialist in Austin, Texas. "I think they're more effective than allergy shots."

Physiologically, the drops, which go under your tongue, work similarly to shots: Repeated exposure to trace amounts of the offending allergen causes the body to build up a natural resistance. When researchers at the Imperial College of Medicine in London recently reviewed 22 study trials, they determined that treatment with allergy drops results in a 34 percent reduction in symptoms, on average. It also significantly decreases the need for additional medications. Some U.S. doctors may be reluctant to prescribe allergy drops, so shop around until you find one willing to consider this option.

STEP 5: TAKE YOUR BEST SHOT

Despite its cartoon-villain name, Xolair could be what rescues you from runaway rhinitis when nothing else can. In a 4-month study published in the *Journal of the American Medical Association*, researchers found that patients receiving a monthly injection of Xolair experienced a 25 percent reduction in their seasonal symptoms.

Here's how it works: During most allergic reactions, our bodies produce an antibody called immunoglobulin E (IgE), which in turn triggers the annoying symptoms. Xolair blocks IgE. "Altering the molecular biology of the immune response is the wave of the future," says Dr. Lockey. Xolair is FDA approved only to treat asthma, but some doctors may prescribe it for other reasons, such as allergies.

NEED TO KNOW

Banish the Burn

Say *hasta la vista* to heartburn: A near cure is now available for acid reflux. Called Enteryx, it involves the injection of a liquid polymer into the valve between the esophagus and the stomach. The substance turns into a spongelike implant, which helps the valve open and close more effectively, keeping stomach acid where it belongs. In a trial of 81 patients receiving Enteryx, 70 percent were able to stop their acid-reflux medication. "It was almost as if they'd never had acid reflux," says James Aisenberg, M.D., one of the researchers. Visit reflux1.com to find a specialist in your area.

No Flu for You

For those of us who prefer to avoid a sharp jab in the arm whenever possible, an alternative to the flu shot is now widely available. Delivered as a nasal spray, FluMist packs all the vaccinating power of a traditional shot, without the wince. It's approved by the FDA for ages 5 to 49 and is being offered at clinics and doctors' offices nationwide.

Not up to Snuff

Individuals taking antibiotics for sinus problems don't recover any faster than those taking a placebo, according to a new Swiss study. So what's the harm in taking antibiotics? Possible side effects, including diarrhea and abdominal pain, as well as an increased risk of producing antibiotic-resistant strains of bacteria. Instead of requesting antibiotics right away, the study's authors suggest that men with symptoms of sinusitis should wait to see if the symptoms abate on their own. If you're still sick after 2 weeks, it's time to go the antibiotic route.

HOW MANY MINUTES YOU SHOULD CHEW GUM AFTER A MEAL IN ORDER TO REDUCE THE RISK OF HEARTBURN: 30

Sick *and* Tired

According to a new study of 300 patients conducted at Georgetown University, people who frequently suffer from fatigue are also up to nine times more likely to have sinus problems than people who aren't chronically tired. So which is a symptom of the other? Researchers are now trying to determine exactly that.

Can't Sleep It Off

Men who habitually snore are twice as likely to suffer from chronic daily headaches as are men who breathe normally while sleeping, according to a study by the National Institute on Aging.

Headache or Migraine?

Don't blame your next blinding headache on stress or your kid's music. A new study by the Headache Care Center in Springfield, Missouri, found that 80 percent of people who thought they were having sinus headaches actually had migraines. "Men are less likely to go to a doctor, and if they go, they're less likely to be diagnosed," says Richard Lipton, M.D., vice chairman of neurology at the Albert Einstein college of medicine in New York City. He developed this three-question quiz to screen for migraines:

1. In the past 3 months, have headaches limited your activities?
2. Does headache pain make you sick to your stomach?
3. Does light bother you?

"If you answer 'yes' to two questions, there's a 93 percent chance you are suffering from migraines," says Dr. Lipton. Many men also are unaware of the availability of treatment.

Triggers. Common culprits are red wine, nuts, bright lights, chocolate, smoke, stress, lack of sleep, irregular exercise, climate changes, and alcohol. But almost anything can set off a migraine, says Robert Kaniecki, M.D., director of the University of Pittsburgh headache center. Your doctor can narrow it down.

Treatment. "Usually a patient just has to pin down the triggers and make minor lifestyle changes," says Dr. Kaniecki. Prescription medications can stop pain soon after onset.

Back in Business

Conventional wisdom says if you have a bad back, sleep on plywood. Conventional wisdom is wrong—a medium-firm mattress is significantly better at beating back pain than a firm one. In a 3-month study of 313 back-pain suf-

PERCENTAGE OF LOWER-BACK PROBLEMS THAT CAN BE PREVENTED BY BUILDING YOUR ABDOMINAL MUSCLES: 75

ferers, Spanish researchers found that those who slept on medium-firm mattresses were twice as likely to experience pain relief as those sacking out on stiff mattresses. "The medium-firm ones adapt better to the curves of the back," says Francisco Kovacs, M.D., Ph.D., the study author. When shopping for a mattress, look for "medium" or "cushion firm."

Pain Got You Down?

If you have frequent back pain, headaches, or muscle pain, you may be dealing with more than what a few ibuprofen can handle. You may be suffering from depression. A new study from Stanford University reports that people with major depression are more than twice as likely to have chronic pain as people who aren't depressed. "It's possible that depressed people feel pain more acutely than other people," says Alan Schatzberg, M.D., the study author. And even if you aren't depressed, a prescription for an antidepressant may help, since many have proven pain-fighting capabilities.

Aspirin and Asthma Don't Mix

Aspirin may look like a medical multitool, but its power can cut both ways. Specifically, aspirin may cause asthma attacks. After analyzing more than 60 studies of asthmatics, doctors writing in the *British Medical Journal* found that 21 percent had experienced an aspirin-induced asthma attack and were also likely to suffer a similar reaction to other pain medications. Changes in inflammation levels may trigger attacks, say doctors. If you have asthma and a headache, grab Tylenol; only 2 percent of those who reacted to aspirin were also affected by acetaminophen, the active ingredient in Tylenol.

Breathe Easier

If you're waiting for us to stop raving about fish oil, don't hold your breath, especially since new research shows that omega-3 fatty acids may help treat a common form of asthma. In a 3-week study of athletes suffering from exercise-induced asthma, University of Indiana researchers found that those who supplemented with 5.4 grams (g) of omega-3s daily had an 80 percent improvement in lung capacity, compared with no change for those taking a placebo. "Omega-3 fatty acids stop inflammation, allowing the lungs to dilate," says Timothy Mickleborough, M.D., the study author. More research is needed, but he speculates that even 2 grams of omega-3s daily—roughly what's in five packets of Coromega—should help someone with exercise-induced asthma breathe easier.

Getting pricked with needles is another way to keep asthma at bay. Researchers in Austria treated a group of asthmatic men and women with acupuncture for 10 weeks. At the end of the trial, more than 70 percent of the group reported a significant reduction in asthma symptoms.

Keep Your Toothbrush to Yourself

New research shows that hepatitis C might be spread through a shared toothbrush. Chia Wang, M.D., from the University of Washington, analyzed saliva of 12 infected people and found that 21 percent of the samples were positive for the virus and that half the subjects left some hepatitis C behind on their toothbrushes. "We think it may be related to having small amounts of blood in the saliva," says Dr. Wang. Kissing and sharing drinks is probably okay, she says, but anytime blood may be involved—such as on a toothbrush—avoid sharing. Remember, there's no vaccine for hepatitis C, which can lead to chronic liver disease.

Become Less Irritable

Irritable bowel syndrome (IBS), a gastrointestinal disorder that affects 1 in 20 men, may now have a mental fix. A new U.K. study shows that hypnotism provides long-term relief to IBS sufferers—meaning less abdominal pain, constipation, and diarrhea. After a dozen 1-hour sessions, 71 percent of patients experienced fewer symptoms and less anxiety. What's more, these benefits lasted for up to 5 years. Researchers believe hypnotherapy may alter muscle movements in the intestines. Go to apmha.com/hypnosishelp for certified hypnotherapists.

Don't Lose Your Lunch

Scientists are getting close to cracking the code on *E. coli.* They say that sprinkling freeze-dried egg yolk on your food could prevent bacteria like *E. coli* and salmonella from making you sick. The powdered yolks come from chickens that have been exposed to food-poisoning bacteria in a lab and thus carry antibodies to fight off the germs. Developer Hoon Sunwoo, Ph.D., of the University of Alberta in Canada, says the egg-yolk "spice," as it's called, is a smart precaution for cookouts and buffets and when traveling abroad. It could be on store shelves within a year.

FAST FIXES

You stock the medicine cabinet with echinacea, wash your hands all the time, and get a flu shot each fall, but you're still wasting sick days being sick. What gives? Actually, you're not alone. The average American gets ill three times a year. We want you to be better than average. Use these 12 tips to stay healthy or, if the bug's already bitten, to feel better fast.

1. Soothe your sore throat. Just a guess: Last time you went to a doctor for a sore throat, Mom drove and you missed a day of school. Now that you're a grown-up, start with this checklist, prepared with the help of Greg Grillone, M.D., an otolaryngologist at Boston University's medical center.

Symptom: Constant ache

What it means: Pain fibers in irritated mucous membranes are reacting to inflammation.

Remedy: If it's severe, see a doctor for a strep test—a streptococcal infection, the most common of bacterial throat infections, may lead to rheumatic fever. Antibiotics can knock it out.

Symptom: Tickle or incessant cough

What it means: Nerve endings are reacting to inflammation or irritation of mucous membranes and are triggering cough receptors.

Remedy: Gargle with salt water and take an over-the-counter medication containing dextromethorphan, which takes effect within 30 minutes.

Symptom: Hoarseness or no voice

What it means: Laryngitis, or swollen vocal cords; commonly caused by a viral infection.

Remedy: Wait it out with aspirin. Viruses can't be fought with meds. And shut up—whispering can be more of a strain than talking.

Symptom: Coughing up phlegm

What it means: Infection, possibly bronchitis. You're churning out thicker mucus than normal to fight the infection.

Remedy: Same as for the tickle. Guaifenesin, an expectorant found in some cough medicines (read the label), will help break up the mucus.

Symptom: Swollen lymph nodes

What it means: An aggressive virus or infection like mononucleosis. Your nodes are working overtime to fend off the sickness.

Remedy: Consult a doctor for a strep or blood test.

2. Stop hacking. Cough drops are appealing—a remedy in a handy, candy package. But a Life Saver is just as good a treatment. "For throat irritation, any lozenge will do," says Jason Surow, M.D., an ear, nose, and throat specialist in New Jersey. Sucking on hard candy produces saliva, which makes mucus, which makes the lining of your throat less irritated. What about menthol? It's just an aromatic compound with no healing properties. The real solution is to drink lots of fluids and avoid caffeine.

A portable cough cure that has a better chance of working is Robitussin CoughGels, which contain dextromethorphan, a proven soother. Or try Chloraseptic Relief Strips with benzocaine to numb your pain.

3. Put an end to your allergies. As the seasons change, so do allergens. The culprits that make your eyes water in the spring aren't the same ones that are bothering you in the fall. Ragweed gets all the publicity (and the Claritin commercials), but watch out for mold and dust.

Buy a dehumidifier. Dust mites and mold thrive in humid homes, says Patricia McNally, M.D. Keep house humidity under 50 percent.

Do laundry. Washing your sheets in hot water once a week is more effective (and much less expensive) than buying an antiallergy mattress cover. According to two new studies, those things are useless. Researchers in the United Kingdom and the Netherlands studied 1,500 people, half of whom slept on beds with mite-proof mattress covers and half of whom did not. At the end of the study, both groups were equally likely to have allergy problems. Meanwhile, researchers at Wright State University in Ohio found that a mix of warm water (97° to 100°F), detergent, and chlorine bleach removes up to 98 percent of dust-mite allergens.

Bag it. Quit procrastinating on the yard work. Leaves and clippings harbor mold that multiplies when it's rainy and damp, explains Dr. McNally. Clear away any brush, leaves, and compost in your yard.

See someone. Consult a specialist. "The treatments for seasonal and year-round allergies are not necessarily the same," says Marianne Frieri, M.D., Ph.D., of Nassau University Medical Center in New York.

Feel you can suffer through? Consider this: Athletes with nasal allergies who exercise outdoors in the fall can develop exercise-induced asthma, says Dr. Frieri.

4. Fend off ulcers. Toss a few extra strawberries or a handful of frozen peach slices into your morning cereal or smoothie. Both are good sources of vitamin C, which may reduce your risk of developing an ulcer or help prevent ulcer flare-ups. In a 7,000-person study, researchers at San Francisco VA Med-

NUMBER OF STRAWBERRIES IT TAKES TO SUPPLY YOUR RECOMMENDED DAILY INTAKE OF VITAMIN C: 6

ical Center found that individuals with the highest levels of vitamin C in their blood are 25 percent less likely to be infected with ulcer-triggering *H. pylori* bacteria. The study's authors theorize that higher levels of C in the blood may boost immunity.

Another way to reduce your risk of getting an ulcer? Reduce your stress. First they said it caused ulcers, then they said it didn't, and now stress is guilty again. Researchers at Columbia University found that people under extreme stress have a greater risk of getting ulcers than people leading less stressful lives.

5. Stay positive. Keeping a positive attitude may help you avoid getting sick, a new University of Wisconsin study reports. Researchers measured the brain patterns of a group of healthy men and women and compared the results with the subjects' levels of viral antibodies. At the end of the 6-month trial, they found that the people with the most activity on the left side of the brain—the region that controls positive moods—also had the highest antibody levels. The more antibodies you have, the stronger your immune system—and the easier it is for you to ward off the flu. Researchers are still working to determine how the variance in brain activity alters immune-system response.

6. Juice up your immune system. Want to help boost your immune system in 10 seconds? Chug 12 ounces of V8 juice, preferably the low-sodium kind. German researchers recently found that men who drank tomato or carrot juice daily enhanced immune-cell functions, including those of natural killer cells, by up to 25 percent. These men all started out with low blood levels of the carotenoids lycopene and beta-carotene, but odds are you're low, too; only 4 percent of American men say they're eating the recommended number of daily servings of fruits and vegetables. To ensure that your liquid produce has punch, drink it with a meal. "A certain amount of fat is required for the efficient absorption of carotenoids," says Bernhard Watzl, Ph.D., the lead study author.

7. Don't get caught by surprise. You know to wash your hands and disinfect your office doorknob with Lysol after Hacking Jack departs. But you probably don't know about these surprising places where nasty health threats hide.

Cubicle. Sick of work? There's a good reason. Employees without a window are 23 percent more likely to call in sick probably because of breathing in stale, germ-ridden air. Until you brownnose to a corner office, step outside periodically or take breaks near a window.

Toothbrush. Flushing the toilet can throw fecal bacteria up to 20 feet. How far away is your toothbrush? Sanitize your brush with mouthwash or at least put the seat down before flushing. Bonus: Your girlfriend will mistake your caution for sensitivity.

Contact-lens case. Solutions may not kill all forms of acanthamoeba, a common tap-water amoeba that can cause a potentially blinding eye infection. It breeds quickly in lens cases, so rinse yours only with lens solution.

Garden hose. Standing water in a hose can soak up lead and other chemicals, so buy one labeled "safe for drinking." Let the water run for a minute anyway.

8. Don't pull the trigger. Some herbal supplements and headache medications don't mix. According to a new study from the University of Utah, common migraine medications can interact negatively with such herbs as ginkgo, ginseng, St. John's wort, and valerian. Worse, the herbs may actually trigger migraines or intensify symptoms. "More than 30 million Americans suffer from migraines, and up to 40 percent of Americans take herbal supplements, so this could be a huge problem," says Carla Rubingh, Pharm.D., the study author.

9. Shed some light on your pain. The most effective pain reliever may be in your fridge. In a study of 150 people, University of Minnesota researchers found that 93 percent of those with persistent musculoskeletal pain had low blood levels of vitamin D. The deficiency weakens bones, allowing painful deposits to form under their surfaces. "It could be easy to mistakenly attribute the pain to an old sports injury," says study author Greg Plotnikof, M.D. Fortunately, the fix is simple: Get 15 minutes of sun exposure each day. Live in Seattle? Drink low-fat fortified milk daily and make sure your multivitamin contains at least 200 to 400 international units (IU) of vitamin D.

10. Sit down or shut up. Talking on your cell phone while walking ups your odds of lower-back pain, according to Australian researchers. "During walking, the deep-trunk muscles remain active to control the spine. The activity of these muscles is reduced while you're breathing in to speak," says Paul Hodges, Ph.D., the study author. If you have back pain but must talk and walk, keep it brief.

11. Heat things up. New adhesive low-level heat wraps hide under your clothes, give you hours of stealth warmth, and provide comic relief when your girlfriend rips off your shirt. The wraps warm up when exposed to the air (it's chemistry, man). The journal *Spine* reports that low-level-heat-wrap therapy worked better on lower-back pain and stiffness than ibuprofen or acetaminophen. The pain relief can speed your rehab because you'll be more likely to move around and stretch. Leading makers of the wraps are ThermaCare (three for $7), Sunbeam (three for $8), HeatZone (four for $13), and Grabber ($2 each).

12. Make a speedy recovery. If you've had knee surgery, cut down on recovery time and painkiller use by taking nonsteroidal anti-inflammatory drugs called COX-2 inhibitors. Researchers at Chicago's St. Luke's Medical Center studied 70 knee surgeries and found that patients receiving the drugs pre- and postop healed faster and needed 25 percent fewer painkillers than the placebo group. Knees fine but the back bad? "[The findings] could probably be utilized for other kinds of surgery," says study author Asokumar Buvanendran, M.D.

OUR FINAL ANSWERS

Head Off a Migraine

What's the best way to attack a migraine?

—G.R., Honolulu

Preemptively. Aspirin defeats run-of-the-mill headaches, but it's pretty much powerless against migraines—that is, unless you take it before the headache hits. In a Harvard study, men who took 325 milligrams of aspirin every other day were 20 percent less likely to have recurring migraines than those who rarely used aspirin. Researchers believe aspirin's blood-thinning properties may reduce levels of migraine-triggering serotonin in the brain.

The Frat-Party Fix

When I'm hung over, why does having an alcoholic drink make me feel better?

—S.B., Vancouver

It's certainly not the alcohol. When you have a hangover, your brain cells are dehydrated and your blood vessels are dilated, so more alcohol—a very efficient dehydrating agent—won't help, says Frederick Freitag, D.O., associate director of the Diamond Headache Clinic in Chicago. It's probably the other stuff in your concoction that heals you: the fructose, electrolytes, caffeine, or water. "Fructose helps the liver regenerate necessary energy sources for the

PERCENTAGE OF AMERICANS WHO ADMIT TAKING MORE THAN THE RECOMMENDED DOSAGE OF OVER-THE-COUNTER PAIN MEDICATION: 44

NUMBER OF PEOPLE WHO DIE EACH YEAR FROM PAIN RELIEVERS: 16,500

enzymes that break down alcohol," says Dr. Freitag. Caffeine eases the dilated vessels, and with the help of fluids, brain cells are hydrated and jolted from their temporary inhibited phase. Dr. Freitag recommends sports drinks, water, or tomato juice (high in fructose) with a side of Excedrin (aspirin and acetaminophen formulated with caffeine).

Come In from the Cold

Can you really catch a cold if you go outside with wet hair?

—F.H., Dayton, Ohio

No. "You could go outdoors with wet hair every day and you wouldn't catch a cold—provided you're a hermit," says Jack Gwaltney Jr., M.D., professor emeritus of internal medicine at the University of Virginia. You catch colds from people, not the elements. Even if you're physically cold and shivering, there's no greater chance of getting sick than if you're warm and comfortable.

Cough It Up

I'm baffled by the choices in the cough-medicine aisle. What's the magic ingredient?

—W.F., San Diego

Take a shot of something containing dextromethorphan (like Vicks 44 Cough Relief or Robitussin Maximum Strength Cough Suppressant). A British study of 710 coughing adults found that those who took 30 milligrams of this drug hacked 12.7 percent less than those who took a placebo. If that fails, mix a glass of hot water, a tablespoon of honey, and the juice of one lemon, says Bristol University's Knut Schroeder, M.D. Sip it slowly, like a cup of tea. The honey can soothe your throat, and the lemon may stimulate your salivary glands to produce extra fluid to ease your cough, Dr. Schroeder says.

Wake-Up Call

Which getting-out-of-bed pains are warning signs?

—P.R., Birmingham, Alabama

All of them. "If you're in pain, something's wrong," says Allan Levy, M.D., team physician for the New York Giants. Here's his diagnosis:

Sore muscles. When you put your muscles through a rigorous workout, they shorten to protect themselves, and as you sleep, they stiffen. It's the lengthening to their normal size that causes the discomfort. Lessen the ache by stretching after exertion, while your muscles are still warm.

Achy knees or ankles. Bad form puts undue tension on the joints. Next stop: the DL. So find a good podiatrist who can troubleshoot your wonky stride and the pain that goes with it.

Stiff neck. It could be your massive head. "A lot of people get arthritis because their heads are heavy. The vertebrae in your neck are small, so there's wear and tear on your spine," says Dr. Levy. One of those C-shaped neck pillows might help, as could lowering or raising the position of your current pillows. Experiment.

Let 'em Take a Crack

Can I really trust a chiropractor with my aching back?

—B.W., Stamford, Connecticut

Chiropractors may be a satisfying choice to manage acute back pain. According to a 2002 study funded by the Agency for Healthcare Research and Quality, a third more patients are satisfied with the back treatment and advice they get from chiropractors, compared with medical doctors. You can safely play those odds for one to three sessions, according to Jens Chapman, M.D., professor of orthopedics and neurological surgery at the University of Washington, as long as you're not experiencing any other disturbing, doc-worthy problems—weakness in your legs, incontinence, or sexual letdowns, for example.

Choose your chiropractor carefully; you can give a pass to any who advertise free evaluations (they're fishing for suckers) or take loads of x-rays (they're padding the bill), says Stephen Barrett, M.D., a retired psychiatrist and head of Quackwatch. "If you've simply stretched or strained something and you know it happened that way, there's no reason to take an x-ray." And don't be too quick to call in reinforcements. "The vast majority of back pain resolves itself if you simply take it easy for 2 or 3 days," says Dr. Chapman. Some mild, low-impact exercise, like stretching and walking, along with a heat pack and over-the-counter anti-inflammatories, may save you from both back and wallet pain.

Comparison Shopper

Are the pharmacy- or grocery-store-brand medicines just as good as the brand-name stuff?

—Emil B., Orlando, Florida

Yes, generics and store brands are just as effective and cost about one-third as much as the brand names. But this applies only to over-the-counter drugs.

Prescription medicines should always be dispensed as written unless your doctor says otherwise.

Pick Your Juice Wisely

Can grapefruit juice really mess with your prescription medicines?

—B.G., Lincoln, Montana

Yes. Grapefruit juice inhibits the gut enzyme that metabolizes some medications, so your body absorbs more of the drug. That might ramp up the side effects. OJ is okay; it leaves the enzymes alone.

Don't Get Stung

I went through a desensitization program for bee stings 10 years ago. When will my immunity wear off?

—H.J., Miami

Never. "Once you've received your series of shots, you'll be 97 percent protected for your entire lifetime," says Brian Smart, M.D., an allergist and spokesman for the American Academy of Allergy, Asthma & Immunology.

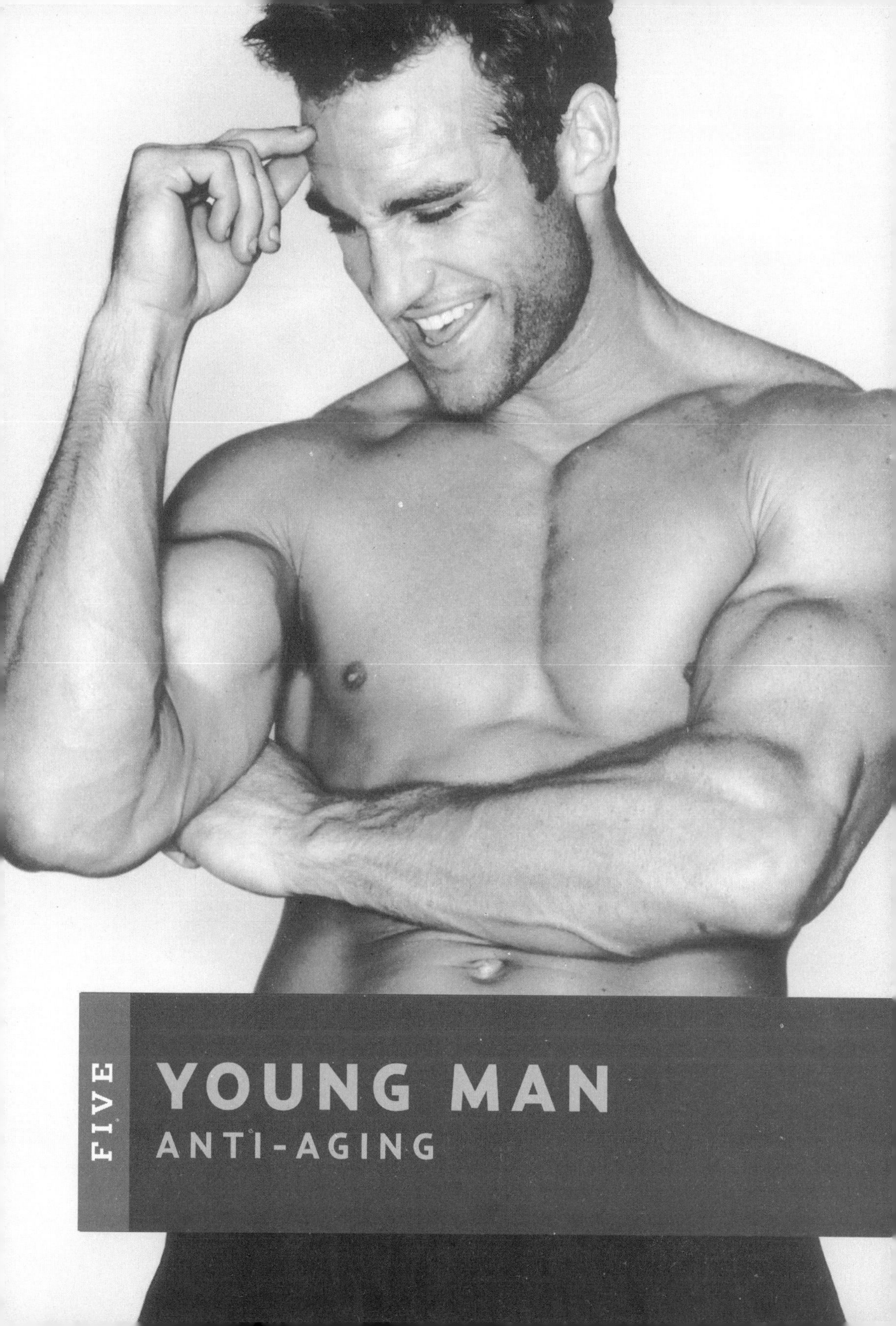

FIVE

YOUNG MAN

ANTI-AGING

MUST READS

The Fountain of Youth

The Vitality Project for Men promises to make you feel 20 again. But the substances prescribed by its doctors, namely testosterone and growth hormone, are controversial. Should you take them to slow aging?

By Donovan Webster

I was about to become a guinea pig. And on that sun-shot morning two years ago, as I walked through the door of a low, adobe-style building in Scottsdale, Arizona, I was unsure how I felt about it.

The building is headquarters to a burgeoning health-care industry aimed at 35-year-old-plus guys just like me. Launched in January 2003, it's called the Vitality Project for Men. The idea is simple: Give men a one-stop shop where they can upgrade their lives. After paying a $1,000 to $1,500 "club fee" that covers the first visit, you spend the day getting your life shaken down and rebuilt by health-care and lifestyle professionals. There are medical assessments of your health and diet, discussions about vitamins, supplements, and (if necessary) Viagra, suggestions about skin care, and even a consultation with a cosmetic surgeon to discuss possible facial tweaks.

But there's another attraction. The Vitality Project offers something that most medical providers rarely consider. It believes that restoring youthful zest may involve elevating your level of testosterone.

This isn't as reckless as it sounds. As the Vitality folks are quick to point out, they're merely returning this compound to the level it was when you were in your 20s. (Testosterone declines naturally with age.) And science has shown that low, supplemental doses can reduce overall body fat and increase lean-muscle mass. The results of these studies have been published in such respected periodicals as the *Journal of the American Medical Association.*

NUMBER OF MEN WHO UNDERWENT A NONSURGICAL COSMETIC PROCEDURE IN 2002: 627,234

But these reports also advise that further studies on larger groups of men need to be done before testosterone replacement becomes standard practice. And yet, there I was, walking toward the front desk of a fully legal clinic devoted to administering this unproven treatment.

TO TURN BACK TIME

I didn't really need a major overhaul, I told myself. I was only 44 at the time, I exercise daily, get ample sleep, and try to eat right. Even so, this testosterone-replacement therapy was certainly alluring. What middle-aged guy wouldn't want to feel like he did in his 20s? Although no one can put a precise figure on how many men are using it, Stanley Slater, M.D., deputy director of the National Institute on Aging, says the treatment's popularity is "growing with exponential speed."

Once inside the doors, everything about the Vitality Project put me at ease. The waiting room had a leather couch and armchairs; several TVs tuned to CNN, ESPN, or a movie; shelves stocked with guys' magazines and nutrition books; plus a glass-fronted refrigerator filled with cold bottles of water. Even the receptionists were male. "If a guy calls and, for instance, wants to talk about Viagra, he won't have to tell a woman about it," explained Jim McGuire, the Vitality Project's founder. "That's just one of a hundred ways we've designed our business exclusively for men."

My first appointment was with staff nutritionist Teri Crenshaw. She led me into an exam room and pulled out two strange-looking devices. One resembled a big Breathalyzer; the other, a pair of paddles. The Breathalyzer-like device was called a Body Gem, and it found my resting metabolic rate by measuring my breathing through a removable plastic fitting. The "paddles" computed my body composition by sending a low-level electrical current through me. The time it took for this painless charge to travel from one hand to the other determined my level of internal body fat.

"It measures visceral fat—the fat around your organs—as well as subcutaneous fat, which is what the old-style fat calipers calculate," said Crenshaw. "So it's very accurate."

Ten minutes later, Crenshaw finished. I was already learning new things about myself. I have a resting metabolism that burns 2,640 calories a day, which is important to know for the purpose of losing weight, and my body fat came in at 22.6 percent.

"You're healthy," she said, "but these days, with as much as we know about preventive medicine, we can change the future if we start working with what we know today."

Next, I got a complete physical from clinical director Stewart Mischelof, P.A.C. This ranged from the classic "turn your head and cough" to the dreaded greased-up finger. Pronounced healthy once more and back in my street clothes,

I was led into a conference room where Eli Hammer, M.D., was waiting to critique my blood work. (Ten days before my visit, as it does for all patients, the Vitality Project sent a licensed phlebotomist to my house to draw several vials.)

First, though, Dr. Hammer wanted to tell me how he came to the Vitality Project. Sometime during the 1990s, he said, medicine as practiced in America "stopped making sense" to him. To make money for his employer, a large community medical center, he was forced to see more and more patients. "Before long, I was spending only 5 or 10 minutes with each one. That was a fundamental problem for me," he said. The stress caused him to gain 40 pounds and become depressed. Eventually, despite having four kids to support, he decided to quit.

During his soul-searching respite, Dr. Hammer began reading about testosterone and human growth hormone (HGH) supplementation as a way to slow aging in men. By 1996, when HGH was approved by the FDA for use in adults with deficiencies, he was already setting up the Hammer Institute for Anti-Aging. His prescription included exercise, good nutrition, and, when appropriate, drugs such as testosterone-laced skin cream and injectable HGH. (Although the Vitality Project does not support the use of HGH, Dr. Hammer provides it as a service to his patients through his anti-aging institute.)

"What I'm doing is getting their body chemistries to optimal levels. Women have had these kinds of treatments for decades. But when men lose libido, gain weight, feel depressed, and/or start having unexplained difficulties in work or marriage, they've had nowhere to go. I wanted to fill that void."

MY BODY IN NUMBERS

Dr. Hammer and Mischelof began addressing my life by examining my four-page blood workup. The experience was methodical and remarkable. The lab's numbers—the mysterious components of my blood—were explained in a way that for the first time made sense to me. At each line on my report, I was told why this measure is important, what's an acceptable range, and what happens if the number is too low or too high. We discussed triglycerides; HDL and LDL cholesterol; uric acid (an indicator of gout); prostate-specific antigen, or PSA (an indicator of prostate cancer); homocysteine (an indicator of heart disease); and dozens more test results. They all looked pretty good.

Finally, we got to the all-important HGH and free-testosterone levels. For my age, both of the readings were a trifle slim. The acceptable range for HGH is 90 to 360. My level was 111. The acceptable range for free testosterone is 50 to 210. My reading was 121.

"You're a little on the low side," said Mischelof, "especially for a guy of 44. But you're not exhibiting any signs of deficiency, so I wouldn't advise any treatment right now."

Dr. Hammer had a different opinion. "I'd like to put you on low doses of both HGH and testosterone," he says, "just to bump you up and see if there's any appreciable change in your life."

He leaned back in his chair and smiled. "I've been taking supplements of both for some time. Initially, I tried them to see what my patients were experiencing. But I tell you, for me the results have been terrific. I'm 43, and I feel 22 again.

"I have more energy and less joint stiffness. I've lost weight. I feel great. And as a result, I'm a better husband and father. It's really remarkable."

A SECOND OPINION

Some experts, however, don't think so.

According to Thomas Perls, M.D., director of the New England Centenarian Study at Boston Medical Center, "Any doctor dispensing these compounds with the intention of slowing aging should have his license revoked. It's quackery. There is no evidence to show these treatments are effective or safe, and there could be dangerous outcomes that we haven't had time to detect."

For men with undiagnosed prostate cancer, for example, elevated levels of testosterone may speed the cancer's growth. Elevated levels of HGH can carry the threat of joint pain, carpal tunnel symptoms, and possibly cancer. (Consider Lyle Alzado's deathbed proscriptions against hormone use.) Also, because of the way HGH was once manufactured, some users were in danger of contracting Creutzfeldt-Jakob disease, the human version of mad-cow disease. Thanks to better manufacturing procedures, this danger has all but disappeared.

"But here's the thing," said Dr. Slater. "We just don't know enough about these two treatments to approve or disapprove. Even if they're prescribed and monitored by a physician, do we know there's no long-term danger? We do not. The only thing we know is that in men who have lost their pituitary glands or testicles, supplemental testosterone or HGH has benefits. That's proven. But are these treatments beneficial for 'normal' people? The results are unknown. Still, since the hormones have FDA approval, there are doctors who are going ahead and prescribing to 'normal' men."

NUMBER OF MEN WHO WOULD SAY "NO, THANKS," TO A PILL THAT WOULD ALLOW THEM TO LIVE FOREVER: 2 in 3

Which is why at the Vitality Project, I was feeling a little uneasy as Dr. Hammer and Mischelof awaited my decision on whether to join their program. They reassured me I would have new blood work done every 3 months to make sure PSA and other cancer indicators didn't rise. And they also reassured me that if I suffered any side effects, I could stop treatment without experiencing medical complications, and my body would basically return to normal (a point that Dr. Slater agreed with).

So why was I hesitating? Two reasons: First, I wasn't sure I wanted to rub testosterone cream on my body every morning. Second, the whole program is expensive—$250 to $350 per month. And because it's considered an "experimental" treatment, my insurance won't cover it. That computes to $4,200 per year for the rest of my life.

And yet, listening to Dr. Hammer and other happy customers at the Vitality Project, I had to wonder: How good do they feel compared to me?

So I stalled. I told them I'd like to think it over. Anyway, my visit wasn't over.

MORE IN STORE

I headed for another consultation with Crenshaw, who had taken the typical daily and weekly diet I provided and, based on my test results, drew up a menu plan designed to help me shed some troublesome pounds. She recommended that I eat 178 grams (g) of protein daily, 304 g of carbohydrates, and 79 g of fat. Attached to her plan were several pages of sample breakfasts, lunches, and dinners that meet this criteria.

Then I was off to the "treatment room" with Michelle Caleb, the director of skin care, where I got my first skin evaluation and facial. It wasn't too bad. When the hour-long, $150 treatment ended, I walked out with an appreciably smoother and less lined face (though the effects were short-lived). As the Vitality Project's aesthetician, Caleb also offered to assist me with redoing my wardrobe. Judging from her put-together look, she'd probably do a great job accompanying me to Nordstrom and helping me trade my blue jeans and fleece tops for clothing that makes me look more, in her gentle words, "like a full adult."

My last stop, after 5 hours of clinical care, was with Marc Malek, M.D., a cosmetic surgeon. Like everyone at the Vitality Project, Dr. Malek, who not only does cosmetic surgery but also reattaches limbs at the University of Arizona Medical Center, is credentialed and certified. Plus, he's an articulate, funny, and reasonable guy. "In your case," he said, "I'm not going to advise anything. You've got some smile lines around your eyes, but I can see you're a happy guy.

"What we're doing here," he added, "is restoring guys' health and self-image. Aging has always been harder on men than we want to admit. We're about making men's lives better and giving them that extra boost—be it with one of several different medical treatments or a little plastic surgery."

Then, once again, I found myself back in the conference room with Dr. Hammer and Mischelof. They inquired tentatively about my day's experience. Did I think the Vitality Project for Men is a good idea?

And I had to answer yes. There's a world of men out there who for one reason or another can use the kinds of support they're offering. There's the recently divorced guy who at age 50 has let himself go and needs to update his life and get himself back into shape. There's the guy needing Viagra. There's the older businessman who in this more competitive world is looking to find a useful edge through better skin care, a little surgical tuck, or some advice on what to eat to lose unwanted weight. All these things, it seemed amply obvious to me, the Vitality Project supplies.

On the subject of supplemental testosterone and HGH, however, I chose not to sign on. I decided that, as it relates to my peace of mind, medical science hasn't given either treatment enough study. Adding to that is the expense. To their credit, neither Dr. Hammer nor Mischelof pushed it. And that professionalism, more than anything else, piqued my interest.

Strangely, as I drove off toward my hotel, I kept wondering if—just maybe—I shouldn't join in and schedule another quarterly visit for 3 months from then. Instead, I decided to keep watching the medical literature. And my patience may have paid off. The results of a series of large National Institutes of Health studies on hormone-replacement therapy are, in fact, due out later this year.

After all, I'm now only 46.

Lift Fast, Age Slow

If you aren't flinging the weights around at least some of the time, you're missing out on the most powerful benefit of strength training

By Lou Schuler

The first time I let go of the weight, I felt as if the clouds had parted and shown me a mountaintop I'd never known existed. It was a mountain I knew I was destined to climb. I was trying an exercise I'd seen a trainer doing with an athlete on ESPN—a one-armed lateral raise in which you heave the weight into the air as you lift it past shoulder height. I was instantly hooked on this new way to train. Now almost every workout I do includes exercises in which my feet leave the floor or a heavy object leaves my hands.

But it gets even better: As I began to look into the science of fast lifting, I learned some very good reasons to go ballistic. It's not just fun; it's vital to your health and longevity. Here's why: Your muscles are designed to work at all speeds. What you don't use, you lose.

If you don't train your muscles to move fast—a quality generally referred to as "power," to distinguish it from pure strength—they lose the ability to do so. "As we age, the ability of our muscles to generate power decreases much faster than strength," says Rob Newton, Ph.D., an exercise researcher at Edith Cowan University in Australia.

Power is the last thing you want your muscles to lose. In middle age, muscle power helps you make that quick step to the left to avoid eating the bumper of a speeding taxi. The older you get, the more crucial it is, Newton says. One ill-timed slip or stumble can mean a broken hip, which for many seniors is truly the end of the road. Power is the difference between catching yourself after that stumble and hitting the pavement like a sack of liver-spotted potatoes.

Moreover, fast lifting is a highly underrated way to build muscle. A recent study in the *European Journal of Applied Physiology* shows something that contradicts almost everything you've read in fitness books and magazines: Fast lifting may produce greater gains in muscle mass than slow lifting. In this study, two dozen people lifted either fast or slowly, and each group focused on eccentric training (lowering a weight against resistance) with one arm for 8 weeks, then on concentric lifts (raising the weight) with the other arm for 8 more. The arms that lowered weights fast got the biggest gains in strength and muscle size.

One of Newton's studies showed another reason why fast lifts may build more muscle, especially if you let go of the weight or leave the ground. Newton compared two types of bench presses—throwing the bar at the top of the lift, and holding on to it. He found that the triceps work 44 percent harder when you let go of the bar.

So now it's time to throw, and grow.

POWER UP YOUR WORKOUTS

As you've probably guessed, there's more to fast lifting than walking into a gym and tossing some iron around. If you don't hurt yourself with your random flings, you'll probably hurt someone else. Some guidelines:

Beginners. Work slowly and deliberately most of the time. You'll learn the exercises and see substantial increases in strength and muscle size. When you incorporate fast lifts into your program, keep them simple: Try the medicine-ball throw shown on page 185, along with jumps (without any added weight) onto a step or box. (It's best not to jump down off the step or box until you're in pretty good shape; instead, step down carefully between jumps.)

Intermediates. You can try some of the fun stuff, including jump squats (one of my favorite images is of a 90-year-old woman doing jump squats in one of Newton's studies) and ballistic bench presses. Most of your training should involve fairly heavy weights, and you should always handle them with care. One combination I like: Do several (five to eight) sets of three repetitions of a ballistic exercise with a fairly light weight. Then do the conventional version of the exercise with a heavier weight. I tried this and found that I could do twice as many repetitions as I expected with the heavier weight.

Advanced lifters. Do fast lifts requiring more skill and coordination, such as the jumping clean and the single-arm snatch. You might divide your workouts so you separate fast lifts with light weights from slow lifts with heavy loads. A sample schedule:

Monday	Tuesday	Thursday	Friday
upper-body lifts with heavy weights	fast lower-body movements	fast upper-body exercises and throws	lower-body moves with heavy weights

If you choose to do fast and slow lifts on the same day, do the fast ones first, right after your warmup (at least 10 minutes of movement; you don't want to lift fast with cold muscles). That's when your muscles and nervous system are freshest. Follow that with heavy, slow lifts (after a secondary warmup in which you do several sets with progressively heavier weights). Then do your least important exercises—curls, extensions, and so on—with moderate weights and at normal lifting speeds.

Whichever exercises or techniques you try, rest assured that fast lifting is safe. Many of the studies proving its effectiveness were done on people old enough to be your parents, or maybe even their parents. The object of the research was to help the seniors gain more control over their muscles and, by extension, their lives. But if you employ the movements to build a bigger, stronger body for no reason beyond your desire to have it, more power to you.

WE HAVE LIFTOFF

You're cleared for handling this six-pack of ballistic exercises.

OVERHEAD MEDICINE-BALL THROW

Strengthens shoulders, chest, lats, triceps, abdominals

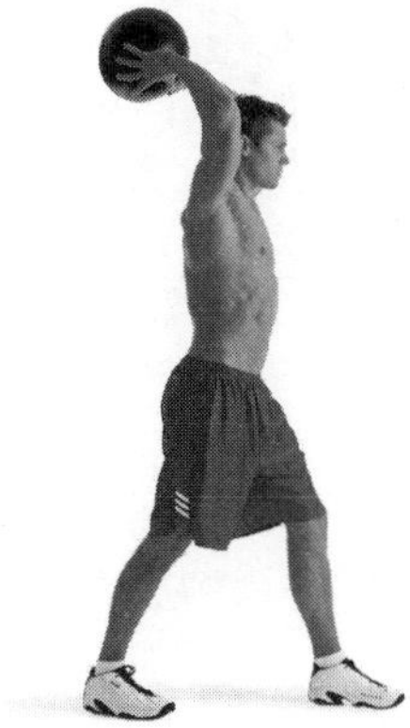

Grab a medicine ball with both hands and stand facing a cinder-block wall or something similarly solid. Stand about two paces away, with one foot in front of the other.

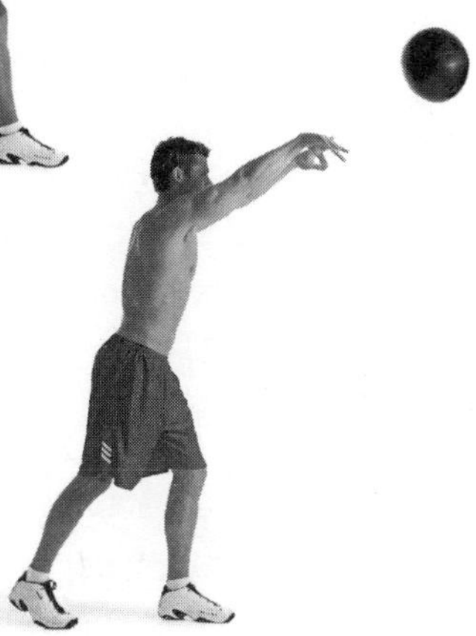

Fire the ball overhead (as if you were throwing a soccer ball in from the sideline) to a spot on the wall just above your head. Catch the ball, recoil, and throw it again as fast as you can, always trying to hit the exact same place on the wall. You know you've hit the sweet spot when the ball comes straight back to your hands without your having to move. Do one or more sets of 10. You can also throw to the wall from the side, from your chest, or even underhand to work different core muscles.

JUMP SQUAT

Strengthens entire lower body, with emphasis on quadriceps

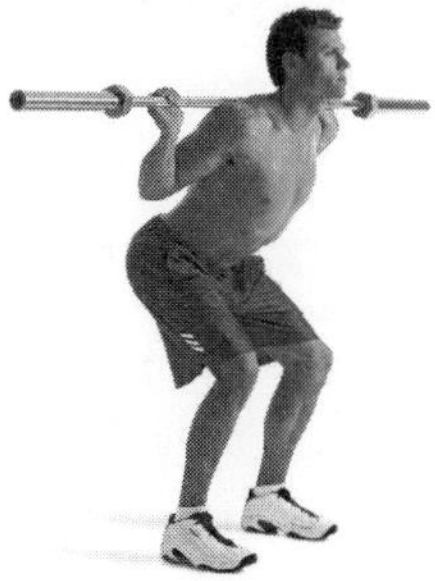

Stand in a squat rack and rest a light barbell across your shoulders. Step out from the rack and set your feet shoulder-width apart. Dip your lower body so your knees are bent at about a 60-degree angle.

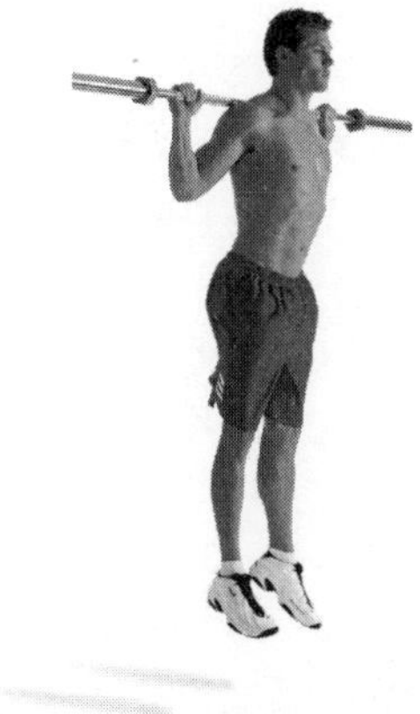

Jump so your feet come off the floor. Land with soft (slightly bent) knees, immediately dip your lower body again, and repeat. Do three to five sets of four to six repetitions.

BOX JUMP

Strengthens entire lower body, with emphasis on hamstrings and gluteals

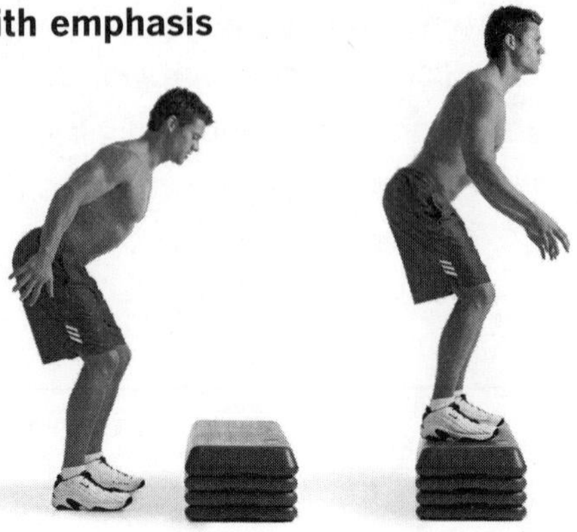

Set up a box or step that's about 12 to 18 inches high. Stand in front of it, throw back your arms, dip your lower body, and jump up onto the box.

Land on both feet, stand upright, then step down and repeat. Do three to five sets of five to eight jumps.

More challenging: Stand with one foot on the step in front of you, the other on the floor. Push down hard with the heel of the foot on the box, catch air, and switch legs so the opposite foot lands on the box. Do three to five sets of four to six jumps with each leg.

SINGLE-ARM EZ-CURL-BAR SNATCH

Strengthens hamstrings, gluteals, lower back, trapezius, rear shoulders

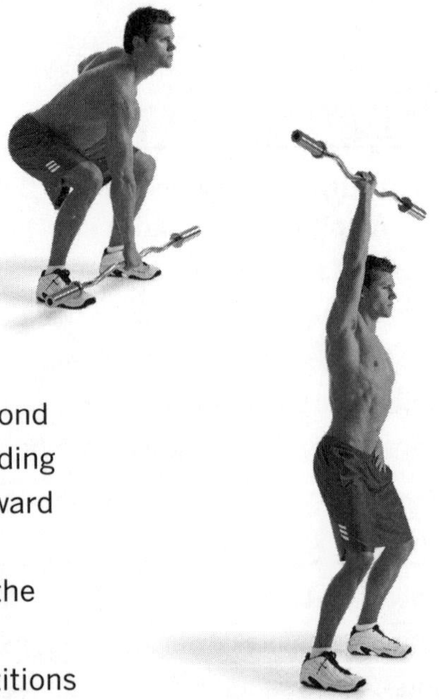

Hold an unloaded EZ-curl bar with one hand in the middle of the bar, between your legs and near the floor. Bend your hips and knees as if you were about to jump.

The move has three parts, which happen in a couple of seconds. In the "first pull," you rapidly pull the bar to your midthighs while keeping your arm straight. In the "second pull," you jump off the floor while bending your elbow and "throwing" the bar toward the ceiling. In the "catch," your arm straightens overhead as your feet hit the floor and your knees bend slightly. Do three to five sets of one to three repetitions with each arm.

MEXICAN JUMPING CLEAN

Strengthens entire lower body, trapezius, shoulders, biceps

Grab a pair of light dumbbells, stand in front of a box or step that's 6 to 12 inches high, and hold the dumbbells at your sides. Dip your lower body and allow your arms to drift back behind your body. Then thrust your arms forward as you jump up onto the box.

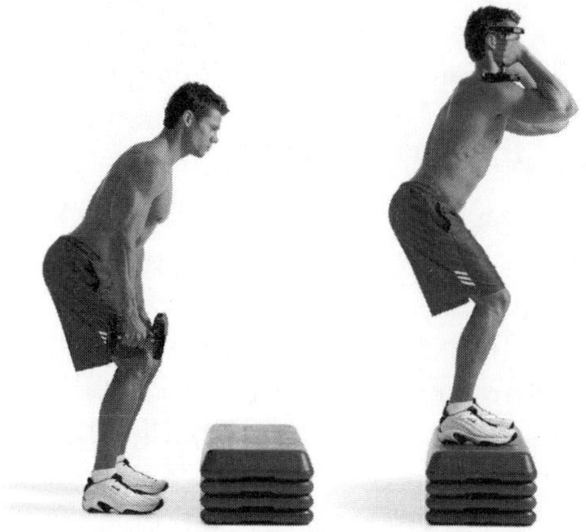

As you jump, pull the dumbbells up and rotate your arms to make the dumbbells land on your shoulders. At the end of the movement, your upper arms should be parallel to the floor and the ends of the dumbbells should rest on your shoulders. Do one to three sets of up to six jumps per set.

BALLISTIC BENCH PRESS ON SMITH MACHINE

Strengthens chest, front shoulders, triceps

Lie on a flat bench under the bar of a Smith machine so the bar is over the bottom half of your chest. Grab the bar with an overhand grip, just beyond shoulder width. Roll the bar's hooks off the restraints.

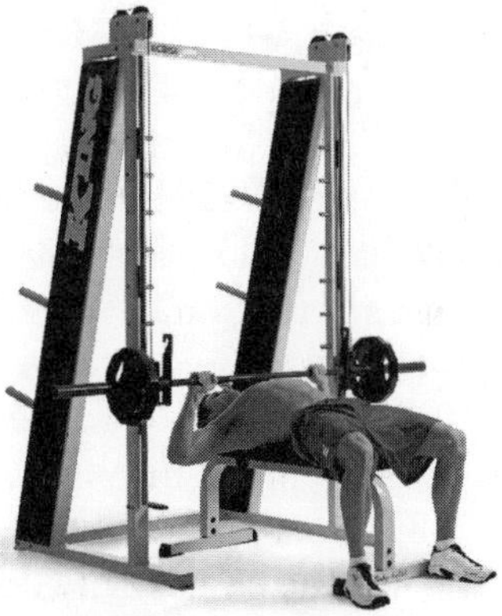

Quickly lower the bar and push it off your chest as hard as possible, letting go at the top. Catch it on the way down, immediately lower it to your chest, and repeat the action. Do five to eight sets of three repetitions.

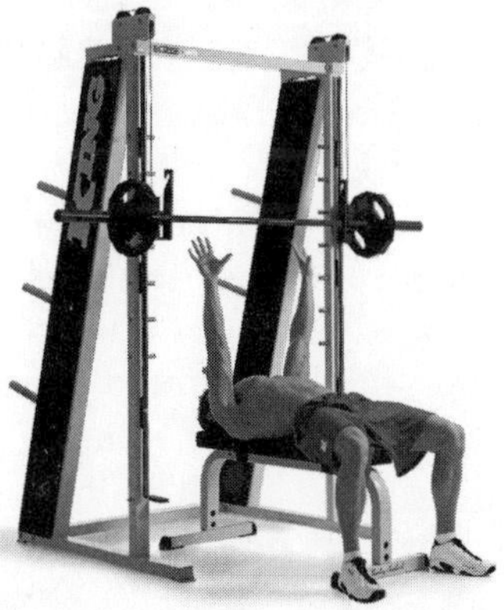

Never Need a Toupee

His noggin was bare. He wanted hair. All he had to do was spend a week in sunny Florida—and let a doctor cut 2,200 holes in his head

By Douglas Dechert

My vacation plans were set: a week in a nice hotel in beautiful Boca Raton. But while other guys would return from such a trip with golf scorecards and stealth bikini photos, I'd be coming home with the ultimate souvenir—a full head of hair. Or the seeds of one, at least. I'd decided that I was done being bald, so I signed on for a $10,000 procedure called follicular-unit micrografting, a new surgery that lets you treat your scalp like a wheat field and grow your own.

My intended crop: hair. Lots of it.

I was nervous, of course. A lot could happen. My seedlings could die in the field. It could look terrible. It could hurt. (The doctor told me I'd be awake the whole time.) Nursing these anxieties, I sat in the lobby of my hotel, jittery, waiting for the Town Car the surgeon sent for me. Then I ran a hand across my smooth scalp and smiled. It would all be over soon. My indecent scalp exposure, that is.

Here's what the first day of my vacation itinerary included: After numbing my skull with lots of anesthetics and some quality drugs (a great selling point for any surgical procedure), the doctor would peel a long, thin strip of hairy skin off the back and sides of my scalp—a flat eel of flesh with one greasy yellow side and one long, hairy, buzz-cut side. Medical technicians would then separate every tiny, egg-shaped hair follicle from this "donor" tissue. Next, the doctor would incise thousands of $^{3}/_{16}$-inch-deep slits in my scalp. Then the surgical team would plant 4,800 of my own healthy, productive hair follicles into the open wounds, one, two, or three at a time.

The more I thought about it, the more I thought that sending a driver was the least the clinic could do. A cigarette and a blindfold might be more like it.

SERVICE WITH A SCALPEL

The sterling service continued when I arrived in the wood-and-earth-toned lobby of the Bauman Medical Group. A pretty, redheaded nurse brought me water and Valium. (Should I have tipped?) Smooth jazz dripped from speakers. After I was shown to Dr. Alan Bauman's office, I realized that he was Valium in human form—so calming, experienced, and reassuring. Plus, he'd assembled a team of two M.D.'s and four nurse/technicians to work the assembly line of my head. And this is the guy who is a nationally recognized leader in microsurgical hair restoration, including eyelash transplants. My head is the Capitol dome in comparison. How could he miss?

Dr. Bauman made sure that I'd adhered to the preop regimen of abstinence from alcohol and aspirin (blood thinners) and had refrained from strenuous exercise. (Impact workouts can hinder clotting.) Why the precautions? Well, you've heard about how head wounds bleed. In the name of progress, Dr. Bauman was about to inflict thousands of them.

The next step was for me to sit back with my head in a machine that used tiny, high-pressure water jets—like a brushless carwash—to cleanse my hair and scalp in an antibacterial rinse. It felt nice. So did the Valium. Kickin' in. Yeah.

I was then seated in a surgical lounge chair with a tape of *Hannibal* playing on the TV across the room. Wait, didn't Anthony Hopkins perform some interesting scalp procedure on Ray Liotta in this one? The drug buzz wouldn't let me care. Dr. Bauman strapped a band around my head. Dozens of tiny needles embedded inside delivered continuous doses of painkillers into my scalp.

I smiled dreamily. "Give me the highest dosage . . . and some more Valium, please."

I was feeling no pain as the doctors went to work behind me. The surgical team's small talk distracted me from the fact that something major was happening. Then I heard a tearing sound. It was the thin tape of skin being peeled off the back of my head for the donor follicles.

Dr. Bauman immediately went to work suturing the wound. Meanwhile, several medical technicians using microscopes and microscalpels extracted and transferred thousands of gelatinous, seed-shaped hair follicles from the fleshy eel to petri dishes.

Now it was time for Dr. Bauman to put the "scalp" in "scalpel." His weapon of choice: a shiny, custom-made blade with an angled tip, like a slim X-acto knife. This is the truly artistic phase of the procedure. With deftness and precision, he made several thousand incisions in a randomized pattern through the bald areas of my scalp—all the while taking into account the natural direction and density of each follicle as he made the cuts. This would determine how natural my new hair would look once it sprouted.

My mantra: Relax, he does eyelashes!

ROUND TWO

After lunch (I recommend the meatball sub), they converged on me once again—a combination of at least two doctors and/or technicians filling Dr. Bauman's incisions with my uprooted follicles, which looked like servings of

PERCENTAGE OF MEN WHO WEAR TOUPEES: 4

fish-egg sushi. They hovered over me for hours with tiny forceps, plucking, poking, pushing. Slowly, all the sites in my scalp were filled. The drugs continued, and I happily munched Doritos while watching incomprehensible images flicker on the TV screen in front of me.

I didn't lift a finger, but when it was finished, I was exhausted.

THE IMPLANTABLE MAN

Cosmetic surgery for men is growing—and so are the many body parts that can now be enhanced

We've always believed that the best way to get bigger muscles is to work hard for them in the gym. But in an age when fast food dominates diets and overnight delivery is the rule in work and commerce, it's only a small wonder that instant muscle is achievable as well. Here's the list of body parts now available for sale. But if you want to boost your self-respect, you'll still have to earn that on your own.

Abs

Using liposuction tubes, the surgeon "liposculpts" horizontal and vertical lines of fat from your belly, forming faux abs. The effect appears to be permanent (long-term studies don't exist yet), but there are limitations. "You can't take somebody who needs to lose 50 pounds and give him a six-pack," says Mark Solomon, M.D., spokesman for the American Society of Plastic Surgeons. Another option: dropping in silicone ab implants, in which plastic substitutes for low body fat and thousands of crunches.

Number of procedures done each year: Probably only a few hundred
Cost: $2,000 to $4,000

Biceps and Triceps

A solid silicone implant is inserted in a pocket between the muscle and the *fascia*, a layer of strong, fibrous tissue that covers the muscle. J. Howell Tiller, M.D., a plastic-surgery veteran practicing in Miami Beach, is one of the few surgeons to do these operations. In his opinion, they entail the lowest risk of complications of all implant procedures.

Number of procedures done each year: Fewer than 100
Cost: $5,000 to $8,000

Butt

The doctor makes an incision in the midline of your buttocks and slips the implant (one per side) in a pocket beneath the gluteal muscle. The sitting factor increases the risk of implant migration and dimpling and also increases the pain. "During the first 2 or 3 days, patients swear they won't make it through," says Dr. Tiller. "After a week, though, they're pretty comfortable."

Number of procedures done each year: 100 to 150
Cost: $6,500

Around 4:00 in the afternoon, Dr. Bauman did his final examination, using forceps to push back the occasional recalcitrant seedling that had popped up out of its little furrow. Then it was back to the washing machine for one last antiseptic bath.

My debriefing consisted of an introduction to the special postoperative

Calves

Calf augmentation has been around for 30 years, says Dr. Solomon. But it's still not common. "I do two a year," he says. The calves have thin skin, which ups the risk factors. The surgeon makes an incision in the crease behind the knee and inserts two silicone implants within each calf to simulate the two sections of muscle. Recovery time for this procedure is minimal. There will be scarring behind the knee and some temporary or permanent loss of feeling in the calf.

Number of procedures done each year: Fewer than 100
Cost: $5,000 and up

Chin

The surgeon cuts between the lower lip and gum. The skin and tissue are stretched to form a space for the implant. Short-term risks are minimal, but the silicone could eventually regress, requiring a new implant.

Number of procedures done each year: 4,000 or more
Cost: $1,500

Pectorals

Doctors go in through the armpit, installing solid, custom-fit implants beneath the chest muscle and on top of the ribs. Patients can usually go home an hour after surgery, but, says Dr. Tiller, "this is one of the more painful procedures."

Number of procedures done each year: 650 to 700
Cost: $4,500 to $5,500

Penis

To lengthen the penis, the doctor snips the ligament that anchors it to the pubic bone, allowing a 1- to 2-inch section that's normally inside the body to slide out. Afterward, the patients are often required to wear external weights taped to the penis in order to maintain the length that was achieved during surgery. Girth enhancement (up to 30 percent) can be achieved through a graft of material from a tissue bank.

Number of procedures done each year: 900 to 1,000
Cost: Lengthening, $4,000 to $6,000; widening, $7,000 to $8,000

See "The Risks of Implants" on page 192.

take-home kit I'd be using for the rest of my vacation. No bandage was placed on my scalp. Instead, I was issued gauze pads and liquid-filled packets. My instructions: Soak the gauze in the solution and place it on my head for an hour, twice a day. The solution was a hydrating treatment containing an infusion of copper peptide that would help heal my skin. "Copper is an essential nutrient for healing skin cells," said Dr. Bauman. "The more you use it, the sooner you'll heal." There was also a set of shampoo and conditioner full of similar compounds. And, best of all, they gave me a series of little manila pill packets: Percocet and Motrin (for pain), prednisone (to reduce swelling), and Propecia (to prevent future loss of my untransplanted hair).

Dr. Bauman nodded at my shredded head and gave me a satisfied grin. "Six months from now, you won't believe how much hair you have."

THE DAY AFTER

The next morning, I woke up with spotty smears of blood and other effluents on the sheets and pillowcases. (Note to self: Tip maid.) I gingerly washed and conditioned my hair. The streams from the showerhead felt like individual flamethrowers, and after I dried off, the general, viselike pressure all over my head was worse. But that's what the Percocet was for.

I reviewed some notes I'd tapped into my laptop the night before, under the influence of my whole prescription cocktail: "My scalp is a tight, hard helmet, both numb and prickly at the same time. As I contemplate the rending of the hairy strip of flesh from the head, it occurs to me that the appropriate metaphor is 'adult circumcision.'"

But in my case, I'll have more to show for this cutting, not less.

Later that day, Dr. Bauman gave me another computerized scalp wash. Then I was introduced to a new machine: the Low-Level Laser Therapy Hood. It looked like an old salon hair dryer, but retrofitted by Q: Inside were

THE RISKS OF IMPLANTS

Seroma: A collection of fluid other than blood around the implant. It's usually reabsorbed naturally, but if it persists, the doctor will have to remove it with a needle or surgery. *Risk:* About 15 percent; common with buttocks implants

Displacement: Implants can shift. Surgery may be required to remove, replace, or fix. *Risk:* Approximately 5 percent

Infection: Devastating if it occurs (usually within 2 months of a procedure). You'll need surgery to remove the implant, then possible hospitalization and intravenous antibiotics. *Risk:* Less than 2 percent (more likely with buttocks implants)

Hematoma: Internal bleeding can collect around the implant after surgery. If the hematoma's large enough, you'll need surgery to remove it. *Risk:* 1 to 2 percent

rotating red laser projectors that stimulated scalp cells and hastened healing of the thousands of mosquito-bite scabs.

A daily field trip came onto my vacation schedule: I was to travel across town to Integrative Therapies, a sports-medicine clinic, where for the next 5 days I'd spend an hour a day in a hyperbaric chamber—you know, the kind of oxygen tent that Michael Jackson slept in (before being sent to the big house). It looked sort of like an inflatable, clear plastic coffin. Once I got inside, they pressurized it to a few times normal atmospheric pressure and fed in pure oxygen. The pressure forced oxygen into my lungs and even into my pores to accelerate healing.

Afterward, I felt pretty good, but there was absolutely no improvement in my moonwalk.

The rest of my vacation flew by. After 5 days, I was off pain meds entirely and feeling pretty normal. Dr. Bauman told me that all was well. The implantation scabs would fall off in about a week; the stitches would dissolve soon after that.

He lent me another cool gadget—a LaserComb, which worked like the laser helmet I'd been using in his office. "Run it slowly over your entire scalp for 15 minutes every other day," he said. He also told me that in 9 out of 10 cases, the spiky little shoots that I could feel sticking straight up like a crew cut would fall out, and those roots would go dormant for a few months, then gradually—yes!—regenerate hair.

He shook my hand and said, "This will be the longest 6 months of your life. Be patient and then enjoy your new hair."

One year later: The results are nothing short of miraculous. I've gone from Costanza to Kramer—a Chia Pet on Miracle-Gro. Every week that's gone by has brought noticeable improvement. It's a pleasure to look in the mirror. My whole life has improved—the person I always felt like on the inside is now visible on the outside. And he's one hairy guy. My current girlfriend—young, beautiful, fun—is unfazed by it all. She likes my full head of hair. Her only response to the work I've had done is, "When do I get my implants?"

NEED TO KNOW

The X Men

Researchers at the University of California at Davis have identified a new health risk for men. Called fragile X–associated tremor/ataxia syndrome (FXTAS), the disease targets men over 50 who carry a defective "fragile X" gene. Symptoms include tremors, anxiety, and balance problems. Researchers hope this discovery will lead to better diagnoses and treatments.

Alzheimer's Research

New evidence suggests that Alzheimer's disease starts in middle age. By creating the conditions of Alzheimer's in a simulated brain, UCLA scientists have found the lesions that lead to the disease in people as young as 40. They hope to discover how to slow the breakdown of myelin, the fatty membrane in the brain, which leads to the lesions.

One promising treatment is the athlete's-foot drug Clioquinol, which helps dissolve the A beta-amyloid plaque believed to cause Alzheimer's, say Australian researchers. Patients in later stages of the disease showed significant improvement after taking the drug in a clinical trial. Larger trials are planned.

No Wrinkles, In Time

Forget Botox and collagen. If you want to eliminate wrinkles, liquid silicone may be the way to go. In trials, researchers at the New York University medical center have found a way to safely and permanently eliminate major wrinkles by injecting silicone into the skin and basically "filling in" the creases. FDA testing is under way.

Strange Relief

What the bacteria used in Botox treatments is good for: It may help improve bladder function and other symptoms of an enlarged prostate, Italian researchers report.

Cataract Clues

The traditional treatment option for asthma may have a serious side effect: According to a new U.K. study, the steroids in some forms of asthma inhalers may significantly increase individuals' risk of developing cataracts as they get older.

Speaking of cataracts, after studying more than 100 eyes, scientists at the University of Washington at St. Louis found a link between the development of cataracts and the degradation of a gel that lies between the lens and the retina. Next step: Find out why the gel degrades and how to prevent the process.

Lose Your Glasses

Bifocals may be part of your father's future, but they don't have to be part of yours. A group of U.S. scientists has found a way to remove the fluid in the eye and replace it with a new manmade gel that smooths and softens the "aged" lens, improving its ability to focus and eliminating the need for bifocals.

Dodge Dentures

A fruit or vegetable a day may keep dentures away. A recent USDA study found that men with the worst diets are also the most likely to be missing teeth after age 50. Researchers attribute the men's lack of choppers to their diets' lack of beta-carotene, folic acid, vitamins A and C, and fiber.

Stay Grounded

Sticking vibrating insoles into a pair of shoes could help improve your balance, as well as reduce an elderly person's risk of falling and breaking a hip. According to a new study from Boston University, vibrations improve the transmission of nervous-system signals from the feet to the brain. The more effectively these signals flow, the more sure your footing becomes. A vibrating shoe insert is now under development for consumer use.

FAST FIXES

When it comes to growing old, well, we'd rather not. That's not to say we're willing to check out at a young age. It just means we'd prefer to become more distinguished with age, like a fine wine. We hope to be turning heads and wooing women like Sean Connery as 007. Not to mention we want to be physically strong and mentally sharp so we can save the world, if need be—not tethered to a nursing home hospital bed and drooling. With that in mind, we culled together these 10 ways to slow the hands of Father Time, so you can become better with age. Now sit back with a martini (shaken, not stirred, of course) and read on.

1. Rub out wrinkles. Got a furrow in your brow? Or laugh lines, but you're not laughing? Prevent further damage with an extract of white tea leaves that may help fight wrinkles and keep your skin looking young, according to a Case Western Reserve University study. "Chemicals in the tea appear to protect your skin from sun-induced stress, which can cause the cells to break down and age prematurely," says Elma Baron, M.D., the study author. To put white tea to use, try rubbing on a lotion containing white-tea extract before you apply your sunblock. A lotion with white tea extract, called Origins White Tea Skin Guardian, is available from origins.com.

2. Get a face-lift. If the damage to your skin has already been done, here's some good news: Looking young into old age may be a lot easier, thanks to a new type of nonsurgical face-lift recently unveiled at an American Academy of Dermatology conference. During the new procedure—called a radio-frequency face-lift—physicians zap wrinkles with a blast of high-powered radio waves, causing skin to contract and tighten. As the skin tightens, it helps erase fine lines and wrinkles and lifts sagging facial muscles. "The procedure generally takes less than an hour and is much safer than a surgical face-lift," says David Goldberg, M.D., dermatologist at Mount Sinai school of medicine in New York City. Radio-frequency face-lifts are currently available at select medical centers across the country. (Prices range from $1,000 to $2,000 per session.)

3. Never need a hearing aid. Concertgoers, rejoice. Studies have shown that the antioxidant N-acetylcysteine (NAC) can protect the ear from permanent noise damage. Research is now being put to the ultimate test—rifle training with the Marines—in the hope of developing a hearing-loss pill. The Marines are taking 900 milligrams of NAC (available at health-food stores) three times a day, but even a single dose after noise exposure could substantially reduce hearing loss, says Colonel Richard Kopke, M.D., the study director.

4. Stand tall. Women aren't the only ones who need to worry about becoming hunched over as they get older. A new report from the National Osteoporosis Foundation found that men over 50 are at greater risk of breaking a bone as a result of osteoporosis than of coming down with prostate cancer. In fact, up to 2 million American men already have osteoporosis, while an additional 3.6 million suffer from low bone mass—an immediate precursor. The best prevention? Making sure you get the recommended 1,000 milligrams (mg) of calcium a day from milk, cheese, and yogurt. Some research has shown that too much calcium may actually increase the risk of prostate cancer, but the vitamin D in dairy products can offset that risk.

5. Check your vitamins. If you're taking supplemental vitamin A, it's time to reconsider. Researchers in Sweden found that getting too much vitamin A in your diet may increase your risk of broken bones as you get older. In a 30-year study of 2,300 men, researchers found that men who took more than 25,000 international units (IU) a day were two to three times more likely to break a bone. Eating foods that are naturally high in A (carrots, spinach, mangoes) is still the best way to supplement your A intake, the study's authors report.

One vitamin you may need more of: vitamin E. The recommended intake for men under 50 is just 15 mg a day, but a Tufts University study says older men who bump intake to 200 mg may be better able to fight off cataracts, heart problems, and Alzheimer's disease.

6. Enjoy the lean times. If you have big plans for your retirement, try to avoid gaining weight as a middle-aged man. According to a new study from Finland, men who put on the fewest pounds during the middle years of their lives have the best quality of life during old age. Researchers studied 1,600 men over a period of 25 years and found that those who gained the least weight as they got older also had the lowest risk of chronic pain, illness, disability, and mental or emotional problems later in life.

BIRTHDAY THE AVERAGE GUY WOULD LIKE TO LIVE TO SEE: **100th**

CHANCES HE ACTUALLY WILL: **0.8%**

Another important reason to consider dropping those excess pounds: Being overweight could increase your risk of developing Alzheimer's disease. After tracking the health of two groups of people for nearly 20 years, researchers in Sweden found that for every 1-point increase in body-mass index (BMI), your risk of Alzheimer's may increase by more than 30 percent. Cut just 125 calories from your diet each day, and you'll lose a pound a month, enough to seriously lower your BMI—and Alzheimer's risk—in less than a year's time.

7. Stay on the move. We've known anecdotally for years that working out can improve the health of the ol' gray matter, but now researchers at the University of Illinois have come up with physical proof to show that exercise does indeed make your brain stronger. After analyzing brain scans of 55 people over the age of 55, researchers found that men who regularly worked out lost significantly less brain tissue as they aged than men who exercised rarely or not at all. "This is further proof that working out can help keep your memory strong and prevent the loss of cognitive function as you get older," says Arthur Kramer, Ph.D., the study author.

8. Butt out. Reason number 45,678 to give up smoking: It's bad for your memory. London researchers found that men who smoke heavily are more likely to start losing their memory during their 40s and 50s than men who don't smoke.

9. Keep your blood pressure in check. A study from the University of Pittsburgh reports that high blood pressure may increase your risk of becoming more forgetful as you get older. High blood pressure appears to impair the flow of blood to the brain, making it harder to perform memory tasks.

10. Take some sage advice. Taking a sage-oil capsule may improve your memory, according to new research from Northumbria University in the United Kingdom. In a study of 44 adults between the ages of 18 and 37, researchers found that individuals who took 50 microliters of sage oil performed consistently better on a memory test than those who swallowed placebos. "It's possible that sage may even help treat Alzheimer's disease someday," says Nicola Tildesley, Ph.D., the study author. Sage oil is available at most health-food stores.

OUR FINAL ANSWERS

Rise to the Occasion

I'm already noticing I'm not, um, up for the job as long as I used to be. What do I have to look forward to as I get older?

—D.L., Spokane, Washington

Let's just say there's something to be said for the quickie. Back when you were in your twenties, you lasted some 54 minutes. Ah, the good old days. At age 50, it's already down to about half that: 29 minutes. By age 70? You'll be stiff about 7 minutes. Of course, you'll probably be stiff other places all the time.

Down on Your Knees

My knees ache all the time. How can I tell if it's arthritis—or just time to quit playing basketball?

—C.L., Parris Island, South Carolina

Only your doctor will know for sure. "It's important to see a health-care provider at the earliest warning signs of arthritis so he can begin treatment to prevent joint damage and disability," says John H. Klippel, M.D., medical director of the Arthritis Foundation. "More often than not, an x-ray is required to try to determine any changes in or loss of cartilage or bone."

AGE-RELATED CHANGE IN HIS PHYSICAL APPEARANCE THE AVERAGE GUY DREADS MOST: **SHRINKING**

RUNNER-UP: **GOING BALD**

If you're diagnosed with arthritis, the two best ways to fight back are to control your weight and, no kidding, keep exercising. For every extra pound you shed, you'll reduce the load carried by each knee by 3 to 4 pounds, says David Felson, M.D., head of the arthritis center at the Boston University school of medicine. Strength and flexibility exercises—especially low-impact and nontwisting types—will beef up the muscles that surround your knees, which will provide better knee support, thus reducing pain. It will also help slow the pain's progressive worsening over time, Dr. Felson says.

Gray Matter

Can stress really turn your hair gray?

—S.T., Denton, Texas

No. According to John F. Romano, M.D., professor of dermatology at Cornell University, pigment-producing cells are genetically programmed to stop producing hair pigment at a certain age, regardless of how much (or little) stress you have in your life.

The Bald Truth

My older brother is going bald. Will I?

—T.L., Detroit

Did you see those pictures of the Bee Gees when Maurice died? One Bee Gee brother was bald, one was hairy, and the third was a little bit of both. The same odds could kick in for you. To see if they will, dig out a photo of your brother at your current age; a compare-and-contrast exercise should reveal whether you two are in lockstep, genetically. In general, these rules apply: The first signs of male-pattern baldness occur by the early 20s. If you're losing it on top, in front, or especially over the ears at that age, prepare for the Willis look. The later the thinning starts, the more likely you'll retain some coverage.

Brain, Down the Drain

I constantly lose my car keys. Is this early Alzheimer's?

—D.C., Missoula, Montana

You're probably just forgetful, not doomed to the circular ward. "Every day, I forget which floor I parked my car on and have to search for it," admits

Steven DeKosky, M.D., director of the Alzheimer Disease Research Center at the University of Pittsburgh. If he's not worried, you shouldn't be. But if your lapses disrupt your life, see a doctor.

To spark your memory, Jon Keith, author of the book *Everyday Memory Builder*, recommends using the POP system:

- Keep a Positive attitude, which feeds your natural memory (as opposed to a negative approach, which causes stress).
- Observe your environment.
- Picture and think about where you place your keys as you set them down. "If you take that 1 additional second to look at the action, that will help your absentmindedness," Keith says.

Grouchy Gramps

Are old men grumpy by nature?

—R.J., Eugene, Oregon

No. On personality tests scored like the SAT, men who were in their 50s scored 30 points higher in agreeableness than men in their 20s, according to the researchers behind a study in the *Journal of Personality and Social Psychology*. The reason: Older guys become more caring because they're raising children and grandchildren and forming closer bonds with their loved ones. Both factors lead to a better outlook on life.

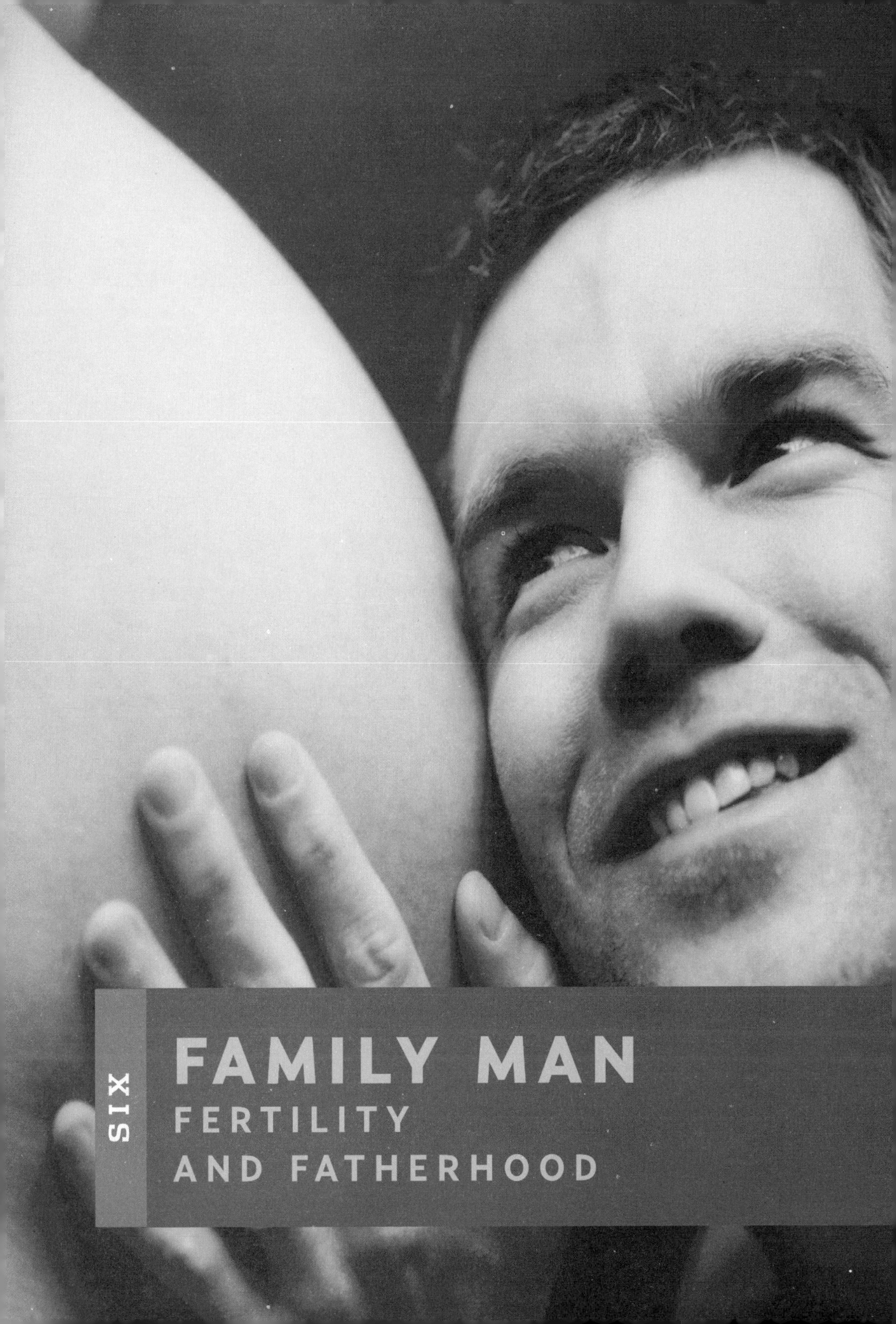

SIX

FAMILY MAN

FERTILITY AND FATHERHOOD

MUST READS

Are You Ready to Reproduce?

Rate your parenting preparedness with this test of the most important qualities for any dad-to-be

By Liesa Goins

1. What's the status of your relationship?

A. Married, thank you very much.
B. Not married, but we're solid.
C. We're still figuring it out.

Research shows that living apart from his father means a kid is two to three times as likely to have health and emotional problems, use drugs, drop out of school, or end up in jail as those who live with two parents. Before you combine DNA, try to combine households.

2. What else do you do with this woman?

A. We have plenty of shared interests.
B. Becoming parents is our main focus.
C. Practicing the art of conception is enough.

"Possibly the most important determinant of a father's relationship with his kids is his relationship with the mother of his children," says Roland Warren, president of the National Fatherhood Initiative. Having common interests strengthens your bond, so develop activities outside the bedroom.

3. Can you skip regular trips to Circuit City?

A. As long as I can still look at the sale ads.
B. Do I also have to skip visits to Home Depot?
C. How will I know if there's a new Sims out?

"If you're not prepared to sacrifice something, whatever it is, you're not ready to become a parent," says Corey Donaldson, author of *Don't You Dare Have*

Kids Until You Read This. A good start? Volunteering. Ladling out soup is much easier to deal with than predawn diaper changes.

4. How often do you have to cancel plans?

A. Almost never.
B. A couple of times a week.
C. All the time.

Kids require quantity time as well as quality time. "A kid needs a father's presence, attention, and time more than anything," says Warren. Now's the time to practice keeping appointments. If work is your time suck, check into office policy on flextime and telecommuting.

5. Do you have an extra $9,650 to spend?

A. If I had to, yes.
B. Who does?
C. There's no way, unless I sold a vital organ.

According to parenthood.com, it costs about $9,650 to raise a kid for the first 2 years. Then it gets expensive: You'll spend $181,480 for the first 18 years, not including college. See what expenses you can cut—saving cash and giving up indulgences puts you on the path to parenthood.

6. Are you a favorite uncle?

A. I'd like to think so.
B. Does a few hours a month qualify me?
C. I remember birthdays; what more is there?

Lousy dads typically have a bad attitude before becoming parents, Donaldson explains. Enjoying other people's children is a good indicator of how you'll feel about your own. Do some babysitting, or visit friends with kids for a weekend to see how you hold up.

7. Do you ask for directions when you're lost?

A. Only after I've tried a couple of "shortcuts."
B. Depends on your definition of "lost."
C. I always find the way on my own.

"This may sound trivial, but your willingness to ask for help can be a big indicator of how well you can handle parenting," says Maurice J. Elias, Ph.D., author of *Emotionally Intelligent Parenting.* Having a support system you tap into increases your odds of raising a well-adjusted kid.

8. Do you enjoy hanging out with your dad?

A. Definitely.
B. Depends on how many beers I've had.
C. I try to avoid it.

Studies show that if you had a good relationship with your dad, chances are good that your kid will have a good one with you. If you're at a loss, recruit a parenting mentor. Talk to people you know who have solid relationships with their kids or with their parents, and find out what they do.

Scoring A = 3 points, B = 2 points, C = 1 point

18–24 points Congratulations. You're ready to start procreating. "The most important part of being a good dad is wanting to be a good dad," Warren explains. Enjoy the conceiving.

10–17 points Chances are you'll do fine. But it wouldn't hurt you to work on some of your weak areas if you want a "#1 Dad" mug.

9 points or less You're not quite there, but these are all factors you can improve. Get a puppy, and take this test again in a couple of years.

Tipping the Scales

The epidemic of childhood obesity is fast creating a national health crisis. Here are 10 steps you can take today to keep your kid slim and healthy

By Peter Moore

"**A**nd the sins of the father shall be visited on his children, and his children's children unto the third and fourth generation . . ."

As a source of weight-loss inspiration, the Bible is pretty much overlooked.

But there's tons of useful stuff: fasting, high-quality aerobic activities like wandering in the wilderness, and manna from heaven, the ultimate low-fat snack. And God's warning from the book of Exodus is tailor-made for dads: Just conjure it up the next time you're hoisting a greasy load toward your slavering gob while your kids look on. And, oh yes, they're watching. Very closely. The American Dietetic Association says that parents are kids' number one role models (40 percent cite them as such), far outpacing the next-closest finisher: those bad boys of work-release, professional athletes

(8 percent). Seventy percent said they turn to their parents for information on nutrition and healthy eating. So if you can set a good example with your forksmanship, you have a fighting chance at countering the 30 billion dollars a year the food industry is spending to sell a chubby lifestyle to you and your kids.

So far, the marketers are winning. One in seven American kids is currently overweight or obese, a jump of 50 percent in the past 20 years. That's nine million Whopper Jr.'s spilling out of their buns, growing to full Whopperhood. (Researchers at NYU have correlated the plump jump to the invention and marketing of the supersized meal in the late 1970s.) At the rate we're going, by 2011 the fat kids on the playground will be banding together and making fun of the few remaining skinny ones. At least, until the large generation succumbs to diabetes, heart disease, colon cancer, and other diseases associated with too much flesh and not enough action. The USDA figures that kids consume around 1,900 calories a day, even though they need only 800 to 1,300. Urp.

Kind of makes the Happy Meal stick in the throat, doesn't it?

"A lot of parents tell me, 'My kids don't like healthy foods,'" says David Katz, M.D., associate clinical professor of epidemiology and public health at the Yale medical school. "Well, 'finicky' is not an excuse. You never hear a parent say, 'My child doesn't like to look both ways before he crosses the street.' They tell him to do it. They should do the same thing with dangerous foods. More of today's kids will die of complications from bad foods they eat than they will from tobacco, drugs, and alcohol."

Even slim kids are at risk of heart disease and cancer. And exercise habits and dietary smarts are the way to avoid them. You, more than anyone else, can help your kids do that. Yeah, you.

Here is where you can take a page from the Old Testament playbook: Throw some commandments at 'em. Okay, so you're not God. But with the help of the smartest people in the weight-loss game, you can keep the whole family out of caftans.

1. THOU SHALT MOVE THINE ASS.

According to a University of Buffalo study, a kid's risk of obesity doubles for every hour of television he watches every day and drops 10 percent for every hour of exercise he gets daily. And given that the average kid watches television for 21 hours a week, that's a lot of doubling going on—and not just in chins. Michael Levine, M.D., pediatric endocrinologist at the Cleveland Clinic's children's hospital, notes: "It's very difficult to eat while you're playing football; it's easy when you're just watching it on a screen." Perhaps your kid sips an extra sugary drink or two while he mashes the remote; each additional soda increases his risk of obesity by 60 percent, according to a study done at Children's Hospital in Boston.

Now might be a good time to show equal parts backbone and understanding, Dad. Make a deal: For every hour they spend on the GameCube, the computer, the Xbox, the Game Boy, or the tube, they have to put in an hour of physical activity. You can easily track their tech time and buy cool stuff, too. A new line of TVs from RCA is equipped with KidPass, a system that lets you set the number of minutes each kid can watch. When the time

SEPARATE WHINING FROM DINING

Your little angels can turn into head-spinning monsters when they crave their fat fix. James U. McNeal, author of *Kids as Customers,* has identified seven whining strategies they use. Maurice J. Elias, Ph.D., author of *Emotionally Intelligent Parenting,* provides the snappy aisle-nine comebacks that just might save their lives. Or at least their waistbands.

Pleading, Persistent Whine

"Please, Dad, puh-LEEEEEZE!"

Dad comeback: First rule of whine response: Always stay calm in public. Elias suggests saying, "You can ask me 1,000 more times and my answer will be the same. Be sure to keep count. When you get there, ask me again and I'll tell you the same thing."

Forceful Whine

"I've got to have it!" or "I'm gonna ask Mom!"

Dad comeback: Never debate with Mom in front of the whiner; parents should present a united front even if you disagree, says Elias. If the kid has already executed the end-around, say, "It may be okay this time, but Mom and I will be talking about this, and it may not be okay next time."

Threatening Whine

"I'm not gonna move until you buy that for me!"

Dad comeback: Self-control is key here. Elias suggests taking away privileges: "If you're not moving in 2 minutes, there will be no Xbox for 2 days." The more they stay put, the more privileges lost and for longer.

Sugar-Coated Whine

"Ple-e-ease? You're the best daddy in the whole world!"

Dad comeback: "Quite right, son. It's because I care about you so much. And that's why I won't let you do anything that's harmful to your health."

Emotionally Threatening Whine

"I'll hate you forever!"

Dad comeback: You are not giving in because you care, and because you care, you cannot give in. Stay firm and never debate. A little guilt never hurt, either: "I wish you didn't hate me, because I love you."

Pity Whine

"But everyone will tease me if I don't drink Harry Potter Coke!"

Dad comeback: Go ahead and sympathize, then bring down the iron hand. And turn it into a lesson about how to handle being teased. If the kid can stand up to the needling, the teaser will pick a different target.

is up, the box shuts down. It might be the best tech investment you make this year or in his lifetime.

The best way to monitor exercise time, of course, is to be a sports hero: Play with your kid. "The *Men's Health* Family Workout," on page 212, gives you an exercise plan that (a) is fun and (b) can make the entire family healthier.

2. THOU SHALT HONOR THY BMI.

By correlating height and weight, body-mass indexes (BMIs) give adults a clear picture of where they ought to be (BMIs between 18.5 and 24.9), where they're starting to get in trouble (25 to 29.9), and where they've crossed a big fat line (30 or higher). It's vitally important to measure BMI in kids as well. The sooner you and your kid stop and reverse any weight gain, the less likely she is to be permanently stuck on the down side of the health teeter-totter. You can calculate your kid's BMI and yours at menshealth.com. A score that puts her above the 85th percentile for her age means she's on the wrong side of a weight shift of historic proportions.

3. THOU SHALT KNOW THINE ALTERNATIVES.

"A healthy diet isn't about deprivation," says Dr. Katz. "Parents need to know the best foods in every category—chips, cookies, juice—that their kids are going to want to eat."

Dr. Katz has supplied just such a list in his book, *The Way to Eat* (Sourcebooks, $22). Some of his kid-zone selections:

Cold cereals. Post Raisin Bran, Multi-Bran Chex, Life

Cookies. Barbara's, Frookie, Health Valley

Snacks. Stonyfield Farm low-fat drinkable yogurt, Health Valley granola bars, Jell-O fat-free pudding

Frozen desserts. Nonfat frozen yogurt, fruit-juice bars, fat-free Fudgsicles

4. THOU SHALT GUARD THE GATES.

You have the power to shut out bad foods. If a food is high in refined sugar or high-fructose corn syrup, don't let it into your car or the front door of your house. Children won't be able to bug you for junk that isn't in the cupboard, and you won't guiltily snarf it when they're in bed, either. Along those lines, it's never too early to limit saturated fats and trans fats (partially hydrogenated anything on the label), which are arterial disasters for everybody you care about. Conversely, if a food is acceptable, there's seldom any reason to control portions, so the food battles fall, right along with everybody's BMI numbers.

5. THOU SHALT NOT CREATE UNNECESSARY FAT CELLS.

One doomsday scenario has it that our current nine million fat kids will find love, have nine million supersized weddings, and produce in excess of

18 million obese children, causing the collapse of beds, shoe arches, and civilization as we know it. It could happen, in fact, but it doesn't have to. "You can change the way inherited genes will act," says Dr. Levine. "The environment overrides the gene template." One way it does this is through fat-cell creation. Sometime early in a child's life—it could be the first few years or even the first few months—your kid begins forming fat cells, with the total number being determined by the kinds of foods he's eating. If he's overstuffed as a baby, he'll have more fat cells. And that's like laying in a big supply of luggage before a long vacation: Your wife will fill every bag. So it is with those infinitely expandable fat cells. It's never too early to watch the ingredient lists. Another key to a healthy, lean baby: breast milk. And it comes in such attractive packaging. (Studies show that babies fed with formula are more likely to become overweight as kids.)

6. THOU SHALT NOT DRIVE THRU.

Researchers at Brigham Young University doled out pedometers to 1,954 children in three countries. The tallies: Swedish boys average 18,346 steps a day, Australian boys take 15,023, and American boys take 13,872. You'll never guess who the fattest ones are. One lesson: On the rare occasions when you eat fast food with your kid, at least commit to hoofing it from car to restaurant. Once you reach the counter, fight the national obesity trend by ordering from our special edition "Eat This, Not That" on page 214.

And now that you've established the principle of one-foot-in-front-of-the-other, find excuses to interject it into other aspects of your kid's life. He can walk to the neighbor's house, ride a bike to school. If he doesn't love his bike, skateboard, inline skates, or scooter, buy him the coolest one you can afford. Foot and bicycle power appeal to kids' sense of independence, and while they're escaping you, they fill up their lives with exercise.

7. THOU SHALT NOT TAKE THY SCHOOL-LUNCH PROGRAM IN VAIN.

According to the *Journal of the American Dietetic Association,* 77 percent of principals said their schools had contracts with soft-drink companies—virtually floating most school activities on a sticky brown tide. And just consider the fact that Coke has signed on as a "sponsor" of the National PTA and has a seat on the board. Can the Coca-Classroom be far behind? "Vending machines are like Superfund sites with push buttons," rages Dr. Katz.

He advises that a few shrill parental voices can go a long way toward bringing around the principal, school board, and local politicians on the matter of scouring the schools of crap food and crap-food advertisements. Be a part of the trend to detoxify cafeterias.

You should also take an interest in your kid's school-lunch choices; in with the whole fruit, 1 percent milk, baked chips, and peanut butter, out with the

(continued on page 214)

THE *MEN'S HEALTH* FAMILY WORKOUT

According to a new survey by *Prevention* magazine, 76 percent of all children ages 10 to 17 say they'd like to exercise with their parents. So get moving. We asked Michael Mejia, M.S., C.S.C.S., advisor to the Center for Sports Parenting, to create age-specific father-kid workouts designed to be as fun as they are effective. Do them 3 days a week to form a lasting habit.

Ages 6 to 8

Benefit to your kids: Builds fitness, improves body awareness, and increases flexibility.

Benefit to you: Cures treadmill boredom.

How to do it: Perform exercises in succession.

1. Jumping Jacks: Do 10.

2. Zigzag Sprints: Cover a total of 40 yards by running 10 yards, then changing directions and running another 10 yards.

3. Body Weight Squats: Do 10.

4. Bunny Hops: Jump forward, keeping your feet together, for 10 to 15 yards.

5. Pushups: Do as many as you can.

6. Monkey Run: Shuffle sideways for 10 yards and back, two times. Turn around and repeat, leading with the other foot.

7. Squat Thrusts: Do 5 to 10, just like in junior-high gym class.

8. Rest for 2 minutes, then repeat.

Ages 9 to 11

Benefit to your kids: Improves speed, agility, quickness, and strength.

Benefit to you: Burns fat and increases your pickup-game draft value.

How to do it: Cardiovascular training first, then strength training.

Cardiovascular Workout

Complete each exercise before moving on to the next.

1. Rabbit Race: Allow your kid a 5- to 10-yard head start for a 40-yard race, chasing him from behind. Rest 90 seconds, then repeat five times.

2. Driveway Shuttles: Place six tennis balls at the end of the driveway. Take turns sprinting to retrieve them. Rest 90 seconds; repeat three to five times.

3. Tag: Mark off a 20-foot-by-20-foot area and play tag. (You're it!) Go continuously for 60 seconds, then rest for 60 seconds. Do five rounds.

Strength Workout

Perform each pair of exercises as a superset, doing one set of each exercise before resting for 90 seconds. Do a total of two or three sets of each.

Superset 1

1. Broomstick Overhead Squats: Hold a broomstick with arms straight above your head. Keep your body as upright as possible and squat as deeply as you can. Do 6 to 10 repetitions.

2. Pushups: Lower your body until your upper arms dip below your elbows, then push yourself back up. Do 6 to 10 reps.

Superset 2

1. Single-Leg Phone Book Touches: Place a phone book in front of you, stand on your left leg, and squat to touch the phone book with your right hand. Do six repetitions, then switch legs and repeat. That's one set.

2. Bridges: Get into a pushup position, but bend your elbows and rest your weight on your forearms instead of your hands. Pull in your abdomen. Hold for 20 to 30 seconds. That's one set.

Ages 12 to 16

Benefit to your kids: Builds speed endurance and improves balance and core strength.

Benefit to you: Works muscles you didn't know you had in a high-intensity fat-burning session.

How to do it: Do cardiovascular followed by strength one day, vice versa the next.

Cardiovascular Workout

Complete all sets of each exercise before moving on to the next.

1. Rundowns: You sprint for 5 to 10 seconds. When you slow, your kid sprints until he catches you, then slows to your pace. Repeat. When your kid catches you five times, you've completed one set. Do two sets each, and build up to four.

2. Timed-Suicides: Sprint as fast as you can for 5 yards, then turn and sprint back to the starting line. Do this continuously, increasing the distance to the turnaround by 5 yards each time. Cover as much ground as you can in 30 seconds. Then rest while your kid runs. Repeat two to four times each.

Strength Workout

Perform the exercises as straight sets, doing two sets of each exercise before moving on to the next. Rest 90 seconds after each.

1. Single-Leg Deadlifts: Stand on your left leg holding your right leg in the air, bent 90 degrees. Slowly lower your body until your left thigh is parallel to the floor, then push yourself back to the starting position. Do six repetitions.

2. Swiss-Ball Back Extensions: Lie chest down on a Swiss ball, your arms in front of you and your feet braced on the floor. Raise your arms, shoulders, head, and chest as high as possible. Pause for 2 seconds, then return to the starting position. Do 10 to 12 repetitions.

3. Swiss-Ball Leg Curls: Lie on your back on the floor and place your lower legs on a Swiss ball. Push your hips up so that your body forms a straight line from your shoulders to your knees. Without pausing, pull your heels toward you and roll the ball as close as possible to your hips while keeping your body in a straight line. Roll the ball back to the starting position. Do six to eight repetitions.

4. Traveling Lunges: Stand with your feet hip-width apart and step forward with your left leg. Lower your body until your left thigh is parallel to the floor and your right knee nearly touches the floor, keeping your torso upright. Push off your left leg so that your body is in the starting position again. Then repeat, lunging forward with your right leg this time. Continue to alternate legs until you've traveled 20 yards.

doughnuts, soft drinks, french fries, and mystery meats. One small change can produce a big difference: The Center for Science in the Public Interest points out that kids who drank a cup of 1 percent milk instead of 2 percent each school day would cut almost 19 pounds of fat during their school careers. If your kid uses a swipe card for cafeteria purchases, tell him you'll be checking on what he buys; many schools offer printouts.

8. THOU SHALT NOT BE A SLAVE TO THINE HYPOTHALAMUS.

Picture yourself at the Thanksgiving table, having stuffed yourself in the usual way. You push back, give your belly a pat, and say, "What's for dessert?" That's your hypothalamus in action, according to Dr. Katz. Here's how it works: The gland at the base of your brain contains hunger regulators for the main flavors that make up a diet: sweet, salty, bitter. At one point, it drove *Homo sapiens* to sample a lot of different foods; when you filled up on one, you stopped eating and sought another, thereby ensuring a good variety of nutrients. Now the huge food companies do our grazing for us, and their food scientists combine sweet and salty flavors within single foods; Cheerios have nearly as much salt as pretzels, but it's masked by sugar. As a result, you'll just keep on eating, because you'll never exhaust your taste in any single area. "Every processed food has chemical flavor enhancers to keep you eating," Dr. Katz says.

EAT THIS (INFREQUENTLY)	NOT THAT (EVER)
Burger King 4-piece chicken tenders, fries, and milk Kid's Meal: 510 calories, 22 g protein, 22.5 g fat (7 g saturated)	Cheeseburger, fries, and soda Kid's Meal: 710 calories, 22 g protein, 28 g fat (11 g saturated)
McDonald's Hamburger, fries, and milk Happy Meal: 590 calories, 23 grams (g) protein, 22.5 g fat (7 g saturated)	Cheeseburger, fries, and soda Happy Meal: 650 calories, 18 g protein, 24 g fat (7.5 g saturated)
Wendy's Chicken nuggets, fries, Frosty, and milk Kid's Meal: 730 calories, 24 g protein, 31 g fat (10 g saturated)	Cheeseburger, fries, Frosty, and soda Kid's Meal: 814 calories, 24 g protein, 27 g fat (9.5 g saturated)

There are a few ways to avoid becoming hypothalamic slaves:

- Eat just one snack at a time, so you'll tire of it and close the box.
- Buy foods with short lists of simple ingredients to cut down on chemical hypothalamus bafflers such as sodium chloride, sodium benzoate, sodium bicarbonate, monosodium glutamate, and artificial flavors.
- Plan meals around flavor themes so you know when to lay down the fork. For example: citrus on the chicken and in the salad.
- Eat whole fruits, grains, and vegetables, not their superprocessed Frankenstein cousins.

9. THOU SHALT AVOID FAD DIETS.

Don't succumb to every crazed weight-loss notion that floods the airwaves. If you're on cabbage soup one week and the alphabet diet the next, and in the meantime yo-yoing between guiltily overweight and grumpily lean, your kids will think that food is complicated. It shouldn't be; more often, it's a matter of simplifying choices. "It's not an arcane story," says Dr. Katz. "Kids can get used to a healthy diet. That's what parents do for their children." The key: Train them in bedrock principles they can sustain for a lifetime.

10. THOU SHALT ACT AS A FAMILY.

If you want to help your kids eat better, exercise better, live better, they can't go it alone. You have to do it with them. If the kitchen is filled with junk and one shelf is nutritional nirvana, the result is preordained: Junk wins. The same goes for junk diets, junk lethargy. Bad currency drives out good. So does what dads do best: Launch a good-food-and-exercise crusade, but with a spirit of adventure, a sense of humor, a lust for discovery, and, above all, a policy of togetherness. If you pitch it right, the whole gang will sign on. The sins of the fathers will most assuredly be visited on their children, but here's the beauty part: So will their righteousness.

Hold On to Your Kid

Headed for divorce court? The system is stacked against you. Here's how to make sure the children don't leave along with the house and the car

By Bill Stump

Larry Hellmann was waiting for a flight at New York's LaGuardia Airport in 1988 when he phoned his wife and daughter. Within minutes he had a new destination: divorce. "My wife told me not to come home," Hellmann says. "I was shocked, and I had no idea what my rights were as a father. Worse, because of that, I almost lost my daughter."

Hellmann eventually gained custody of his child, but only after years of emotional and legal torment. Now the secretary for the National Congress for Fathers and Children, he works to spare other men the same ordeal.

Fathers have gained some legal rights in the past decade, but they're still at a disadvantage when negotiating custody in a divorce. "Even though almost all states recognize men as equal parents with equal rights to custody, some judges, psychiatrists, and social workers favor keeping kids with their mothers,"

THE SINGLE FILE

Seven ways unmarried fathers can protect their rights

Arranging a custody deal during a divorce is brutal enough, but trying to protect your rights as a father if you're not married to the mother is harder still. One in three children born in the United States is the child of unwed parents, and the number of single fathers is rising. If you're one of them, it's vitally important to know what your rights are so you can stay involved in your child's life.

"Traditionally, single men have yielded all control and decision-making to the mother, but that's slowly changing," says Dave Bruer, executive director of the Fathers Resource Center in Encinitas, California. "Men want to be fathers to their kids, but they need to know how to assert their rights."

Here are Bruer's suggestions for single dads:

- If you're living with the child's mother or with an expectant mother, continue to do so.
- Put in writing and share with the mother your intentions regarding custody, living arrangements, support, and access to the child.
- Accompany the mother on visits to the doctor.
- Even if the mother refuses to acknowledge you as the father of her child, make every effort to contribute to her emotional, physical, and economic well-being until paternity tests can be done. Document all your efforts.
- Insist on sharing all costs, and set up a bank account for the child, even if the mother refuses your help.
- Establish your father-child relationship legally. If you're the father of a newborn, sign the birth certificate and make sure that the child has your last name.
- Contact a fathers'-rights or parents' organization that offers support and attorney referrals. A good place to start is the Fathers Resource Center, (760) 634-3237.

says Jeff Atkinson, an attorney with the American Bar Association and author of the *American Bar Association Guide to Family Law.* Successfully battling this bias is a matter of knowing which actions to take and which to avoid.

Don't leave home. Maybe it's the nagging, or the fighting, or the personal trainer's trunks you find in the hamper. You pack a bag and take up residence on a buddy's couch.

You've just made your first big mistake.

"The instant you leave the house, you yield a major advantage when it comes to gaining custody," says Henry James Koehler, a fathers' rights attorney in Beverly Hills, California. The court, which will impose its own custody arrangement if you and your wife can't agree on one, may look at your decision to leave as a sign that your wife is the real custodial parent. What's more, your departure gives your wife a chance to prove that she can go it alone. "Don't underestimate the court's emphasis on the children's current situation," says Atkinson.

It can turn ugly. "Some women will charge abuse and persuade a judge to sign an order of protection," says Jeffery M. Leving, a Chicago attorney and coauthor of *Fathers' Rights.* "It's frequently a tactic to force you out of the house and away from the kids and to characterize you as an unfit parent. Hire a lawyer to fight it immediately."

Beware of temporary separation agreements. "Often the terms of a temporary separation agreement become the final terms of divorce," says Mary Reed, a legal writer in Austin, Texas, and coauthor of *Divorce for Dummies.* "Don't sign a deal believing that you can easily renegotiate the custody arrangements later."

Call a marriage counselor. Even if your marriage is beyond saving, seeking counseling may help you in a custody fight. "Find a marriage counselor who testifies often in custody cases in your local court system. Make an appointment for you and the kids, then invite your wife," Koehler advises. "If your wife comes, the psychologist can hear both sides, and you get credit for initiating the meeting. If your wife doesn't show, you can tell the court she wasn't willing to cooperate. Either way, you win points."

You also win by being fair and reasonable when talking about the divorce in front of your children. Explain that the issues are between you and their mother and that the split isn't their fault. Don't fight with or criticize your spouse in front of them. Remember that they love her, too.

"If a father tells his kids the only reason for their pain is that Mommy doesn't love Daddy anymore, that's a big strike in my court," says Judge James W. Stewart of the Santa Clara (California) Superior Court, Family Court Division.

Find the right lawyer. Finalizing a divorce and determining custody usually takes a minimum of 6 months, so hire an experienced, supportive attorney to be at your side throughout the process. Word of mouth is the best way to find candidates, but don't choose a lawyer solely on someone's recommendation. Ask prospects how often their custody cases go to trial. If the percentage is higher than the national average—less than 10 percent of cases make it that far, according to Atkinson—ask why. "Some unethical lawyers allow proceedings to drag on without a resolution so they can bill more hours," says Leving. Also be wary of attorneys who discourage you from pursuing court-approved mediation. They may have their eyes on a new Ferrari and not on your future.

Know what custody arrangements you want. If you haven't been an active parent, are you sure you'll be able to be one in the future? How can you convince the court of that? If work or poor health is going to affect the time you can spend with your kids, will you really be able to handle primary custody? When deciding what role you want to play in your children's lives, be realistic and keep the kids' best interests in mind.

Let your wife know you're not a pushover. Although the court must approve any custody arrangement, in most cases you'll be better off reaching a settlement with your wife before you go in front of the judge. "When you let the courts decide, you must deal with a judge who has his or her own prejudices," Reed says.

That doesn't mean you have to accept whatever proposal your wife and her attorney dangle in front of you, however. Take the time to prepare your own custody plan, and show that you're ready to battle for it. "If they see that they have a fight on their hands, they're more likely to back down from extreme demands and cooperate with you," Reed says.

Gather evidence to support your case. If your case goes to trial, you'll have to convince the judge that you're an active, effective parent. You'll need references—teachers, the pediatrician, neighbors—who will vouch that you are closely involved with your kids.

And alert the court if you can guarantee a strong female presence in your children's lives—your mother, perhaps, or a stable girlfriend. "The courts are concerned about the atmosphere they're sending the children into," Stewart says.

Another tip: Sign up for a parenting class through a local agency—before the court orders it. There are classes that cover all age-groups and subjects: how to defuse a temper tantrum, when to buy your daughter a training bra, and lots more. "Taking a class like that impresses me tremendously," says Stewart.

Gather evidence against your wife. You have to assume that if your case reaches the trial stage, it will get nasty. Your wife will bring evidence that will portray you—at best—as an ineffective father. Be prepared to produce any proof you have that your wife isn't suited for the custody arrangement she's seeking. If she has alcohol, drug, or psychiatric problems, for example, or if she has engaged in risky sexual behavior, you'll want to produce medical records or witnesses.

Be on your best behavior. If you've been a good husband and father during your marriage, don't ruin it now by dropping a bundle at the track, organizing a buddy's lewd bachelor party, or being arrested for DWI. "Assume that your wife's lawyers will be watching everything you do," says Koehler. "No matter how harmless it may be, any action can be misrepresented to the court."

Don't let your wife bait you into bad behavior, either. "If your wife lays into you, maybe poking you in the chest for emphasis, be careful," Koehler says. "She could be trying to lure you into losing your temper." Succumbing to anger, even for a second, will cost you.

Learning How to Be a Part-Time Parent

Marriages end. Fatherhood continues

By Colin McEnroe

When my son, Joey, was 4—a tiny kid racing along a trail in a woodsy park—a dog darted across his path and the two collided at a 90-degree angle, the boy flipping over the animal's back. When I caught up with him in the dust, it was clear he'd had the wind knocked out of him. I picked him up. There was one lone tear.

"You're going to be okay in about 30 seconds," I told him.

Silence.

I held him in my arms. "It's okay to cry," I told him on that day 10 years ago. He just glared at me. His hero was Hawkeye from *The Last of the Mohicans*. You don't show the Hurons your fear, your uncertainty.

He has been Hawkeye ever since. Warlike when provoked. Independent. Protective. He guards his mother, my ex-wife, like a one-man secret service.

Our divorce, last March, elevated the level of alert. Yellow when we were still together, red now that we're apart. One day last October, I was washing the very stinky "family" dog, slopping water all over the deck of my ex-house. Joey was throwing his backpack into the car—I drive him to school to make sure I see him every day—and he became distressed about the water.

"It could freeze. Mom could slip on it."

"It's October!"

"It's dangerous. I need to warn her." He barged back into the house to protect his mother from this high-risk situation. Neurotic? A little. But it was also a pleasant reminder of who he really is. He dresses like 50 Cent—chains and football jerseys and bulky jeans that weigh as much as a pygmy deer. He looks and acts as if he's packing, ready to rumble, a gangsta. The truth is, he couldn't have functioned at school if he'd thought his mom might slip and hurt herself. Warning her made him free to concentrate on getting as little as possible out of American public education.

Since our family broke into two households, I've been in school, too. Single-Dad School. It's a new set of skills, and then . . . it isn't. It's just the old set. The things that make you a good married dad also make you a good single one.

When I say "school," I'm speaking metaphorically . . . mostly. In our state, the law requires divorcing parents of minor children to take a 6-hour parenting course. You sit in a room with 13 other men and women, all bound together by the common thread of having shanked the marriage ball into the rough. The first thing the facilitator does is to write, on a huge piece of paper on an easel, the names and ages of everyone's kids, from newborn Nicole to 17-year-old Tyler, because it's "important to keep them all here in the room with us."

I quickly realized I was surrounded by people who were doing everything wrong: insisting that their kids were "just fine" (no kid going through a divorce is just fine), letting hostilities escalate in front of the kids, haggling over little stuff, letting the new girlfriend into the picture too fast. (Two people in the class were, I was pretty sure, some kind of couple, getting out of their respective marriages and attending the mandated class as a date.)

Thank God, I thought, I wasn't doing anything wrong.

But then I heard my voice saying to the circle, "My son asks me all the time to explain why I left. I try to answer the question, but I don't know how. And he presses me, and I tell him if I explain, I'm going to sound like I'm finding fault with Mom; and I never want to do that."

"But isn't that kind of sneaky?" said one of my mates in the Fellowship of the Ringless. "You're implying that there is something negative about your wife just by refusing to say it."

"Uhhhhh," I rejoined.

"Couldn't you make it something negative about yourself?" asked another Fellowshipper.

"I'm not sure I could explain to anyone why my marriage broke up," said a third. "Why are you even trying?"

I called my ex-wife the minute I got out of the class (which she had already taken).

"We should fall down on our knees and be thankful we're both such nice, reasonable people," I told her.

There was a gentle but dead silence.

"I . . . should . . . fall down on my knees, anyway," I told her.

"Bingo."

Okay, so maybe I had a few blind spots of my own.

Here is what I do know: There is just no substitute for contact with your kid. My first promise to Joey, when I left his mom, was "I will see you every day." He pretends that this is a nuisance, complains that his other friends see less of their fathers than he does. But I notice that his last words, whenever we part, are always the same, almost ritualistic: "When will I see you next?"

Of course, contact will be more difficult if there's acrimony between you and your ex. So there must not be. At least not much. My friend Peter is my guru on divorce. He handled his own divorce and remarriage so gallantly that one night his ex and his current wife went to see *The First Wives Club* together. Without him. You want to listen to that guy.

When I moved out, Peter said, "You're doing what you want to do. Now find out what everybody else wants and make sure they get it."

Peter's other advice: "Swallow (almost) any bitter pill. Pretend she's right when you know you are."

He's right, and I do it. Because I still care for her, and because I know Joey will feel that much safer if his parents are cooperating instead of bickering. And because how I treat his mother will become a Rosetta stone for how he treats women later in life.

It also helps you think of others more when you've participated in a major screwup yourself. Look, you failed. To whatever degree you have (mis)represented yourself as The Man, the guy with the right answer, the wielder of domestic justice, you now have to concede that you didn't have everything figured out. The family is busting up, so how much of a genius were you, really?

On the other hand, you're still the alpha male, and don't forget it.

"You're not even around anymore!" Joey likes to tell me when I'm attempting to discipline him, especially when I'm attempting to discipline him on behalf of his mother.

"That doesn't change anything. I'm still your father," I tell him.

Sometimes I have to make this point a little more forcefully. I don't believe in spanking or hitting, but for most of his life, when I've needed to assert dominance, I've firmly put him on his back—on a couch, on a bed, on the lawn—pressed down on his chest from above, and looked directly into his eyes. He refers to this as "alpha wolfing," and he knows it's serious. I've done it a few times since the breakup, usually when he's tried to use my absence to ride roughshod over his mother. He knows that the alpha wolf is never far away. Justice can be meted out.

That's one side of it. On the other side, there are opportunities, in the time after separation, to experiment with . . . democracy. In certain areas, Joey and I are on oddly comparable footing. For example, we're both about to start dating.

In this department, he has taken it upon himself to become my advisor. For example, there was the 29-year-old woman at the health-food store who kept asking me out. (I'm 49.)

"Gina," I told her sweetly one evening, "I have jackets that are older than you are."

"Are you out of your mind?" Joey demanded when we got back to the car. "You think that's going to happen a lot? A woman her age asking an old fart like you to go out with her?"

And the early restirrings of my romantic (if that's the right word) life have defrosted a few insights I might not have remembered to give him as he makes his first foray into the world of women.

"All that macho stuff on your rap CDs about bitches and hos and cars and bling-bling? It doesn't really work with women," I told him one night. "They want somebody strong and confident and a little tough, maybe, but they also want the flowers, the poems, the tenderness, the consideration. You're good at talking to people and noticing their feelings, much better at it than I am. And that's what's going to get you women. Remember Hawkeye? He would do anything to find Cora and save her. That's what women want. A hero who adores them."

Whether he heeds this bit of advice is an open question. He also gets a glimpse when I crash and burn, with the cameras rolling.

"What's wrong with you?" he asked one night. We were in the car at a red light.

"Nothing."

"Something's wrong. You look sad, and you're kind of mumbling to yourself under your breath."

A pause. He's very attuned to people. It's almost pointless to lie to him.

"If you must know, there was a woman I was kind of hoping to have a relationship with. And now it feels like it's not going to work out. And I'm sad about that."

"Is this about Ed Levine's sister?"

"What makes you say that?" I startled like a horse. I'd had no idea he knew.

"Look. You're not the first person in the world this ever happened to."

This is the way it goes for us now. Our old life lies behind us, in smithereens, but we get to build something new out of the rubble.

But you have to preserve a thing or two from the old world, as well.

Nine months after the separation, Joey still yearned for the Christmas Eve party his mother and I always gave. So we gave it again. We split the cost and the errands. The night was a success in every way, especially the most important one: Our kid saw that some of what was precious could be recovered from the storms of last spring. At the end of the evening, I gave my ex-wife a long hug and told her I was proud of what a beautiful party she had thrown. These days, her hair is blonde, and she has new contact lenses.

The booklet they give you at the state parenting class is called *Putting Children First.* When you do that, the adult wounds have an odd way of healing faster, too.

NEED TO KNOW

Babe Magnet

One out of five couples suffers from some form of infertility—and between 30 and 50 percent of the time, those fertility problems involve the man. Would-be fathers take heed: Yale researchers have developed a technique that uses a "magnet" to attract healthy sperm cells while weeding out lower-quality ones. To separate them, doctors smear a special acid on the bottom of a petri dish. Healthy sperm cells stick to the acid, while inferior-quality sperm are washed away. Samples are then used for in vitro fertilization.

The only drawback? The procedure may affect whether you have a boy or girl. Babies created through a similar procedure are 20 percent more likely to be girls than boys.

There's My Old Man

A sperm cell can kill itself if it has damaged DNA—another way we men keep the species strong. But new research into this process, called apoptosis, shows that as a man ages, damaged sperm cells are more likely to survive. A study in *Fertility and Sterility* magazine shows that men older than 35 are four times more likely than younger men to have sperm with highly damaged DNA. If a DNA-damaged sperm fertilizes an egg, chances are higher for miscarriage, birth defects, cancer, or mental disorders. So men should pay attention to their biological clocks, says study author Narendra Singh, M.D., Ph.D. If you want to be a father at 40, battle sperm damage daily with the antioxidants vitamin C (250 milligrams), vitamin E (400 international units), and selenium (200 micrograms).

Boys in Babeland

Worried about being the last of the Schlobotniks? Time your wife's pregnancy correctly and you may be able to increase your chances of having a son, Italian researchers recently determined. In a review of 14,000 births, doctors found that women are 4 percent more likely to have boys when they get pregnant during the late summer or early fall.

Give It a Shot

Vaccinate your child, tear-free. According to a study published in the *Archives of Dermatology*, a device called a YAG laser used with an anesthetic cream reduced the pain of shots by 61 percent. The procedure, commercially called Epiture Easytouch, is already available.

Like Son, Like Father

If your child has been diagnosed with attention deficit/hyperactivity disorder (ADHD), consider making your own appointment with a psychiatrist. University of Maryland researchers found that parents of children with ADHD often have ADHD and other mental health problems. Researchers tested the parents of 214 children, both with and without ADHD. Parents of kids with the disorder were 24 times more likely to be afflicted than the moms and dads whose children weren't, says study author Andrea Chronis, Ph.D.

Home Is Where the Unhealthy Heart Is

If you're a stay-at-home dad, make sure you take good care of your ticker. According to a new study from the National Institutes of Health, men who stay home and raise their children are 82 percent more likely to die of heart disease than men who keep their noses to the traditional grindstone and work outside the home.

Big Fat Medical Bills

The consequences of the childhood obesity epidemic just keep multiplying. A new study from the University of Southern California reports that overweight children are more likely to develop asthma than their leaner, more active counterparts. Worse, a Yale expert suspects that because of their poor diet, today's children may be the first in modern history to have shorter life spans than their parents.

NUMBER OF MEN WHO ARE STAY-AT-HOME DADS: 105,000

NUMBER OF WOMEN WHO ARE STAY-AT-HOME MOMS: 5.2 MILLION

Family Fun Time

A Game Boy is good for keeping the kids quiet on a car trip, but not so hot for family togetherness. Playing games as a family is a great stress buster and bond builder. Moreover, some games help "develop skills that translate into real life," says Joshua Smyth, Ph.D., professor of psychology at Syracuse University.

DVD technology fuels many games now, including Trivial Pursuit Pop Culture Edition ($40, trivialpursuit.com), which uses a DVD to flash visual questions, and Scene It? ($30, amazon.com), which features real movie clips.

For the little guys in your life, there are games like Mattel's new Break the Safe ($20, amazon.com), which levels the playing field since you all play as a team. Smyth's advice: Change teams periodically so everyone feels he has a chance to win—something that's not an option when you're fighting for the remote.

The Cost of Being an Absent Dad

The number one excuse most men give for not spending more time with their families? Work. Think your kids aren't missing you? A study found that 42 percent of teenagers want to spend more time with their dads. Missing out on time with your kids has a huge hidden psychological—and financial—impact on you and your family. Here's what 6 months of catching up at work rather than playing catch with your kids could cost you.

It'll take . . .	Research shows . . .	You pay . . .
Extra supervision for the kids	Your wife can't watch them all the time, so you'll need day care or a sitter.	$4,550
More allowance	Guilty parents tend to become more generous with allowances.	$480
A tutor	Kids whose parents don't take an interest in them tend to perform worse academically.	$1,010
Couch time of 1 day a week—for the kids	Children interpret an unavailable dad as an unsupportive one—which leads to anger and hostility that a therapist will have to work out.	$3,000
A cell phone with instant messaging and Internet service	An electronic connection to the kids is better than no connection at all.	$970
Two new video games and a shopping spree at the mall	Parents set up latchkey kids with the latest games so they can entertain themselves.	$170
Disney World for a week	It's the classic guilt reliever.	$2,300
TOTAL		$12,480

FAST FIXES

There's no instruction manual to having and raising kids. (Of course, if there was one, we probably wouldn't read it anyway.) But there are some simple things you can do to make the whole fatherhood thing a lot easier. These 11 tips that cover from conception to kindergarten and beyond will help you raise kids with a good head on their shoulders.

1. Grade your guys. Do you know if your sperm are ready to dive into the gene pool? New at-home fertility testing kits can help you find out.

Spermconfirm will give you a sperm count after you send a sample in for analysis. Marc Goldstein, M.D., chief surgeon of male reproductive medicine at Weill Cornell Medical Center in New York City, calls it a first step. "There's no substitute for a thorough physical examination and semen analysis," Dr. Goldstein says. $60, spermconfirm.com

FertilMARQ works like a home pregnancy test: An indicator changes color to tell you if your sperm count is above or below the World Health Organization's cutoff for decreased male fertility. The test can't tell you how far above that level you are or whether the quality of the sperm is good, but at least you'll know if you're carrying a loaded gun. $30, drugstore.com

2. Keep your boys healthy. Get the lead out. A study of 140 couples undergoing in vitro fertilization found that high lead levels in men blocked the receptors that help sperm bind with eggs. Consider cleaning up your act: Study author Susan Benoff, Ph.D., says higher lead levels were found in men who drank, smoked, and weren't active.

Commuting to work with your windows down also could increase your risk of becoming infertile. In an Italian study, researchers found that men who were exposed to car fumes for several hours a day had much-lower-quality sperm than men who hadn't inhaled as much exhaust.

3. Carry a tune. Expectant dads: When your wife goes into labor, bring her favorite CD to the hospital. According to a Case Western Reserve University study, music significantly reduces a woman's labor pains. Researchers say the music soothes women's nerves, causing the pelvic muscles to relax.

PERCENTAGE OF MEN WHO ARE IN THE ROOM FOR THE DELIVERY OF THEIR BABY: 80

4. Pitch in. Taking 15 minutes in the evening to take out the trash and load the dishwasher could improve your home life. In a recent study of 3,500 people, researchers at the University of California, Riverside, found that men who perform the most chores around the house have the best relationships with their children. Helping out teaches children good values. It also makes wives feel loved and more like equals, which increases their interest in sex, says John Gottman, Ph.D.

5. Keep it together. Think kids are better off if an unhappy couple divorces? Think again. A Pennsylvania State University study agrees that while in some cases divorce is necessary to escape a violent situation, more than 70 percent of divorces occur for lesser reasons. Spouses who are constantly fighting but act civilized when it comes to the kids should think twice about splitting. These are the types of divorces that cause psychological harm to the kids in the long run.

6. Butt out. If you're still smoking, quit for your kid. Researchers at the Fred Hutchinson Cancer Research Center found that quitting smoking before your child reaches third grade can reduce his or her odds of becoming a smoker by up to 40 percent. "The period of time between the ages of 8 and 20 is when people are most likely to start smoking," says Jonathan B. Bricker, Ph.D., the study's lead author. However, if kids don't see their parents smoking during this time, there's a good chance they'll never pick up the habit, he says.

7. Turn off the TV and computer 30 minutes before your kids' bedtime. A Texas study found that the bright light from televisions and monitors acts like a stimulant to children's brains and disrupts their sleep—and everyone knows sleepy kids don't do as well in school.

8. Get your kid a guitar. Chinese researchers found that children enrolled in music-education programs have better memories than children who can't play an instrument. The more lessons they had, the better their memories became. Researchers believe that musical training helps develop the left temporal lobe of the brain, which strengthens the brain's ability to remember.

9. Talk to your kids. The teasing, challenging tone that many fathers use with their children readies kids for the outside world, research suggests. Gene G. Abkarian, Ph.D., professor of linguistics at Colorado State University, reviewed studies of "child-directed speech" in *Fathering*. He offers these tips for helping your kids communicate.

Respond to them. Instead of your default "Mm-hmm" response to their stories, ask follow-ups: "Tell me more," or any who-what-when-where-why question.

Challenge them. Use vocabulary they may not know (yet) to expand their grasp of language. You'll be surprised what sticks—and what they figure out.

Joke with them. Good-natured sarcasm forces a child to figure out when you're serious—a valuable lesson in how to read people in the real world.

10. Raise a rich kid. We all want our children to be more successful than we are—maybe become real estate tycoons who can set us up with a villa in Monte Carlo. Here's how to make them clever about cash at an early age . . . so you can think about early retirement.

Buy a railroad. Or maybe Park Place. "The formula for financial success is found right on the board game Monopoly," says Robert T. Kiyosaki, author of *Rich Dads' Success Stories*. Kids learn to invest so they know what green can do for them.

Watch your mouth. Be careful what you say regarding money in front of your children, says Kiyosaki. Never say, "I can't afford it," or "I'll never be rich." Instead, say, "How can I afford it?" This opens their minds to the possibility of obtaining wealth.

Bank it. Start a four-piggy-bank system: one each for spending money, savings, investing, and charity. The amount isn't important, but putting something in every day is.

Encourage growth. Begin paying allowance around age 3, or when the kid starts saying, "I want," suggests Neale S. Godfrey, author of *Money Still Doesn't Grow on Trees*. Base the amount on the kid's age (a 10-year-old earns $10 a week). Godfrey's timetable: By 5, he should have a savings account. At 10, own stocks. By 12, make money outside the home. By 16, be off the allowance system.

11. Read these directions. The dads of *Men's Health* magazine have spent hundreds of birthday and Christmas Eves assembling toys—from basketball hoops to Easy-Bake Ovens. We know the agony of the missing part, of directions translated from Farsi, of batteries not included. Here's what you can learn from our mistakes.

- Always read the directions before starting. We've often found ourselves at step 63, only to realize that the triangle thingies should have gone on the axle doohickeys before the linchpins were inserted into the sprocket slots. Disassembling is guaranteed to take the wind out of your wassails.

PERCENTAGE OF PARENTS WHO GIVE THEIR KIDS A WEEKLY ALLOWANCE: 50

PERCENTAGE OF PARENTS WHO PAY THEIR KIDS FOR GETTING GOOD GRADES: 29

- Have a Phillips-head screwdriver, a hammer, and a pliers handy. No improvising with kitchenware. Using a corkscrew on a bike chain brings no comfort or joy.
- Never assemble under the influence. Bonded bourbon and a box containing 337 plastic parts are a dangerous mix. You can choke on a little plastic dollhouse beagle.
- Spread a white sheet on the floor and arrange the parts in groups. It's easy to lose parts in the pattern of the Oriental rug.
- Don't tighten any screws or nuts until you've finished. A little wiggle room really helps.
- Beware these warning signs: Banging a screw with your heel; turning a bolt with your teeth; sweating profusely; feeling your blood pulse in your temples. Then it's time to put down the Allen key.

OUR FINAL ANSWERS

Ready or Not

My wife is pregnant, and I'm having panic attacks. Am I not ready to be a father?

—K.P., Biloxi, Mississippi

Being a dad is one of the most important things you will ever do, so you should be anxious—and excited. Calm yourself with information. Take a parenting course, read books on fatherhood, and redirect your anxiety by making your wife's situation better. When you appreciate what she's going through, you'll realize you have less to panic about.

No Time Out?

I work all day, and my wife takes care of our 4-year-old and the baby. As soon as I get home, I play with the kids and help get them ready for bed. My wife takes it easy when I get home. Don't I get any downtime here?

—J.K., Columbus, Ohio

We get it. You deal with a nasty boss, high-pressure deadlines, and some real ruthless folks at work, right? And your wife, all she deals with is diaper rash, nuking a few hot dogs, and flicking between Nickelodeon and the Disney Channel? Do this: Trade places for a week, and tell us who needs the downtime. What you have to understand is that when it comes to your home life, your wife's the starting pitcher, and she throws a ton of pitches every day. Be a trouper and close out the game. The more saves you make, the more she'll want to give you a break and throw a complete game herself.

Take Aim

My 6-year-old went to a birthday party where the boys were shooting BB guns. I'm not against guns, but that's ridiculous. What should I do?

—T.F., Red Oak, Texas

There's nothing more embarrassing than parents who fight with other parents about Little League playing or some other stupid crap. This is not stupid crap. These morons put guns in the hands of 6-year-olds. You couldn't have stopped the guns from showing up the first time, but you can stop it from happening again if you call the parents on it now. Do what you hope those kids did at the party: Shoot straight.

Three's a Crowd

> The problem is, my wife lets our daughter sleep in our bed. The kid cries if we don't let her, and it's killing our sex life. What should I do?
>
> **—R.M., Carmel, California**

It sounds like your little girl is playing you like a video game. This is about control—over the kid and over your wife. Do what one guy we know did: He told his wife they were going to go 1 week without giving in. The kid stays in her bed, no matter what. By Wednesday, the girl is sleeping fine, and so are they. So try that. When she realizes that tantrums won't get her anywhere, the habit's broken. And the joystick is back where it belongs—in your wife's hands.

Athletic Support

> My son is a wuss about sports and wants to quit. How can I get him to toughen up?
>
> **—O.T., Fresno, California**

Do you want a happy, well-adjusted kid, or do you want to mold him into something he's not? Forcing him to participate will mangle his self-esteem if he fails. The best thing you can do for your son is respect him. Spend time with him, listen to him, and patiently help him build athletic skills.

Birds and the Bees

> When should I start talking to my kids about sex? And how much detail should I go into?
>
> **—R.J., Los Gatos, California**

Kids can't avoid sexual messages, so as soon as they can talk, be prepared, says Stephen Braveman, a certified sex therapist in Monterey, California. When

NUMBER OF MEN WHO HAVE "THE TALK" WITH THEIR KIDS: 1 in 3

they're under the age of 4, let them come to you with questions. "Don't be afraid to tell too much," says Braveman. "If it's beyond their understanding or it bores them, they'll block it out anyhow." When they're 5 or 6, talk about good touch/bad touch. At 8 or 9, up the chatter—and the detail, he says. Depending on your personal values, talk to the boys about masturbation and how it's healthy and appropriate, within boundaries. As for girls, they must be prepared for their first menstrual period. As kids get older and wiser, encourage their questions and watch for red flags. Are they visiting porn sites? Spending too much time in their room with their girlfriend or boyfriend? Do they get defensive when you broach the subject? This is when you need to jump in and ask for their questions, Braveman says. Before it's too late.

Battle Plan

How do I keep my kids from fighting with each other?

—B.S., Pittsburgh

Fighting isn't all bad: It's relationship practice, and kids need plenty if they hope to function in the dating world and in that snake pit known as "the office." Good negotiating (a.k.a. arguing) skills can even help out in school: Research has correlated cooperation between siblings and academic achievement. So this one's worth working on. Maurice J. Elias, Ph.D., author of *Emotionally Intelligent Parenting,* suggests a system using marbles and a clear jar. "Every time siblings have a conflict, parents put either one or two marbles in the jar for each child. When the conflict is oral, it's one marble each; when the conflict is physical, it's two marbles each. Once 10 marbles accumulate, there's a penalty," says Elias. The kids have to make each other's beds, do each other's chores, go to bed half an hour earlier, or lose an hour of computer time the next week. If they work well together for an afternoon, take out one marble. If one sibling settles a fight before it goes nuclear, one marble comes out. If a week goes by with fewer than three marbles in the jar, hand over passes for a half-hour-later bedtime or credit toward a book or CD. Bribery works. Just ask the jury.

Custody Disagreement

My ex-wife wants to move the kids out of state. We have shared custody. Can she do this?

—G.K., Revere, Massachusetts

Check your divorce agreement immediately. A good lawyer should have made sure this scenario was covered. If the legal papers say nothing, get yourself to court with a new attorney as fast as you can.

"Thank You, Sir"

How can I ensure that my sons (ages 11 and 13) grow up to be gentlemen?

—A.D., Corpus Christi, Texas

If you radiate respect for yourself and others, so will they—and the battle's half won. "If you want to raise a gentleman, you're actually going to have to be one," says Hugh O'Neill, *Men's Health* magazine's Charm School columnist and author of *A Man Called Daddy*. "Remember the Shaker wisdom: Let your life speak." These rules can help your kids add action to your example.

Rule #1: A gentleman thinks before he speaks (or e-mails, or voice mails).

Do this now: Before you send your boy off to his sleepover, ask him, "What are you going to say to Mrs. Jones when you get there?" and "What will you tell Mrs. Jones before you leave?" "This simple exercise helps children put thought behind their words," says John Bridges, author of *How to Be a Gentleman*.

Rule #2: A gentleman is as polished as the silver.

Do this now: Sit down for a family dinner at least four times a week. Paul Hogan, the real-life butler in Fox's *Joe Millionaire,* advises, "Turn off the TV, put on some music, lay a tablecloth, cook a nice meal, and have conversations with your kids." Practice these social-set pieces at home and they'll feel at ease on a first date, in a job interview, at a client dinner, and at your wake.

Rule #3: A gentleman is social Super Glue.

Do this now: Make sure they know how to behave when they're in a crowd. "Team activities can teach kids that in order to succeed, they need to respect the different talents and roles of the entire group," Bridges says.

Rule #4: A gentleman dresses the part.

Do this now: Separate your son's closet into three sections: play, school, and dress-up. "Dressing well means learning how to dress appropriately for every occasion," says Clint Greenleaf, author of *A Gentleman's Guide to Appearance*. Dividing up your son's closet will make it simple for him to come to the right decision on his own.

Rule #5: A gentleman shows appreciation.

Do this now: After dinner, have your kids help with the dishes while the cook relaxes on the couch. "They need to learn when it's their turn to give something back," says Peter Post, director of the Emily Post Institute and author of *Essential Manners for Men*.

Rule #6: A gentleman is defined by how he treats women.

Do this now: Your wife is the ultimate practice dummy. Make her feel like a lady, and your sons are by definition gentlemen in waiting.

Lift the Curse

My son has started to swear like an Osbourne. What do I do?

—E.R., Jersey City, New Jersey

Back in the day, dads used soap and belts. But now, young dads have to use more time-outs than Chris Webber. Any disciplinary tactic will work if you're firm but not fanatical, using a fair system of punishments and rewards. You can try just about anything, except telling the [bleep]er that if he doesn't clean up his little [bleep]ing mouth, you'll take every [bleep-bleep] one of his [bleep]ing video games until he's six-[bleep]ing-teen.

Give Gramps a Chance

My dad worked all the time. Never did anything with us kids, barely grunted when he got home from work. Now that he has time, he wants to be all involved with my kids. I'm not so sure.

—T.J., Phoenix

So your dad blew it. But when it's all said and done, which is more important: sticking it to your old man or giving your kids a chance to get to know their grandpop? Don't you blow it, too.

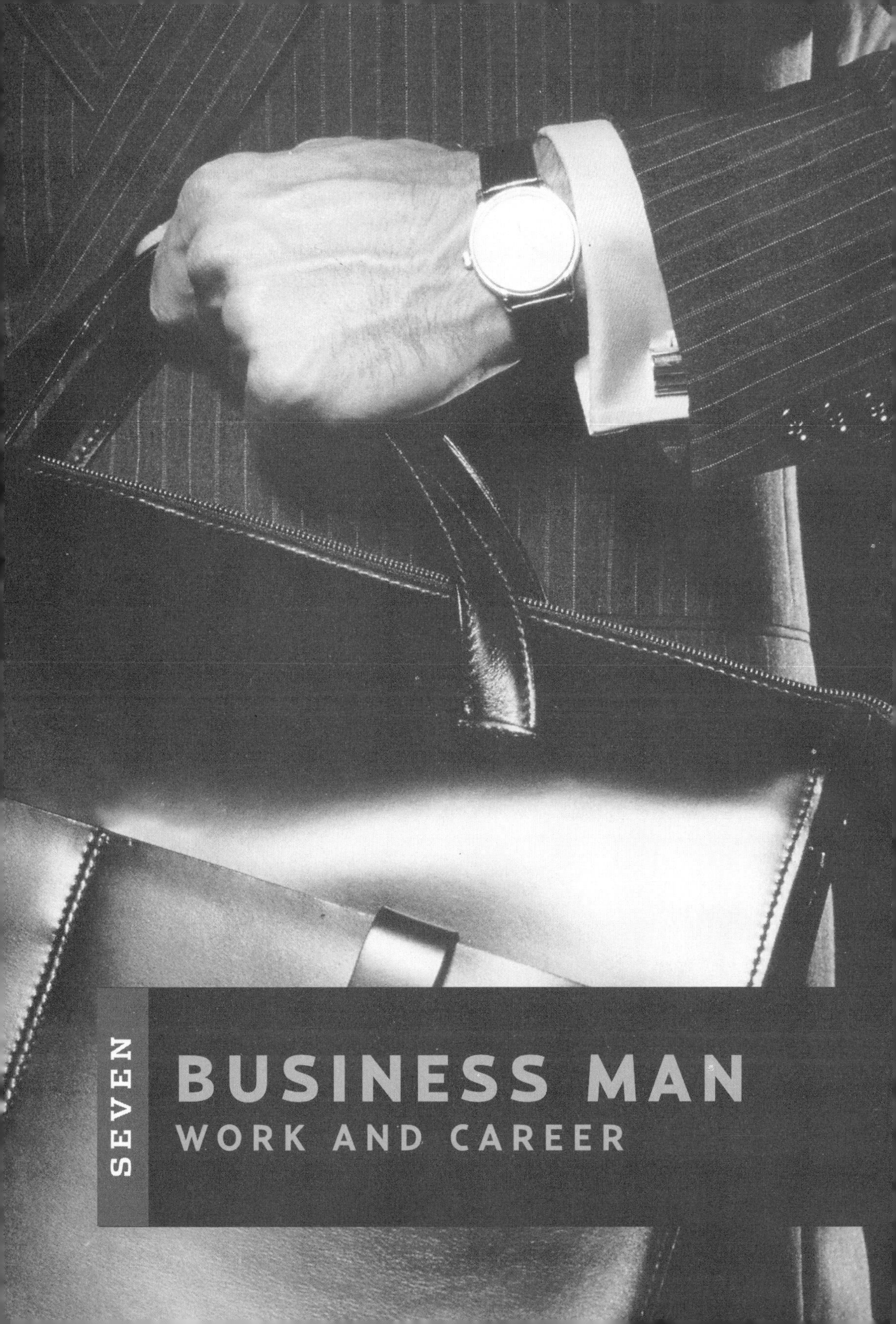

SEVEN

BUSINESS MAN

WORK AND CAREER

MUST READS

Find Your Dream Job

You've been in the same career for 20 years. It's time for a change. Do you dare?

By Christopher McDougall

The List, ultimately, is what ended Herb Lurie's career.

Fifteen years ago, shortly after he started a Wall Street job as a mergers-and-acquisition specialist for Merrill Lynch, Lurie randomly began jotting down things he wanted to do before he died. He was logging brutal hours in those days, sometimes 100 a week, and the List was one thing that helped keep him going. "Someday," the List reassured him, "you'll get more than 3 hours of sleep a night. You'll ride horses and travel and do more to maintain the machine than just swallow food and shower."

At first it was a few quick scrawls on a Merrill memo pad:

Learn to play piano.

Skydive.

Take an African safari.

After Lurie began free-climbing through the Merrill Lynch ranks and earning more downtime, the List grew longer and more complicated—way more complicated:

Research autism.

Get a helicopter pilot's license.

Go on an archaeological dig in Greece.

Seeing Eye dogs—how are they trained?

What kept the List alive and manically evolving was Lurie's success. It wasn't long before he'd broken out as one of the greatest deal-makers of his era. As a brainy tactician, he specialized in big bank mergers; and he masked his sharp eye for vantage points and percentages behind a dough-boyish demeanor and easygoing, storytelling manner. In April 1998, he landed the two biggest bank mergers of all time in the same week: Several days after joining Nations Bank to Bank of America, Lurie united First Chicago with Bank One. Either one of those deals would have made his career. Nailing both made him a legend.

By the time he turned 40, Lurie was cruising toward a cushy management position with Merrill Lynch. The List, however, was still on his desk at home and beginning to nettle him. With time running out, he realized there was no way he could accomplish everything on it in one lifetime. At some point, he'd have to dump a few of his dreams.

Instead, he dumped his job.

"I like this guy already!" erupts Pat Croce, motivational consultant, former president of the Philadelphia 76ers, and author of the *New York Times* best-seller *I Feel Great and You Will Too!* After hearing only the first half of the Lurie story, Croce can't contain himself. He's thrilled by Lurie's unabashed love of learning.

Here's what he means: "Do you know why so many guys hit their professional peaks and feel deflated instead of elated?" he asks. "It's because they've lost their ability to dream up new challenges. For years, they've accepted society's definition of the top rung, and once they get there, they're like, 'Now what?'" Because they were so focused on the practical next step, Croce says, they allowed their imaginations to atrophy. Then a crisis hits—a divorce, a mortality reminder like September 11, 2001, or a good friend's death—and

KNOW WHEN TO CALL IT QUITS

Use these four tests to determine if you should stay or you should go.

1. Develop a mental warning system. Herb Lurie used to say, "I can't imagine anything I'd like doing more than this." Then he caught himself thinking he could enjoy other things just as much. "That's a great technique," says life coach Brian Biro, author of *Beyond Success: 15 Secrets of a Winning Life*. "It gives you a little phrase that can act as a canary in the coal mine to warn you when it's time to get out."

2. Interrogate the witnesses. Before switching careers, ask people in the field you are considering these two key questions: "What does it take to be a success in this profession?" and "Do I have it?" Keep in mind, Biro warns, that some people you respect may be dream-crushers, but listen carefully to what they tell you about the talents and experience needed for their jobs.

3. Do the dental-office test. Imagine that you're in a dentist's waiting room and there are 10 magazines on the coffee table. Nine are about your profession and one is about another subject. Would you choose the magazine about something other than your job? That could be a sign that it's time to go, says Biro.

4. Eliminate your coworkers. Career coach Jamie Fabian suggests you imagine what it would be like doing your job without your current colleagues. Does it seem as if it would be more enjoyable? If so, maybe the problem is the people, not the profession. Consider a lateral shift instead of a career change.

Even if you decide to stay at your job, the process of assessing your situation and making a choice represents assertive action, and that's valuable in itself, says Biro. "You might find that what needs changing is you, not the job."

they feel the urge to make the most of their time. But their "reinvention mechanism" is rusted from disuse.

Lurie, however, was ready for success. He'd unconsciously been preparing for that moment from the day he graduated. "First, he painted a vision," Croce explains. "He didn't care how outlandish it was—all options were on the List. Then, when the time was right, he pulled the old Bugs Bunny trick and found a way to step into the landscape he'd painted for himself."

PRACTICE QUITTING

"Actually," Lurie says, "the first time I tried to quit, I failed." He still loved his work, and his boss jangled his nerves with a few pointed comments: "It's been 20 years since you sat in a classroom. What if you don't like philanthropic work?" And then the killer: "Aren't you going to open the *Wall Street Journal* one morning and be dying to get back into the action?"

This one really hit home. "I was a serious deal junkie," Lurie admits. "For me, finishing a big deal was euphoria. I had some serious worries that I would miss that." So Lurie backed away from his resignation plans, but he didn't abandon them. Instead, it dawned on him that he should apply the same techniques to quitting his job as he had to doing it. Like any other business decision, due diligence was called for.

"I hear from people all the time who spend more time researching their next car than they do their next career," says Jamie Fabian, "the Career Coach," whose advice column for JobCircle.com is based on her 15 years as a human-resources executive. "They're hot for a change, and so they end up making a 'flee from' decision instead of a 'go to.'"

To avoid that, Fabian recommends this essential step: Spend at least 2 days shadowing someone whose career you're thinking of joining. "Learn if your talents and temperament are truly a good match for the job."

IDENTIFY YOUR PURPOSE

The first items Lurie wanted to tackle on the List after quitting his job were to earn a master's degree in psychology and to try to contribute to the treatment and study of acute autism. Lurie had no personal connection to the disorder; he'd simply been intrigued by a documentary he'd seen, and he began reading research performed by one of the top scientists in the field, Bernard Rimland, Ph.D., at the Autism Research Institute in San Diego.

"One day, I received a phone call from a fellow I'd never met," Rimland recalls. He was initially somewhat skeptical about the caller because ever since the movie *Rain Man,* strangers with a highly romanticized notion of autism would call to see how they could get involved. "They don't understand that it's a tremendously debilitating disorder, an excruciating ailment for the victims as well as their families," he says.

Lurie, however, was different. "He was direct, purposeful, and very rational, and I could tell he was highly motivated," Rimland says, and he was so impressed that he put Lurie in touch with David Holmes, Ed.D., executive director of the highly respected Eden Institute in Princeton, New Jersey.

As a psychologist, Holmes feels he understands what pushed Lurie to switch careers. "I think he was very lucky to learn a profound truth at a relatively young age—what ultimately brings us peace is not how much we get, but how much we can share in terms of spirit, knowledge, and encouragement."

STIMULATE YOUR BRAIN THROUGH CHANGE

Gandhi understood that every time you make a change, you discover far more about yourself than you thought was possible," says Brian Biro, former U.S. National Swim Team coach who is now a life coach, helping people work toward goals, and the author of *Beyond Success: 15 Secrets of a Winning Life.*

You can make these discoveries because unfamiliar circumstances stimulate the brain's "reticular activating system," which ordinarily blocks out anything that's not a threat or of value. "It's like a junk-mail filter," Biro explains. "When you're in a comfortable routine, your brain allows only the perceptions that are necessary. But when you're out in the woods, your brain goes on heightened alert."

This primitive consciousness, he says, kicks in whenever you take on a new challenge. Suddenly, you'll find yourself drawing on hidden talents, Biro says, and discovering resources around you that you'd never noticed.

Somehow, Lurie intuited that he would need a lot of challenges, not just a few intense ones. Besides his helicopter lessons, his graduate classes at Columbia, and his work with Eden, Lurie joined the board of the U.S. Equestrian Team, and he and his wife became volunteer dog-walkers at the Seeing Eye Institute in Morristown, New Jersey.

But one man wasn't so eager to receive Lurie's attention. "I was skeptical of him," says Herb Terrace, Ph.D., a professor of psychology at Columbia University and one of the world leaders in nonhuman primate research. "Lots of people say they want to work with monkeys, but they fall by the wayside." Lurie, however, had an interesting idea—he wanted to see if he could combine his work with autistic children with studies in primate communication.

NUMBER OF MINUTES DURING THE WORKDAY THAT THE AVERAGE MAN SPENDS ON THE INTERNET: 61

WHY ARE YOU HERE?

There are hundreds of Web sites and books on how to define your life purpose and find your next career. Our executive summary: Read Viktor Frankl's *Man's Search for Meaning* and ask yourself these 10 questions:

1. What is it that people say you are very good at?
2. What were you doing when you last lost all track of time?
3. How would you answer if a 7-year-old asked, "What are you most proud of in your life?"
4. Who is living the life you most envy?
5. What job would you gladly do for free?
6. How do you want to be remembered?
7. What would you tell your great-grandkids someday is most important in life?
8. What excites you?
9. What angers you?
10. What can you do about both?

This caught Terrace's attention: If Lurie could help link the two disciplines, it could lead to some truly groundbreaking advances.

Still, Terrace was reluctant to give a highly prized seat in his lab to a novice. Finally, one thing won him over. "We were standing outside on a freezing February day," Lurie recounts. "Professor Terrace was still undecided, so he says, 'Look, I've got scientists from all over the world who want time in my lab. Why should I give it to you?'"

Lurie looked around at the miserable Manhattan weather and tightened his coat. "Professor, I could be in the Grand Caymans right now, lying on a beach," he said. "What does that tell you?"

The professor laughed. "You're in," he said.

Epilogue: Herb Lurie finished his first year of graduate school. He has been promoted to the Eden Institute Board of Directors and was elected vice-chairman of the U.S. Equestrian Team. He has nearly all the air miles he needs to qualify for his helicopter license, and he went on safari to Africa last October. But he's proudest of one thing: "He did such a great job in our study that we included his name on our research paper," says Jessica Cantlon, a team leader in the Columbia primate lab. "It's amazing," she adds. "He came out of nowhere, and now he's a major contributor in the field of nonverbal cognition. If there are other men like him on Wall Street, send them to us."

Be Your Own Publicist

Eight ways to network your way into the spotlight

By Mike Zimmerman

Tom Hanks doesn't need anyone's help. Not anymore. Occasionally, at strange hours, when the light is bad and hope is dim, you'll find the reason on cable: *Bosom Buddies*. It ran for 4 years, and Hanks never won an Emmy for it, but he put on that dress and everyone in town suddenly knew his name. Tom Hanks was visible.

Think about your career. Who knows your name? Heck, how many peers even remotely understand your talents, your drive, your potential? If you're not sure, you need a publicist. Not a Hollywood type—just someone who knows you well. Someone like . . . you. What follows is an eight-step, do-it-yourself networking plan, whether you work in a colony of cubes or have your company name stenciled on your pickup. Put it into practice and watch the job offers, promotions, and clients accumulate like interest.

STEP 1: PLANT THE SEEDS

"Good networking is more about farming than about hunting," says Ivan R. Misner, Ph.D., author of *The World's Best Known Marketing Secret*. "It's about cultivating relationships with other business professionals." He used that theory when founding BNI (Business Network International; bni.com), a referral service with more than 54,000 people in all fields trading contacts around the globe. The point being, you don't track down the big elephant. You plant some tasty grass, lure him in, and let him go back and tell the rest of the herd. Then you'll have elephants in your field for years.

STEP 2: ACCUMULATE TRUST

"People do business with people they trust," says Misner. "Until you establish trust, you're not effectively networking." Heed Tim Robbins's example in *The Shawshank Redemption*. With one ballsy gesture—helping the bull guard with his taxes and asking only for a few brews for his fellow inmates in return—he planted the seeds of a network that would bring him freedom.

So sow. This week, make one selfless gesture toward someone in your office, like offering an 11th-hour hand to a project team on deadline. Then repeat every week for a month. That's four seeds scattered, four trusts gained. Just remember . . .

STEP 3: BE SELFISH ABOUT YOUR SELFLESSNESS

Don't help just anyone; who are the four people in your company (or industry, if you're self-employed) who need to know you? This roster is different for every field, says Misner, but some classics never fade: your boss's boss, a key human-resources contact, the guy who organizes the corporate golf tournament. Look for opportunities that play to your strengths. To get the ball rolling, simply use what Misner calls the four magic words: "How can I help?"

STEP 4: BECOME A DOORMAN

What if the tollbooth guy collected business cards instead of quarters? How many contacts would he have in an hour? The best networkers have mastered this philosophy. "Put yourself in the doorway that potential clients will naturally walk through," says Lynne Waymon, owner of Contacts Count.com. She tells the story of a 28-year-old financial planner who specialized in retirement strategies. He took up ballroom dancing and met so many 40- to 50-year-olds that his doorway quickly became jammed. Where do your potential targets congregate?

STEP 5: PARTNER UP

Networking gurus call them symbiotic or synergistic relationships: You partner with a compatible, noncompetitive peer and exploit each other shamelessly for mutual benefit. "Put a lawyer, CPA, financial planner, and banker in a room for an hour and they're going to do business," says Misner. So if you're a plumber, every contractor, electrician, and building inspector in town should know how good you are. If they don't, why not?

STEP 6: DITCH YOUR PRIDE, SHYNESS, AND FEAR

They're the Three Deadly Sins of networking. The prideful guy scoffs at using contacts for blatant ladder-climbing. He's going to make it on his own, damn it. "Those people end up in the unemployment line," says Misner. "Very few people become successful in a vacuum." As for shyness and fear, they can cripple otherwise ambitious, talented people. But even if you're shy, says Waymon, "you can learn a few networking skills that you can turn on at any given moment." She cites film director Mike Nichols (*The Graduate*), who refers to himself as a "site-specific extrovert." To shyproof yourself in social situations, prepare yourself to answer the two inevitable questions:

"What do you do?" Too many people take a humble approach: "Oh, I'm a CPA." Show love for your work—there's a difference between bragging and branding. "First, give them your best talent or skill," says Waymon. "Then tell

PERCENTAGE OF JOB SEEKERS WHO SAY THEY FOUND REEMPLOYMENT THROUGH NETWORKING: 61

them a time when you saved the day, solved the problem, or served the client." And everyone, no matter what he does, has a story. A better answer: "I'm a CPA. I negotiate with the IRS." They say, "Wow, that sounds like a tough racket." You say, "It can be, but last year I convinced Uncle Sam that my client's horse farm was a business, not a hobby." You've suddenly become one sexy CPA.

"How are you?" (a.k.a. "What's new?") This query usually elicits chitchat about blown saves and rain delays, which accomplishes nada. Waymon recommends answering with "gives and gets"—what you can give them ("I hear you need more office space") and what you'd like to get ("I'm looking for a new assistant"). This approach makes for a rich conversation. Plus, you now have a reason to follow up later.

STEP 7: MAKE THE CALL

Too many contacts languish in our PalmPilots. Every Friday for the next 6 months, schedule a quick phone call to someone you should have spoken to in the past 6 months. Yes, schedule it. Otherwise you won't do it. Neglect is the turf toe of a networking plan—even if it doesn't end your career, it'll certainly slow you down. "Remember," says Misner, "it's not net-sit or net-eat. It's network."

STEP 8: SAY THANKS

Misner's team recently asked 2,000 business pros if they were satisfied with the number of referrals they receive. Eighty percent said no. Then they were asked whether they gave any kind of gift or thank-you when they received a referral. Only 20 percent said yes. "I don't know about you," says Misner, "but that feels like a possible correlation." Thank-yous take different forms—a handwritten note, a lunch, a beer, a small freebie—but each goes a long way toward cementing a business relationship. Misner sums it up with two words: "Givers gain."

Impress the Boss

Real-world bosses tell how employees scored points without brownnosing

By Mike Zimmerman

Sucking up is as loathsome as it sounds: an act of bottom-feeding desperation that leaves a man's soul in pawn and his nose stained cordovan. Problem is, history has taught us that it works. Like toadying to the don or caddying for Judge Smails, kissing ass is as longstanding a tradition as backstabbing, stripper-expensing, and paper-clip stealing. To the puckered goes the prize.

Well, no more. Time to grab some *honorable* recognition, gentlemen. We went to the people who are in a position to give such recognition: real-life, big-game bosses who demand results from guys like you every day. Listen to their stories of employees who knocked them out of their loafers with unsolicited acts of competence, fearlessness, and passion. Then see why these strategies worked. But remember—impressing the boss is just step one. The rest of the ladder is up to you.

THE KNIFE MAKER'S TALE

C.J. Buck, president of Buck Knives

"Some years ago, we were redesigning our manufacturing facility. The project was just so huge that it kept getting bogged down. Our maintenance manager at the time had a talent for asking questions in such a way that I could go, 'Oh, by all means, we need to move that machine to the right.' See, as the boss, I'm called upon to juggle multiple projects and keep the scope of those projects clear in my mind. So what really impresses me is when someone organizes the decision process and then clarifies what they need from me before I'm even on the scene. That maintenance manager has since become our V.P. of operations."

Why It Worked: This man did what all employees are supposed to do but so rarely accomplish: Take pressure away from the boss so he can focus on the widescreen view. "My job is to be the tiebreaker in a lot of these smaller issues," says Buck. "To have people who can really clarify the key points and help me make those decisions, I think, is the most valuable. They're not wasting my time."

THE BEER MAN'S TALE

Jim Koch, founder, Boston Beer Company

"Let me tell you about a woman I interviewed 13 years ago for an entry-level job selling beer in Pittsburgh. At the time, Michelle was a fund-raiser for one of the symphony orchestras there. About 15 minutes in, I laid it out: 'Michelle, you've got a great résumé. But what the hell do you know about the beer business?' She lowered her voice and said, 'My mother told me not

GET WHAT YOU ASK FOR

Try this on your boss: "I'd like to take a comp day on the 12th, 14th, or 21st." Put your preferred choice last in a series of three, add an upward lilt to your tone, and nod your head slightly up and down as you say it. He'll not only agree but think it was his idea—and repress the fact that your budget project is due to him that morning.

to put this on my résumé, but I've been a bartender at Friday's for the past 5 years.' Hallelujah! That changed the whole character of the interview. See, I know that to be a bartender at T.G.I. Friday's you have to be very organized and very professional, and you gotta have pizzazz.

"I hired her on the spot. Thirteen years later, she's our national director for bars, restaurants, and hotels."

Why It Worked: Everyone's first instinct is to purge the résumé of any job experience that might come off as menial or low end. "But," says Koch, "she sensed what the boss wanted." If you can provide whatever expertise is needed, don't worry about where or how you got it. Just deliver it.

THE DENIM TRADER'S TALE

Robert Hanson, president of Levi's Brand, U.S.

"I was president of the Levi's brand in Europe from 1998 to 2001. When I first got there, I had to assemble my leadership team, and I'd heard a lot of impressive comments about a guy working for us in the United Kingdom. I'd also heard we were at risk of his leaving the company. So I went to see him, and after some brief pleasantries, he looked at me and said, 'You've got 30 minutes to prove to me why I should stay and work with you.' I thought, Okay, this is an interesting approach. A reverse interview. But what he did in that time was articulate his passion. He wanted the brand to be successful so badly that I had to convince him why I was the right man for my job, or he was out the door. In a half-hour conversation, he showed me how deeply he understood what we had to do to be successful.

"Three years later, when I moved back to the States, he replaced me as president of the Levi's brand in Europe."

Why It Worked: He walked the fine line between confidence and cockiness—no easy trick. He pulled it off because his passion for the work kept his motivations pure. Hanson wishes more employees had that kind of fearlessness. "When people are operating from a place without fear, that's when you get the best work out of them," Hanson says. In other words, silence is deadly. If you know your job, know your business, and have a great new idea, you have nothing to be afraid of. Sound off like you've got a pair.

THE IRON MAN'S TALE

William K. Thierfelder, Ed.D., president of York Barbell Company

"Over the years, the employees who impressed me most were the ones who have been able to take on a task, really own it, and say, 'I'm going to get it done no matter what it takes—even if that means staying over and sleeping on a couch.' They could've said, 'Hey, I can't get this done for another 3 days,' and that would've been fine. But they understood the importance of the project to the company and decided, 'I'm willing to make this sacrifice even though I haven't been asked to do it.'

"I've had employees stay over weekends to get things done; and the kicker is, I heard about it through the grapevine on Monday morning. They never came to me and said, 'Hey, do you know I stayed here all weekend for you?' They just went out on their own initiative and got it done."

Why It Worked: It's easy to stain yourself with elbow grease. It's much harder to wait for your boss's offer to pay the dry-cleaning bill. But that's the right move, says Thierfelder. "It's more impressive to me when someone does something and then doesn't immediately put his hand out, expecting a reward." That makes the boss more prone to put his out, offering a bonus or comp time.

THE HAWG FARMER'S TALE

Jeffrey Bleustein, chairman and CEO of Harley-Davidson, Inc.

"The thing that always gets my attention is a person willing to tell the boss that he's wrong. Recently, we were going to develop a new program to teach

MAKE YOUR BOSS YOUR LACKEY IN SIX EASY STEPS

You've impressed your boss. Now it's time to up the ante—to seize his power for your advantage. Looking for a big raise next year? Here's how to get it.

1. Show up early for meetings. Get there before him and look prepared by bringing a notebook, a cool pen, industry journals, or other props that suggest you know the subject inside and out. Be "working" when he arrives—even if you're actually playing Tetris on your PDA—and insist that the meeting end on time. You have more pressing matters, after all, and can't just chitchat with him.

2. Initiate every handshake. Again, this sends a subtle signal that you decide when his interaction with you begins and ends. Make the shake strong and short, but don't squeeze.

3. Stand closer. If your boss tends to stand 3 feet away when talking to you, take a half step closer. Hold a pen or your glasses in front of you to maintain your comfort level. He'll feel slightly awkward but won't know why.

4. Handle with care. Touching the man is risky (don't try this with a woman), but your hand on his shoulder when making a point says, "You report to me, big guy."

5. Expose him. In his office, sit on a couch or chair that's unblocked by his desk—he'll have no place to hide. Also, put something (a PDA or file folder) between him and his phone to scuttle any escape. Ideally, you want a window or lamp behind you, so that he's forced to look into the light. If there's a window behind him, sit kitty-corner so you're not looking directly at it. Above all, don't sit near a wall—you want his back up against it, not yours.

6. Shut up. Silence is one of the most powerful manipulative tools. He'll feel obliged to fill the uncomfortable voids with things like "Sure, you can have the corner office."

people how to ride. I insisted we start with a clean sheet of paper and develop one that was uniquely our own. The team came back to me 3 months later and said, 'No, that's not the right way to do it. There's an existing program out there that's really quite good. We should link up with this organization, pay them for their program, and add the things that we'd like to do.' I just never expected that result. But in retrospect it was absolutely the right thing to do. The path I sent the team on would've led to unending problems."

Why It Worked: First Amendment rights? At work? "A lot of people think [speaking up] is very risky," says Bleustein, "and I guess in some organizations it is." So eliminate your risk. Bleustein's team spoke up with intelligence, respect, and, best of all, an alternative solution—essential ingredients in a bloodless, if momentary, coup.

THE FLY-FISHERMAN'S TALE

Perk Perkins, president and CEO of the Orvis Company

"A couple of years ago, when a young salesman was calling on one of our retailers in Nashville, a woman and her son entered the store with an Orvis backpack. The strap had broken. She said, 'Can I get this fixed? My son starts school tomorrow, and he really wants to use this pack.' The retailer didn't have another one. Well, the salesman happened to use the very same backpack instead of a briefcase—and he literally gave it to her off his back. He said, 'Here, your son can take this one to school. I'll get his fixed and send it back to you.' The retailer told this story at a sales meeting, and it trickled around the company. When I heard, I thought, 'Well, that's very cool.' Understand, we have salespeople bending over backward all the time. But the curious part to me is how these stories get back to the boss without it's looking like brownnosing."

Why It Worked: Let others sing your praises for you—and yeah, it's okay to ask them to, says Perkins. "If I did something like this and wanted it to get out, I'd find a way to leak it to my peers. I'd say—without being burdensome—'Hey, I wouldn't mind if you'd share this with people back at headquarters.' That works."

Get Focused

Seven ways to drive away distraction and get the job done

By Laurence Roy Stains

"His cardinal sin was a failure of focus." I read that line in the *Wall Street Journal* the other day, and a little shiver of recognition ran up my spine.

How about you? Ten or 15 years from now, will people be so dismissive about you? Very few men are endowed with the sort of concentration that allows them to cut through clutter and get the job done. Most of us are overwhelmed screwballs who need to learn what this focus thing is all about.

Athletes are always striving to perfect their focus. "You have to pay attention to the most task-relevant cues," says Robert M. Nideffer, Ph.D., a performance psychologist in San Diego and president of Enhanced Performance Systems. "You've got to separate signal from noise"—like the wide receiver, for example, who ignores his coverage to focus on the eyes of the quarterback in that split second before the pass. If you're going to advance your game and post a win, you can't get distracted—by the noise around you or the noise inside your head. You have to pinpoint what's important and execute accordingly.

It's the same at work. Identify the "big plays." Don't get distracted, like the poor bastard whose alleged lack of focus was klieg-lighted in the *Wall Street Journal.* His name is John Battelle. At age 31, he became the publisher of the *Industry Standard,* a dotcom newsmagazine that reportedly made $200 million in 2000. Two years later, it was dead. Now a book has been written about this gigaflop. It's called *Starving to Death on $200 Million.* The author says Battelle lost interest in the magazine by the middle of 1999. From then on, he indulged in "fantasies" of turning its subscriber lists into a marketing treasure trove, while ignoring the fact that the magazine was struggling to find and keep those subscribers. Oops.

The enemy of focus is distraction. Only during an Internet bubble could a distraction be so pie-in-the-sky. Usually it takes the form of the work that has to be out the door by 5:00 P.M. When that workload reaches inbox-busting proportions, it sucks up all your attention. The result? You get so caught up in what's urgent, you lose focus on what's important. That crucial distinction was made by Stephen Covey in *The 7 Habits of Highly Effective People,* and it is, for my money, the best part of that best-selling classic. If you spend your days reacting to the urgent but often unimportant priorities of others, your career will consist of putting out fires. You may be efficient—but will you be effective? Your top priorities, the things that will help you keep focused, should be your long-term goals—the projects that will define you, advance your career, and maintain your passion for your line of work.

Only your boss gets the luxury of concentrating full-time on what's important. And we all know why he's able to do that—he delegates the urgent stuff to you. If you're dizzy with conflicting demands on your time, how can you keep your eyes on the prize? Here are some smart ways.

Think by the week. Most planning tools—calendars, daily planners, and to-do lists—help you be more efficient. But you're only prioritizing your crises each day. Covey's cure-all: a weekly worksheet. Organize your life on a weekly basis; this allows you to schedule time for your top priorities and the actions that prevent crises.

Tell people to leave you alone. "It takes the average person 2 to 15 minutes to recover from each interruption," says Joy Baldridge, time-management coach of Baldridge Seminars International. "Interruptions are the biggest time robbers and focus busters." To minimize an interruption, she recommends her "plus, plus, dash" trick. Say two nice things (the plus, plus, or + +), then dash (—) off. Example: "Hey, great to see you. I wish I could talk now. Right now isn't good, though; let's talk at 3:00."

Clear off your desk. Is your desk a mess? I hope so. Psychologists have discovered that messy desks are a necessity in a wide variety of careers. They're also distracting. Although we're barely conscious of it, we all have the same method to our madness. We keep a "hot" pile of papers, probably next to the phone; a "warm" pile or two toward the edges of the desk; and various "cold" piles atop the filing cabinet and every other square inch of horizontal space. These last are mostly completed projects or "just in case" materials. Their presence may ratchet up your sense of being overwhelmed. "As emotional arousal increases, focus becomes more difficult," says Nideffer. So take a rainy Saturday to stash or trash that stuff.

Straighten out your life. If your output is down but your workload is the same, maybe something is bugging you. "One of the hardest things to realize is when your own emotions are slowing you down," says Jeffrey P. Kahn, M.D., a psychiatrist in New York City and president of the consulting firm WorkPsych Associates. "Listen to what people tell you. If they ask, 'Are you

PUT YOURSELF ON THE MAP

Get something big done by high noon

It's lunchtime already, and you haven't done diddly. How many times has that happened? Time-management coach Joy Baldridge recommends a road map that'll guarantee you'll cross six significant things off your to-do list every day.

Draw the letters M, A, and P on a piece of paper for the morning, and do the same for the afternoon.

M stands for the task you must do before lunch (or the end of the day), no matter what. You do not allow yourself to move forward or do anything else before that goal has been accomplished.

A is your advanced goal—work on a project that's due down the road a bit.

P is a premium task, something that isn't a priority but would be great to get a jump on. "A and P are things you do today that will further your success tomorrow," says Baldridge.

Besides planning your day with a MAP, Baldridge suggests you stay focused on what's important by frequently asking yourself, "Is what I'm doing the best use of my time?"

okay?' it's appropriate to say, 'I'm fine,' but then ask yourself, 'Am I okay?'" If, on the other hand, you feel frazzled, but everyone admires your ability to juggle a zillion tasks, then give yourself some credit: You're multifocal. "I see that a lot, particularly among very successful people," says Dr. Kahn.

Respond right away. "In high-pressure situations, people tend to rush," says Nideffer. You've done this, I'm sure—you get an e-mail or memo, and because it requires a moment of thought or the retrieval of more information, you set it aside. Later on, you come back to it (when you're even more rushed) and spend time trying to figure out where you left off. Try not to pick up the same piece of work twice. "Read it and respond," says Dr. Kahn, "rather than put it aside and think you'll respond later."

Carve out time. If you're feeling overwhelmed, break it down. Ask yourself, "What is it, exactly, that I'm not getting to, and how can I get to it?" Doctors need to return phone calls, contractors need to take care of paperwork, salesmen need to sit down and make long-term plans. They all need to carve out an hour or two for these tasks. "Protect that time," advises Dr. Kahn. "Then you don't have to worry about it while you go about your day."

Pick the low-hanging fruit. In the end, your workday will inevitably be a hodgepodge—a crazy salad of big projects, short deadlines, interruptions, distractions, and surprises. Roll with it all, but make sure to do what Dr. Kahn calls "picking the low-hanging fruit—tackling the easy tasks that you can get done quickly. That helps you feel like you're on track."

NEED TO KNOW

The Sexiest Jobs

You don't need to be a model to catch the eye of American women, but having a big hose helps. Firefighters were considered hottest by U.S. women in a ranking of the sexiest jobs. For American men, models were tops. The Durex Global Sex Survey 2003, polling 150,000 people in 34 countries, found that worldwide, both men and women ranked modeling as the sexiest job.

Jobs women consider sexy:	Jobs men consider sexy:
Firefighter: 27%	Model: 20%
Pop/rock star: 17%	Doctor/nurse: 13%
Soldier: 13%	Actor/actress: 9%
Massage therapist: 6%	Teacher: 9%
Model: 5%	Pop/rock star: 8%
Police officer: 5%	Massage therapist: 8%
Doctor/nurse: 5%	Secretary: 7%
Lawyer: 4%	Flight attendant: 7%
Others: 18%	Others: 19%

Success Comes at a Price

If you're on the fast track to the corner office, you might want to take a long lunch today. People who experience success at an early age are much more likely to die young. So say researchers at the University College of Cape Breton in Canada, who charted the life spans of a group of U.S. governors, presidents, Oscar winners, and other notable achievers and found that success early in life often signaled a premature death. "A strong desire to succeed will not increase your risk of dying young," says study author Stewart McCann, Ph.D. Instead, it's the stress of trying to achieve your goals that may be harmful, McCann believes.

HOURS OF HIS LIFE THE AVERAGE GUY WILL SPEND WORKING: 85,725

Dying for a Corner Office

A University of Texas study found that men with repetitive, passive jobs and few decision-making powers are 43 percent more likely to die during a given time period than people with more demanding careers, who make decisions all the time.

Not-So-Happy Hour

University of California researchers studied 1,800 men over a 5-year period and found that individuals who drank more than 10 drinks after work each week were more likely to suffer on-the-job injuries than workers who drank less often.

Blinded by the Light

Unfiltered fluorescent overhead lighting is one of the leading causes of eye problems for office workers, according to research from the Southern California College of Optometry. But the remedy is simple: Stick a tinted UV filter over the lights in your office and you may eliminate any eyestrain you've been suffering. In a test, researchers placed tinted UV filters over the lights above 49 computer users' desks. Within weeks, the workers claimed to have significantly less blurry vision, eye fatigue, and sensitivity to light than they did before the trial. To reduce the glare in your office, look for a prismatic, tinted fluorescent-light cover designed to mimic natural sunlight.

Clean Up Your Act

Yours may be a dirty job, but it doesn't have to be, according to a study in the *Lancet*. Researchers found that placing ultraviolet lights in office-building ventilation systems made workers feel better—they reported a 25 percent decline in watery eyes and noses. "UV works by disrupting DNA in bacteria and molds," says study author Richard Menzies, M.D. Until your boss retrofits the building, pick up an Ultra UV air purifier ($200) from www.trueair.com.

Get Off Your Duff

Sitting at a desk for long periods of time could cause potentially deadly blood clots to form in your legs. The condition, which doctors in New Zealand have named e-thrombosis, occurs when blood cells collect in the legs and start to stick together. (A similar condition can occur during long airline flights.) Getting up and moving around every couple of hours will help keep the clots from starting.

Do a Stand-Up Job

Having a stand-up desk installed in your office can save your back. If you work standing up, you'll cut the stress on your lower back by 50 percent, says Margit Bleecker, M.D., Ph.D., director of the Center for Occupational and Environmental Neurology in Baltimore. "You'll dramatically decrease the pressure you put on your neck, shoulders, and back, and you'll increase circulation, which will bring more oxygenated blood to your muscles and help you work with less fatigue," Dr. Bleecker says.

Pick a desk that has a flat surface for your computer and a slanted surface for reading and writing. The desktop should be even with your elbows when your arms are relaxed by your sides. And be sure to prop one foot up about 4 inches above the ground when you're standing, to take pressure off your lower back.

Want to shop around? Try these online suppliers: http://users.erols.com/standup or www.standupdesks.com. Prices range from $1,000 to $3,000-plus.

Escape the Mouse Trap

Your mouse isn't as user-friendly as it seems. Desk jockeys who click for as little as 30 hours a week are eight times more likely to develop forearm pain, according to a new study by three Danish hospitals. That goes double for neck pain and triple for shoulder pain.

Ergonomic experts such as David Rempel, M.D., recommend taking a 5-minute break each hour and using a mouse that doesn't require dragging.

Logitech's sleek MX700 ($80) solves the problem with a contoured grip for precise cursor pointing, Cruise Control scrolling device for leafing through documents without lifting a finger, and built-in buttons for Web-browsing commands—one of the most common causes of mouse rolling. Gyration's Ultra Cordless Optical Mouse ($80) works in midair like a remote control, thanks to motion sensors.

PERCENTAGE OF MEN WHO DEVELOP CARPAL TUNNEL SYNDROME FROM HANDLING A MOUSE: 5

FAST FIXES

No matter what a guy does for a living, he wants to be a success in the work world. You can trace it back to our mammoth-hunting roots. We wanted to be the guy to bring the woolly thing down and feed the tribe. Now the beast is less woolly and more bully. Follow these tips to win over anyone standing in your way to success, be it your interviewer or your boss. In the end, you'll get the job offer *and* a raise.

Land the interview. Your job search is doomed if your résumé includes any of these:

"References available on request." "Of course they are," says Mark Oldman, founder of Vault, Inc., a career-information service. "It just takes up space."

Career objective. If you must, put it in your cover letter. "I want to gain experience in this business" is too vague; "I want to earn $40,000 as a midlevel assistant in marketing" is too limiting.

A casual e-mail address. An address like KeggerDude@hotmail.com leaves a bad impression.

An Internet link. "You're saying you're so important that they have to stop everything they're doing and go to your Web site," says Allison Hemming, author of the job-hunting book *Work It!* It's a turnoff.

Weird fonts or a gray block of text. "This tells me I will have zero joy reading this," Hemming says. Use bullets to break it up.

Your SAT scores. Or college activities (unless you're a recent grad). This often "disturbs or puzzles the audience," says Oldman.

Get the job offer. Beware the smiling faces that greet you for a job interview. The trend is toward a new style of questioning designed to make you think on your feet, says Brian O'Connell, author of *The Career Survival Guide.*

Old Question: Why should I hire you?

New Question: What can you do for us that someone else can't do just as well?

Your move: Be specific. He's trying to create self-doubt. Repeat the job description (which you've studied) and explain how your talents match it perfectly. "Your ad said you wanted someone who can keep costs down. In my last job, my department was under budget 4 years running."

Old Question: What do you know about our company?

New Question: So, how about our performance last quarter? Wasn't that something?

Your move: Respond with information from the numbers you studied the night before. He's testing your interest and homework habits. Read newspaper clips, annual reports—and news about the competition. "I was impressed with your revenue bump while everyone else was treading water."

Old Question: Why did you leave your last job?

New Question: I've heard some horror stories about your old company. Geez, what was it like?

Your move: Keep your tone positive. He's testing your loyalty and ability to stay discreet. "It was better than you've read."

Old Question: Anything else you want to add?

New Question: Thanks for coming. We'll be in touch.

Your move: Ask for the job. He won't hire a limp wimp. "I want this job. It's a great match."

Scope out the company. You charmed them in the interview; they want you. Now go undercover and find out if you really want to work for them. "Researching the working environment is one of the most important aspects of job hunting," says John Kador, author of *201 Best Questions to Ask on Your Interview.*

Stake it out. "If you see a mass exodus the minute the clock strikes 5:00," be wary, says Kador. You want to see enthusiasm, not clock watching.

Test the atmosphere. See how employees interact; look for family photos and other clues that indicate it's a friendly place, says Maura Belliveau, Ph.D., professor of business at Texas A&M University.

Linger in the restroom (without attracting security). Listen to conversations. "You'll get a feel for the office politics" and a sense of the work atmosphere, says Carole Martin, of Monster.com.

Work networks, such as a business-school alumni directory, to find contacts who work there or who know someone who does. Meet outside the office for a candid perspective, Belliveau says.

Know the lingo. It's your first week on the job. Don't be 404 when it comes to corporate buzzwords. Put this code to use.

Dehire. To terminate. "I hear HR is having a dehire festival next week."

404. Clueless (from Internet error message). "Murphy's 404 about office politics."

Generate warm name flow. Drum up leads from clients. "My cousin's

PERCENTAGE OF EMPLOYERS WHO SAY A POST-INTERVIEW THANK-YOU NOTE CAN BE "VERY IMPORTANT": 48

sorority will generate warm name flow for dates all semester."

Incentivize. To give reason to work harder. "Twenty bucks didn't incentivize my kid in math."

Run with this monkey. Do something with an idea. "This'll take overtime, but I'm going to run with this monkey."

Type-diss. To type while talking. "I thought it was a romantic phone call until I heard her type-dissing me."

Check your voice mail. Quit playing phone tag. Here's how to reach out and touch someone more efficiently.

When Leaving a Message...

Stand out. Everyone says, "Hi Joe, this is Bob." Try this: "Joe! How are you? This is Bob." It'll jump out of the pack and increase the odds of a quick callback, says Nancy Friedman, a communications consultant in St. Louis.

Give your number twice. Slowly. Once at the beginning, again at the end. If they miss a digit, they won't have to listen to the whole thing again, says Elizabeth Danziger, author of *Get to the Point!*

Say when you need a callback. It helps the recipient plan his day, says Terry Wildemann, author of *1-800-Courtesy.*

When Recording Your Greeting to Callers...

Update it regularly. It lets people know where you are and when you might respond, says Lydia Ramsey, author of *Manners That Sell.*

Cut the redundancies. Obviously you're away or on another line. Give useful information, says Friedman, such as, "I'm in the office today."

Stand up. You'll sound more upbeat and confident, says Debra Condren, Ph.D., psychologist and founder of Superiorcareer.com, a career-consulting firm.

Master the memo. Enough with the big words. Keep memos simple. Research at Stanford University reveals that people who use big words when smaller ones will do sound less intelligent. "By making a text more difficult to understand, you are only going to annoy a reader and leave him or her with a negative evaluation of you and your work," says Daniel Oppenheimer, who performed the research as he worked toward a Ph.D. in cognitive psychology. So if you find yourself searching for a bigger word to replace a small one, stop. Your 50-cent words add up to a whole lot of nothing.

Work in a workout. Working out during your lunch hour may be a better career move than working through it. Physically active people accomplish more at the office than their inactive peers, according to researchers in Minnesota. When 683 blue- and white-collar workers reported their work habits and activity levels, the physically active types proved more productive than their sedentary counterparts. "As you exercise, your strength and endurance go up, so you can do more work than someone who fatigues quickly," says Nicolas Pronk, Ph.D., the study's author.

Work late. When you're up against a deadline, it's better to work until the wee hours instead of getting up extra early. Scientists at Stanford University determined that men are more productive when they get most of their sleep early in the morning. The scientists split eight men into two groups: One slept from 10:30 P.M. to 2:30 A.M., while the other slept from 2:30 to 6:30 A.M. After a week, the morning sleepers did better in memory and driving tests, fell asleep more easily, and spent more of their 4 hours actually asleep. "Most of us are programmed by our biological clocks to be owls—working late in the night—rather than early-rising larks," says Christian Guilleminault, M.D., the lead study author.

Get the raise. Annual reviews are like speed bumps—hit them right, you sail right through; hit them wrong, you're out looking for a new subcompact.

"The biggest mistake most people make is not speaking up in their reviews," says career expert Allison Hemming, author of *Work It!* Follow these talking tips to make your way through this crucial confab.

Boss says: "The way you botched the Finkelstein project really put a damper on your year's performance."

You say: "I learned a lot from that experience and used that insight on the Shmedly proposal. That was a valuable learning tool."

Why: You have to put a positive spin on bad news and show how you've proven yourself since, says Hemming.

Boss says: "In what areas do you think you need the most improvement?"

You say: "Since I surpassed my quota in sales and worked on two of the company's biggest money-making projects, I'd like to see if I can exceed that next year."

Why: It's up to you to mention your high points. Bring a list of accomplishments so you don't go blank, says Jeff Taylor, CEO of Monster.com.

Boss says: "We can't promote you at this time."

You say: "Let's make a plan so I can get to the next level."

Why: "Never take no for an answer," Hemming says. Show an interest in growing within the company and ask to meet again in 6 months.

Boss says: "We're giving you a 5 percent raise."

You say: "Is that the best you can do?"

Why: Salary isn't everything; You could negotiate more vacation time or tuition reimbursement—perks that are valuable in other ways.

Boss says: "See you next year, unless you have any questions for me."

NUMBER OF BACTERIA ON THE AVERAGE GUY'S MOUSE AND KEYBOARD: 10 million

You say: "I want to thank you for making my job easier."

Why: Expressing appreciation for guidance stands out—many employers aren't getting basic respect these days, says Andrew J. DuBrin, Ph.D., professor of career development at Rochester Institute of Technology. And don't forget to thank your reviewer for his time and feedback when you leave, DuBrin says.

Time it right. If you're asking for a raise when it's not review time, up your chances of success by picking the right time to approach the boss-man. The best time of day to negotiate a raise? In the early afternoon, right after lunch. Your boss's belly is full and he's simmering in serotonin, the feel-good hormone. "In the late morning he's too busy, and in the late afternoon he's too tired," says David J. Lieberman, Ph.D., psychologist and the author of *Get Anyone to Do Anything*. "A raise isn't always based on your performance, but on how well you get along with your boss. It puts the odds in your favor to catch him when he's in the best mood."

OUR FINAL ANSWERS

Junk Mail

How can I cut down on the number of time-wasting e-mails I get at work?

—M.C., Sugar Land, Texas

There are six basic rules for avoiding unnecessary chatter in your inbox, according to Kaitlin Sherwood, author of *Overcome Email Overload.*

1. Sign off your messages with "No reply needed" to avoid annoying "Great!" and "Wow!" responses.
2. When making a request, finish with "Thanks in advance" to prevent the "Thanks/You're welcome" loop.
3. When completing a response to a request, end with a conclusive statement like, "Hope this helped."
4. Use "FYI" in the subject line to specify that the message is solely informative.
5. Don't write statements phrased as questions, like "Peter and Laura did a great job, didn't they?" Your coworkers will answer them, and you'll have more pointless exchanges.
6. When you receive a CC message and must reply, send your response only to the sender instead of to everybody. Use BCC instead of CC as often as possible.

NUMBER OF E-MAILS THE AVERAGE GUY SENDS EVERY DAY: 32

A Quick Pick-Me-Up

I often get hit with massive, stress-inducing tasks on deadline at work. Got a great 5-minute exercise to help me relax?

—M.K., Raleigh, North Carolina

Cherry picks. A German study found that men with higher levels of cortisol, a hormone produced during stress, performed worse in memory tests than guys with lower levels. That means our brains don't work as well under stress—not when we're in Germany, anyway. Doing stretching exercises—such as the cherry picks described below—forces your muscles to relax, decreasing your stress levels, helping you think more clearly, and sparing you the shame of having to explain the whole stress-cortisol-Germany thing to your boss.

Perform cherry picks like this: Stand with your feet shoulder-width apart, rise up on your toes, and reach as high as you can with your left arm, as if you were trying to pick a cherry off a tree branch that's just out of reach. Hold for a second, lower your left arm, and repeat with your right. Continue this for about 60 seconds, trying to reach a little higher each time. Relax for a minute, then do two more 60-second sets.

Fire Away

How can I safely fire an incompetent employee who filed a harassment lawsuit against her last boss?

—T.R., Tempe, Arizona

The law does not require you to stock your business with incompetents. Document the problems and show the employee the list of failings to lessen the odds a lawyer will be calling you later, suggests Greta Van Susteren, attorney and host of Fox News Channel's *On the Record.* Having evidence that she deserves to be fired should keep you in the clear.

Improve Your Credit

My boss is scum. He takes credit for stuff I do, then blames me for his mistakes. I'm tired of not getting credit. How do I deal with him?

—J.S., Colorado Springs, Colorado

Quick, name your favorite blocking fullback. Can't do it, huh? That's because they get no glory; they just throw their bodies in front of 300-pound defensive linemen so some speedy guy can pick up MVP trophies. It's admirable to be a team player. But if you want to get anywhere, you have to flex a "gimme the ball" attitude. Speak up at meetings, mention ideas in public. Maybe try an end-around: Start talking to other people in other departments. If you're any good, you'll get noticed. And maybe you can work a trade. Bottom line: Don't waste your time on your current boss. Go impress somebody you want to work for.

Beat Boredom

I do the same thing at work, day after day. There's no challenge, nothing new. But I'm stuck because I've been here so long. How do I make my job better?

—D.R., Syracuse, New York

You ever see a roller coaster with all the hills the same size? Of course not; they have one or two huge drops and a bunch of smaller ones, some curves and some straightaways. Wouldn't be any fun otherwise. If you can't change jobs or careers, then you've got to find the twists and turns yourself. Volunteer for new projects, or mentor a kid who just started—anything that gets you out of your rut. And if your boss won't let you do that, get your adrenaline rushes outside of work, like with a ball team or a trip or whatever puts a jolt in your shorts. Because if you don't, your life will feel like you're stuck in a line that's always waiting for the ride to start.

Save Your Reputation

How do I deal with a backstabber at work?

—H.M., Baytown, Texas

Murder still being illegal, just remember that it's your boss's opinion that matters, not your coworker's. But how can you defend yourself to your boss without whining? "Present your case from the perspective of what's good for the organization," says Holly English, former lawyer and head of the consulting firm Values at Work. "If you just complain to your boss, you'll come off as a tattletale. Remind him of your recent accomplishments and tell him how you plan to do even more in the future, and he'll see you as reliable." As for coming by the credit you deserve, do it without making a direct accusation: Pitch a new proposal and take credit for the old by saying, "I thought of this when I had the idea . . . " and leave your coworker's name out of it. Works better than an assault rifle every time.

Stop the Panic

I panic before giving presentations. What's wrong with me?

—C.G., St. Joseph, Missouri

Nothing. Your fear is grounded in eons of evolution—the need to be accepted by the group for survival, says Daniel Amen, M.D., psychiatrist and brain-imaging specialist and author of *Healing Anxiety and Depression.* First take five slow, deep breaths. Anxiety causes shallow breathing, which makes you feel worse. Then kill the ANTs (automatic negative thoughts) invading your brain. It sounds silly, but visualizing destroying those thoughts can work. Positive thoughts release calming chemicals. Try it.

Promotion Pill?

A guy in my office says he's taking the drug Provigil to help him put in longer hours. Should I try it?

—R.T., Taos, New Mexico

If you can find a doctor to prescribe it for you, chances are it will work, but not any better than drinking a couple of lattes. Provigil improves memory and focus, but it's addictive and is prescribed only for narcolepsy, not for getting ahead at work, says John R. White Jr., Pharm.D., professor of pharmacotherapy at Washington State University. The military studied modafinil, the generic form of Provigil, for keeping soldiers alert and awake; turned out 400 milligrams (mg) of the drug was as effective as 600 mg of caffeine. So head to Starbucks instead.

Pecking Order

In a professional setting, when do you shake a woman's hand and when do you kiss her cheek?

—B.T., Marietta, Georgia

"When in doubt, shake hands," says Barbara Pachter, business-communications trainer and author of *When the Little Things Count . . . and They Always Count.* According to Pachter, in the United States the handshake is the proper business greeting, and both men and women should shake hands when they meet and greet. Avoid the cheek kiss in the corporate world. Exceptions: "Once a professional relationship with a woman has been firmly established," she says, "there are times when men and women may break this rule and kiss on the cheek, but it needs to be done cautiously." Or surreptitiously, in the cloakroom.

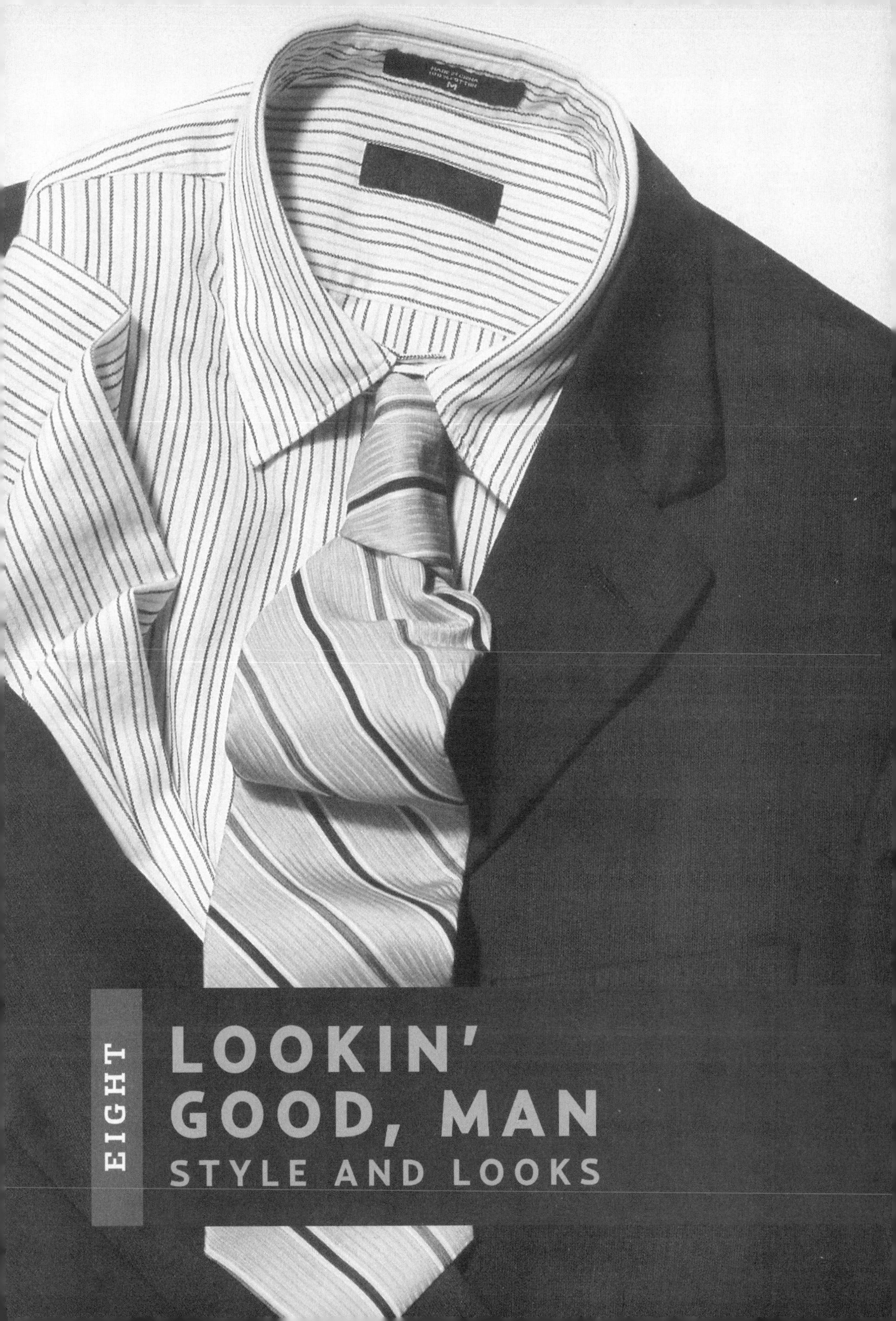

EIGHT

LOOKIN' GOOD, MAN

STYLE AND LOOKS

MUST READS

The 10 Secrets of Smart Style

Everything you need to turn heads and close deals can be found in the following pages. One hint: Nice clothes are just the beginning

By Hugh O'Neill

When circling an account in a skyscraper, he emanates polish and profit. When sucking down scotch in a saloon, he oozes sweet despair. Whether dressed up and gleaming at a gala or dressed down and pitching ball to the kids, he always fits precisely, a bullet in the chamber. He's got that rarest, most coveted of traits—style. Sure, he knows stuff about clothes, about color and cut, contrast and combinations. But he also has a few feelings that are the real engine of his style. Here, once and for all, are the secrets and sentiments that make a man shine.

THE SECRET OF YOU

Start toward style from this sure thing: The world is open to a multitude of male attitudes. Every day, men of every shape, size, taste, countenance, and hue—from wiry utility infielders to mountainous linemen, from trendy fashionistas to guys who still like tweed—turn heads and inspire the masses. You're a beautiful man. Whether you're built for speed or built sturdy, whether strangers think you're handsome or only Mom has noticed, you're fully equipped and good to go. That makes you a beautiful man.

THE SECRET OF YOUR FACE

Your face is your centerpiece of style. Job one is to draw attention to it. Ideally, your face is magnetic by virtue of a little something called a personality. But even absent this, some color and contrast tricks can draw eyeballs to your inimitable mug.

"A man's primary color signposts are his complexion and his hair color," says Alan Flusser, author of *Dressing the Man*. "So the colors of an ensemble should have the same level of contrast as the contrast between his skin tone and his hair color." For example, if you're light-skinned and dark-haired, you should favor the same high contrast between the color of your tie and the color of your shirt or whatever garments you're wearing right below your face. If, conversely, you're a low-contrast guy—say, blond hair and pale skin or dark hair and dark skin—you want low contrast in the shirt-jacket-tie triangle.

Why? Because a high-contrast face surrounded by low-contrast clothes is like a framed painting without the bottom edge of the frame. It encourages her eyes to drift southward, away from the artwork that is your face. If you frame a low-contrast face with high-contrast clothes, her gaze will wander toward the dominant clothes and away from the raw sexual power in your eyes.

Spotlight your face by making shrewd color choices. "Women are always saying, 'I can't wear that color.' You should, too," says Michael Macko, director of men's fashion merchandising at Saks Fifth Avenue. "Hold clothes up near your face to see which colors flatter you." If you've got a pinkish complexion, a red/maroon tie or pocket square will sharpen focus on your face. If your hair is blond or your skin brown, favor warm golds, rusts, browns. Two more tricks: sunglasses, no matter what the season, and scarves, whenever you can get away with them. "Anything around the neck or above will draw attention to your face," says Macko.

THE SECRET OF SLOW

Style never hurries. It doesn't race out to a meeting; it's in command. Oh, it doesn't dawdle, either—there's much to be done—but all its gestures are polished. Or perhaps "finished" is the better word. Want to make a point? Have faith; don't rush it to a conclusion. Take the time to make it. Apply the Sinatra standard: Put on a recording and try to sing along. Note how often you start a syllable just a hairbreadth before the Chairman of the Board does. He always withheld the next syllable until the last possible instant. It sounded as though he was making the lyrics up as he went along. Style believes in itself, thinks it's worth taking a second to shine up life.

THE SECRET OF THE NAKED GREEK GUY

The unmistakable beauty of you notwithstanding, there is an ideal male physique; not for function, but for fashion. The Western icon of maleness is 6'1", 185 pounds, ripped through the middle, with a V-shaped torso. He's Middle Man—tall enough to be a presence in any room but not large enough to frighten the kids. Neither too muscled nor too thin, he's the guy who posed for those statues in ancient Greece. Even as you affirm the wonder of you, keep Mr. Perfect in mind.

If you're shorter and/or heavier than a naked Greek guy . . .

. . . *Wear* garments and accessories that accentuate the vertical and de-emphasize the horizontal. Choose colors with subtle contrasts to unify the length of your body.

Examples: pin-striped suits, V-neck sweaters, sport coats that form a deep V between the lapels, sweater vests, pointed collars, neckties, overcoats worn unbuttoned

. . . *Avoid* contrasting colors north and south, or anything else that guides the eyes across your latitudes.

Examples: big belts or buckles, striped golf shirts, cuffs on your pants, flaps on your jacket pockets, double-breasted suits

If you're thinner or taller than a naked Greek guy . . .

. . . *Wear* clothing that makes you look less long and more substantial.

Examples: bulky sweaters, double-breasted suits, windowpane check suits, crewneck sweaters, jackets that button high, spread collars, wide belts

. . . *Avoid* stretcher-outers.

Examples: pinstriped suits, suspenders, and NFL team jerseys

The move-to-the-middle strategy also applies to the shape of your face.

If you've got a long, John Kerry face, favor crewneck sweaters over V-necks; they round you out. So do spread collars.

If you've got a round, Rush Limbaugh kisser, go with V-neck sweaters, pointed collars, and angular eyeglasses instead of round ones.

THE SECRET OF BIG

Style is generous. On occasion, this means gracefully picking up a check. But the bigheartedness of style isn't about money; it's about affection and attention. Style never forgets that everybody has his story. Style respects each man's path and never blocks another man's light. The world is full of treasure; there's plenty for everybody. The stylish man feels wealthy because he lives in an effusive world.

THE SECRET OF SAME

This style principle is best described in its violation. Imagine a guy turned out formally and fine. He's wearing a gunmetal-gray pin-striped Italian suit, a sweet silk tie, and the just-right gleaming cap-toe oxfords. But when he crosses his legs, he reveals, not a pair of finely woven thin formal socks with some blue threads that refer to his tie, but a thick-textured pair of socks that are barely the right color. This is among the most common style blunders: mixing fabrics or garments or accessories that have no business being commingled. It's like inviting Red Sox fans to a Yankees game: You're just going to start fights. Instead, your formal clothes should all step out on the town together; likewise, your casual duds should carouse at their times and places. You'll save yourself a lot of style heartache if you just remember that smooth cries out for smooth, and rough cries out for rough.

Here's how to sort the high style from the weekend wear in your closet.

Formal clothes generally cluster under these adjectives: smooth, simple, shiny, and one dominant color. Think tuxedo, which is mostly black and subtly gleaming.

Casual clothes are the opposite: textured, thick, patterned, matte finish. Think the L.L. Bean barn coat, which is coarse, featuring zippers, pulls, and rivets.

The exception: Over time, blue jeans, which by rights ought to be casual, have evolved into the ultimate in flexibility. Used with wit, they can work in many different situations. For example, though in most venues you shouldn't wear blue jeans (casual) with shiny slip-ons (somewhat formal), there are certain urban, art-gallery moments and late-summer cocktail-party-on-the-deck situations in which jeans and fancy loafers are okay, assuming of course no socks are involved. Same applies for cashmere sweaters; they can be worn beautifully with denim. Somehow this mix of rough and smooth works. "For spring it's best to wear lighter-weight denim. Spring is all about color, so jeans look great paired with a woven shirt and a linen or navy blazer," says Randy Heil, men's fashion director for Macy's West.

THE SECRET OF YOUR WAIST AND WRIST

Nothing's more expensive than appearing not to give a damn about details. So pop for the perfect accessories for what you're wearing. Again, like cries out for like.

Belts: It's not enough to have one black belt, one brown belt, and the cloth promotional one you got at the golf outing. You need a precise match—in finish and color, and even buckle material—for every pair of shoes you own. When you buy a new pair of shoes, march right over to the belt rack and find their twin.

Watches: Way too many men have way too few watches. You need a sleek silver metal watch, a chunkier silver metal watch, one with a shiny brown leather band, another with a dull brown leather band, and the same two watches in black. You also need a sports watch, maybe two, depending on how adventurous your life is. Over time, build your watch wardrobe so that your timepiece always syncs with the clothes you select.

THE SECRET OF STRIPES

Pattern rules are as follows: When wearing two of the same kind of pattern—two stripes, two checks—make sure they're of different scales. If the pinstripes in the suit are narrow-gauge, the stripes in your tie must be wide, and vice versa. Conversely, if you want to combine two different patterns, be sure they're of the same scale. So a windowpane suit with big squares would require a tie with wide stripes; a shirt with small tattersall checks calls for a tie with narrow stripes.

One more consideration: "A common denominator of color is imperative," says Macko. "If you're going to put a houndstooth with a stripe, make sure they share a color between them."

You can combine three patterns in the triangle where shirt, jacket, and tie meet, but it takes a little something called taste. "If you're mixing patterns, don't be meek," says Macko. "If you have to think too much about it, don't bother." For the brave, here are the guidelines, according to Flusser. Three stripes? The shirt has the narrowest, the jacket the second, and the tie the widest stripe. Two stripes and a check? The stripes should be different sizes, and the check size should correspond to that of the wider stripe.

THE SECRET OF THE SECRET

Perhaps the most powerful ingredient of style is the sense that you have a secret. All men who are raffish emanate a sense that they know something nobody else knows. What is that something? It doesn't matter. It could be which stock is about to triple in value. Or it could be that beyond all the chasing after this and that, beyond all the handsome ties and go-to-meeting suits, all that matters in life is who loves you and whom you love. Either because he's got an edge or because he knows he doesn't need one, the stylish man seems calm and confident about the future. Every time you enter a room, project the quality that you know something reassuring that all the others don't.

THE SECRET OF BREAK 'EM ALL

It's one thing to break rules because you don't know any better. Quite another to scoff at regulations of which you're fully aware. Know that you know them, and feel free to break 'em. If it works, it works. Stylish men never get hung up on a bunch of rules.

Best of All Time

Is your wrist worth watching?

By Jessica Fischbein

A man's watch is typically his main piece of bling, an element essential to his overall style. There are so many watches to choose from, so little time—from platinum mechanicals for black tie to steel chronographs for blacktop. We're firm believers that every man should own at least three: a dress watch, a sports watch, and an everyday watch.

Start with the watch you'll wear most often for work and play: the everyday watch. Only purchase a watch from an authorized dealer at a reputable jewelry store, suggests Mark Wasserman, president of Oris USA. And get a warranty. The good ones will cover buckle-to-buckle repairs for 2 years. Once you're at the jewelry store, look for these details in your next timepiece.

ESSENTIAL

Stainless-steel bracelet. Stainless steel is more practical than leather or rubber in a strap for everyday wear. It's classy enough to complement a business suit, casual enough to wear to the game, and waterproof, so you don't have to take it off to work out or shower. Less practical but more luxurious is white gold.

Water resistance. "It's safe to shower every day in a watch that's water resistant to 50 meters or more," says Wasserman. "For swimming, buy one water resistant to at least 100 meters." Divers' watches must be water resistant to 330 feet or more.

Classic colors. The hottest trend in watches is colorful (blue, red, orange) dials and straps. But for an everyday watch, it's best to go with white, gray, or black—basic shades that will look appropriate in a business setting.

A good fit. The watch should be snug enough that it doesn't slide up and down your arm, but loose enough to move slightly.

OPTIONAL

Luminescent indexes. Glow-in-the-dark guides make it easier to read the time in the dark. With a black or dark-colored dial, they'll stand out even more.

Sapphire crystal. "It's more expensive than mineral glass, which is found on some inexpensive watches, but it's sturdier and highly scratch resistant," says Andy Gilchrist, author of *The Encyclopedia of Men's Clothing.* If you're spending more than a couple hundred dollars, chances are your watch will have a sapphire crystal, but it's always wise to make sure.

Steel (or precious-metal) case. Check the back of the watch or the accompanying documents for the metallic content of the case, says Gilchrist.

TICKER POWER

Watch aficionados prefer mechanical—or automatic—watches to battery-powered quartz watches because of their superior quality, sweeping second hands, and movement powered by the motion of your arm and wrist. The one downside: If you don't wear it for a few days, you'll have to reset it. With good care, a well-made mechanical watch will last more than a lifetime.

That said, every man should have at least one battery-powered quartz watch in his wardrobe. They generally keep more precise time, and they're less expensive. Plus, they're extremely handy after a power outage.

ALWAYS BE ON TIME

- Call (303) 499-7111 to synchronize your watch with the U.S. Atomic Clock.
- For a watch check on your desktop, download free software from boulder.nist.gov/timefreq or http://tycho.usno.navy.mil to automatically set your computer clock to the correct time.
- When you're traveling by air to a new time zone, reset your watch as soon as you board the plane. You'll get accustomed to the time change much more quickly.

Steel is a solid option for an everyday watch. Inexpensive watches are sometimes made with plastic or a resin composite, while some expensive dress watches feature costly precious-metal cases.

Second hand. You want one, especially on your everyday watch. It's also an excellent indicator of quality: On mechanical watches, the second hand sweeps smoothly. On quartz watches, it stops and starts with loud ticks. When you see a supposedly high-end mechanical watch like a Rolex with a ticking second hand, guess what? It's a fake.

Chronograph. It's one of today's most popular styles, though few wearers have a clue about how to use all the functions. Frankly, the stopwatch function alone makes a chronograph worth considering.

Screw-in crown. All diving watches, and many other watches as well, have this feature, which creates a tight seal to make the watch more water resistant. When you unscrew the crown to change the time or date, turn it toward you gently until you feel a light pop. When you screw it back in, don't overdo it. "You just need to screw north until it tightens around the gasket; that's enough to keep it water resistant," says Wasserman.

Into Thin Hair

The average guy has two fears about looking older. The first is that he'll shrink. The second is that he'll go bald. We can't help with the first one, but balding men everywhere can feel a whole lot better following this haircut advice

By Jon Finkel

Why do we say "losing hair" and not "gaining head"? Probably for the same reason we say "losing virginity" and not "finding sex." When it comes to these two sticky topics, looks and performance, men can be so inherently pessimistic.

But if you—yeah, you, the guy with the failing follicles—want to continue to project the same confidence and virility you did when you had a full head of hair (and steam), you need to accept that you haven't changed. Only your looks have. And our looks are supposed to evolve.

To that end, think of your head as a country, with you as president. Your thinning hair is a hot-button political topic. You, as president, can either tell the truth—while putting a positive spin on it, of course—or get caught in a visual web of lies. Positive spin, in this case, is a damn fine haircut. With the right style, you can look smarter and more powerful, even presidential—whether your problem is a receding hairline, a bald spot, or a full-blown "horseshoe." We can't make you president, of course, but we have spoken with a man who can make you look like one: Jeff Sacino, head hairstylist for NBC's *The West Wing*. Take his advice, then smile for the camera.

PICK THE RIGHT SCISSOR HANDS

Barber or stylist? It's pretty much like choosing between Best Buy and Bang & Olufsen. No wrong answer; just different levels of right. Bottom line: "Find the person that does the best scissor work for you," says Sacino.

The barber: Barbershops are assembly lines for haircuts, says Sacino. The less hair you have, the more logical this choice, especially if you just want it simple and short (or if the thought of going to a hair salon makes your testosterone boil). But if you're not sure what you want—or if you want something specific—a barber's likely to disappoint.

The stylist: "Stylists will always choose a hairstyle that fits your face," says Sacino. "They'll take the time to justify the cut and tell you why it'll work for you." Why? They're trained to, and you're paying them a lot more than you would a barber. (Ah, if only balding men could pay by the strand.)

RECAST YOUR HAIRLINE FRACTURES

Men usually try to combat a receding hairline in one of two ways, says Sacino. They grow their hair a little longer and slick it back, or they try to structure their do to look like it used to. Both are mistakes. Instead, strive for volume. "If you want that 'important' aura, with your hair thick in front and strong throughout, use a light gel in your hair and blow it dry while fluffing with a round brush," Sacino says. Your haircutter can teach you how.

If blow-drying goes against everything you stand for, "cutting your hair shorter and leaving it more natural can be best," says Sacino. He points to the cooler style of *Wing's* Bradley Whitford. "His character is not going to look in the mirror and blow-dry his hair. So we keep his hair looking as if he got out of the shower and let it dry on its own." The more conditioned you keep it, the shinier it looks and the more natural it stays. Leave-in conditioners (see "Hair to Stay") keep your hair fluffy and textured, which makes you look as if you have more of it.

Guys who do it right: Nicolas Cage, Matthew McConaughey, Bruce Willis in the *Die Hard* films

LENGTHEN YOUR HAIR BY CUTTING IT

Men often believe that the longer their hair is, the more it covers up their bald spot. "That's absolutely not true," Sacino says. "When you grow your hair long, it separates," creating a valley that goes all the way down to the shiny scalp. Keeping the hair shorter—but not too short—gives it a feathering effect, in which one group of hairs covers the next. "The men with power on our show have short, very clean-looking hair. We're talking about the president's staff. Their look is power."

Also, when your hair gets this thin, avoid styling gels. "They're the worst because they grab too much hair and show more baldness. Stay with creams and texturizing lotions and you'll get a much more natural look," says Sacino.

Guys who do it right: David Letterman, Gene Hackman, Anthony Hopkins

HAIR TO STAY

Whenever possible, feed your hair steak. Clay Cockerell, M.D., clinical associate professor of dermatology at the University of Texas Southwestern Medical Center, recommends products that are high in protein (amino acids), fat (palmitic acid, a lipid), and vitamins, which coat the hair and keep it healthy. Stay away from shampoos that contain sodium laureth (or lauryl) sulfate; both are harsh cleansers. "The most important thing is to avoid excessive damage to the hair," says Cockerell. Our hair-healthy favorites:

Nioxin produces a whole line of natural products specifically designed for men with thinning hair. The potions promote a healthy scalp, which in turn helps keep the hair as thick as possible. Try **Bionutrient Creatives Bliss,** a leave-in conditioner that also provides UV protection. $8, nioxin.com

Redken Extreme's Anti-Snap is a leave-in treatment that fortifies thin or damaged hair and helps prevent breakage, a big concern for men with dwindling hair, says *Men's Health* fashion director Brian Boyé. $15, redken.com

MiN Wash (shampoo) **and Rinse** (conditioner) are safe for guys who color, but they also contain saw palmetto, *Ginkgo biloba,* and panthenol, which improve volume. $14 each, (866) 227-2566

Bumble & Bumble's Gloss gives hair luster while its **Groom Cream** adds texture with lots of vitamins A, D, and E, says *West Wing* hair stylist Jeff Sacino. Groom Cream, $20; Gloss, $13 (800) 728-6253

For styling that keeps hair controlled and soft, Sacino recommends **Kiehl's Crème with Silk Groom,** which contains both palmitic and amino acids, plus vitamins A and E. $17 for 4 ounces, kiehls.com

PUT ON A GOOD FACE

It's long-held dogma that facial hair can look good on a balding man. The key is not overdoing it—think Connery, not Kubrick. "You want to wear a beard that shows your face," says Sacino. "The less you cover a man's facial expressions, the better he looks." Unkempt facial hair is jarring, especially if the hair around your head is clean-cut. A mustache and goatee need to be trimmed to the same length and touched up every couple of days. If you go with a full beard, Sacino points to the way actor Richard Schiff is groomed for the show: "A structured beard with stiff lines does not look good. Use thinning shears to tailor it so there are no hard lines, so it looks natural."

Guys who do it right: Sean Connery in any role without a rug

BANISH THE BALD MAN'S BAD BOOB JOB

That would be the comb-over. If you're left with a horseshoe—little or no hair on top and a lot on the sides—keep it as neat and natural as possible. To be taken seriously, show your extra skin and tailor what hair you have left. With a shorter cut, you take attention away from the hair and put it where it belongs, on your face. "Ed Harris can play any role because it's about his face," Sacino says. "When you see him, you never think about his head. It's about his dialogue, his eyes."

Guys who do it right: Harris, Patrick Stewart, James Gandolfini

SPIT-SHINE YOUR CHROME

Lots of balding badasses—from Willis to Michael Chiklis to Samuel L. Jackson—have shaved their heads clean to great effect. But the question for us not-so-badasses is, can we carry the role? "A shaved head is a tough look," says Sacino. "Vin Diesel shaves to look stronger and have a more dominant presence onscreen. Frankly, I don't think the average guy who wears a suit to work should do it." But you'll never know until you try. Buzz your hair to stubble, then shave with cream and a razor, as you would your face. Don't like it? Don't worry—it'll grow back.

Well, whatever's left will, anyway.

APPROXIMATE NUMBER OF HAIRS ON AN AVERAGE MAN'S SCALP AT AGE 20: 100,000

APPROXIMATE NUMBER OF HAIRS A MAN LOSES BEFORE HE REALIZES HIS HAIR IS THINNING: 10,000

All to Be Tall

Vertically challenged men are paying up to $80,000 to have their legs broken, caged, then lengthened. The gain: 3 inches. The pain: extraordinary

By Joe Kita

The cages surround Jim Conran's legs like little scaffolds. Each has 11 metal pins that screw into his broken bones. Every 6 hours, he must turn these pins ever so slightly in order to tighten wires that pull the bones apart and align them correctly. He has been doing this now for 68 days. And all the time, the pain has been intensifying.

"It's like tuning a violin," he explains. "With each turn of the knobs, the ligaments and muscles and skin come under more tension. Each day everything gets tighter. It's incredibly painful." So much so that Conran won't allow himself to sleep for longer than 3 hours. "I'm frightened I'll miss a dose of medication, and the pain will get ahead of me," he says. Recently, he was given morphine, and that's helped somewhat. But he's still confined to a wheelchair and can stagger only short distances around his Manhattan apartment.

Before you start pitying Conran, you should know that he was not in a horrible accident that shattered his legs, nor does he suffer from a birth defect that's finally being corrected. No, he is an otherwise healthy, 45-year-old, single attorney who is paying $70,000 for this voluntary procedure. In fact, he's been looking forward to this for much of his life. Despite how it seems, he is living his dream.

You see, Jim Conran is 5'5$\frac{3}{4}$" tall. Or rather, he was 5'5$\frac{3}{4}$" tall. In the past few months, he has "grown" 1 millimeter per day (about $\frac{1}{25}$") by turning his 22 pins ever so precisely. And as he's done so, new bone has been steadily forming in the gaps where the segments of tibia and fibula are being pulled apart. When he last checked—and he checks daily—he was 5' 8$\frac{1}{4}$". When he (hopefully) reaches his goal height of 5'9" and this violin tuning ends, he's confident his life will finally be in harmony.

WHEN AN INCH FEELS LIKE A MILE

Short. It's a five-letter word that carries four-letter connotations for men below the national average of 5'9". Unless you're one of them, you don't know how much it hurts to be called that.

Imagine this scenario. You've been accepted at Harvard, West Point, and Annapolis. You're an A student. You've won seven varsity letters, and you nearly qualified for the Olympics. Yet to get into West Point (your first choice), you must meet a height requirement of 5'6". You're slightly below that. So the night before your admittance physical, you have your father repeatedly whack you on top of the head with a textbook in order to raise a bump. Next day, you officially measure in at 5'6$^1/_{16}$". You go on to graduate with honors, serve your country overseas, and eventually end up as an aide to the president of the United States. And you know, your whole life long, that you might have missed all of this—by a quarter inch.

"From a very early age, you start getting clear, institutionalized messages that you're less desirable," says George Holdt, the soldier in question, who, like Conran, is now undergoing limb lengthening. "From the violence you experience in school to the behavior you encounter throughout your social and professional life, the discrimination is always there."

Today, height requirements in any workplace are largely a thing of the past (the military's cutoff is now 5'). But it's an example of the frustration that is the legacy of the diminutive man. And no, it isn't his imagination. Numerous scientific studies have verified the advantages of height. For example, taller men . . .

. . . Are more likely to be hired. When recruiters in one study from Eastern Michigan University were asked to choose between two equally qualified candidates who differed in height, 72 percent chose the taller applicant.

. . . Make more money. Graduating seniors at the University of Pittsburgh who were 6'2" or taller enjoyed starting salaries $4,000 higher than counterparts 5'5" or under. Economists at the University of Pennsylvania even estimate that added height is worth nearly 2 percent in additional income per inch per annum.

. . . Are chosen as leaders. Nancy Etcoff, Ph.D., professor of psychology at Harvard medical school, points out in her book *Survival of the Prettiest*, "the easiest way to predict the winner in a United States election is to bet on the taller man." Of 43 American presidents, only five have been significantly below average height. What's more, Etcoff cites a study of Fortune 500 CEOs that found that more than half were taller than 6 feet and just 3 percent were shorter than 5'7".

. . . Make better first impressions. Surveys by Henry Biller, Ph.D., professor of psychology at the University of Rhode Island and coauthor of *Stature and Stigma*, show that compared with shorter men, guys of average and above-average height are seen as "more mature, uninhibited, positive, secure, masculine, active, complete, successful, optimistic, dominant, capable, confident, and outgoing."

While all of this just colossally pisses off short guys, what really bothers them is how they're viewed by women. Walter W. Windisch, Ph.D., is a psychologist in Towson, Maryland, who evaluates short men considering limb lengthening. "The average patient," he notes, "is 28 years old, male, college educated, professional, of some financial means, the product of parents who expressed concern about height, and, in every case, single."

Indeed, if you read the personals section of your local newspaper or log on to any online dating service, you'll find lots of ads from women listing height preferences. Why are they so particular, especially when they're paying by the letter? Certainly a portion of it stems from the statistics cited earlier—that taller men earn more and enjoy a higher social status. Some of it also comes from Hollywood, where leading ladies routinely look up into the eyes of the tall, dark, and handsome man. It's the romantic ideal. But a good chunk is also based on an almost primitive assessment. Is he a good provider, a worthy protector, a gifted procreator? And on some anthropological level, it's as if she ultimately decides the short man is not. Less than one-half of 1 percent of women marry men who are shorter than they are, according to Etcoff.

"Someone once asked Sigmund Freud, 'What is the goal of life?' and his answer was, 'To love and to work,'" says Windisch. "That's a fairly good summary of what's bugging these guys. They're looking to love and be loved, to work and be valued. It's just that their stature, something totally beyond their control, is keeping them from it."

HOW TO "GROW" 3 INCHES

About 2,500 kilometers east of Moscow, at the western edge of Siberia, is the Ilizarov Scientific Center for Restorative Traumatology and Orthopaedics. Located in the Russian city of Kurgan, in the shadow of the Ural Mountains, it was founded in 1971 by Professor Gavriil Abramovich Ilizarov. Decades earlier, faced with treating a large number of World War II veterans with complicated limb fractures, he began experimenting with "circular external fixators" to keep bones aligned and to speed healing.

Their use as limb-lengthening tools, however, was discovered by accident. While Ilizarov was on vacation, a nurse adjusted a fixator in the wrong direction. When he returned and examined the patient's x-ray, he noticed new bone forming in the gap. This set the stage for a variety of new applications, including the correction of leg-length deformities, bowlegs, anchondroplasia (dwarfism), and, lately, short stature. More than a half century later, the Ilizarov method—as it's come to be known—is still being used in a surprisingly unevolved form throughout the world.

Here's how it works: After taking a series of x-rays to map out the precise dimensions of the bones, the surgeon orders a regional anesthetic and makes two half-inch-long incisions in each leg (usually below the knee). Using a surgical chisel, he then cracks the tibias and fibulas, being careful to disrupt as little of the surrounding tissue as possible. (Note: When a doctor breaks your legs, it's called an "osteotomy.") Next, he attaches the circular aluminum frames. This requires piercing each leg with 11 arrow-sharp carbide pins and pushing them in until they bottom out against bone. The pins are of varying lengths and diameters, with the thicker ones being positioned closer to the breaks for added stability. Once the pins are in position, the surgeon slowly screws them into the hard calcium-and-collagen shell that surrounds the marrow. The rest is comparatively straightforward: Affix the adjustment wires to the pins, sew the two osteotomy incisions shut, treat and bandage the pin wounds. For all that's involved, the entire operation takes just 2½ hours. Patients typically remain in the hospital for 2 to 3 days, after which they can take a dozen or so steps.

But that's the easy part. The frames usually stay on for 3 to 6 months, during which time the bones are gradually separated. This is called the "distraction phase." All but one of the men we spoke with said that, even with heavy doses of narcotics, such as Vicodin, the resulting pain was just on the edge of bearable.

"It will reduce the toughest man to a crying little girl in a matter of weeks," says Jack Turner, a 39-year-old salesman who "grew" 2½ inches as a result of this surgery.

"It's an act of aggression against your own body," adds Conran.

Just as difficult is the helplessness that results. Patients are dependent on wheelchairs, walkers, and the supportive arms of friends and relatives to get around. Most are bedridden except for periodic doctor visits and daily physical therapy. Work is out of the question. This is true not only during the distraction phase but also for 3 months or more after the frames come off and the new bone is hardening. "You need somebody to take care of you virtually all the time," says Rick Morgan, another patient. "Sometimes you can't even reach the bathroom."

THE PITFALLS OF GETTING TALL

Although some doctors make lofty promises, most legs won't tolerate being stretched past 3 inches. It's not the bones that balk but rather the muscles and tendons that surround them. Overall, there's a 25 percent complication rate from this surgery, with the most frequent problem being pin-site infection. That's why patients are given a prescription for oral antibiotics, which they're told to begin taking at the first sign of redness, tenderness, or discolored drainage at the pin entry points. If an infection goes unnoticed, it will spread into the deep leg tissue and then the bone.

A less common but still serious complication is nerve damage. In one study review of 814 limb lengthenings, approximately 10 percent of patients had experienced some form of temporary nerve damage, characterized by chronic pain or impaired motor skills.

But the most catastrophic possibility doesn't present itself until the frames are removed. Even though the doctor will have taken x-rays to gauge structural integrity (the whiter the area, the stronger the bone), there's still a chance that what took months of agonizing pain and tens of thousands of dollars to build will, at the moment of truth, snap. Or the new bone will hold, only to buckle and break weeks later. Either way, doctors call this a refracture; there's a 1-in-12 chance of its happening.

BOOSTER SHOTS

Some doctors believe they've discovered the vaccine for shortness. Is it worth it?

Most short men were short children—while everyone else seemed to be adding inches daily, their own growth spurt sputtered and stalled. What they needed was a way to jump-start their skeletons. Today's short kids have one: human growth hormone therapy.

As the name implies, human growth hormone (HGH) is a substance the body produces to control growth during childhood. It does this by causing the liver to secrete another hormone called IGF-1, which in turn triggers the actual bone growth. Some children have a deficiency of HGH, and until recently, they were the only ones given injections of a synthetic version of the hormone. But in July 2003, the FDA approved HGH therapy for any child in the bottom 1.2 percentile in projected adult height (determined using bone x-rays), regardless of whether he or she has an HGH deficiency. A projected adult height of less than 5'3" for a man or 4'11" for a woman qualifies a child for the treatment.

But it isn't a one-shot deal. In order for HGH injections to have any chance of working, they must be given daily until the child reaches full adult height. This can mean 14 years of needles if started at age 3. And even then, extra inches aren't a given. "The results of growth hormone treatment in otherwise normal short children have been variable," says Ab Sadeghi-Nejad, M.D., chief of the pediatric endocrinology unit at Tufts–New England Medical Center, "ranging from zero benefit to possibly 3 inches." What's more, there's a small chance of side effects later on, such as an increased risk of hip dislocation, diabetes, and possibly cancer.

So is it worth it? "If my child were deficient and were going to end up 4 feet tall, it would be a no-brainer," says Mitchell Geffner, M.D., a pediatric endocrinologist at Los Angeles Children's Hospital. But if it's a question of giving HGH to healthy children who are predicted to become short adults, neither Dr. Geffner nor Dr. Sadeghi-Nejad is ready to sign on. "In addition to the fact that it's not guaranteed to be effective and has potential side effects, the question remains," says Dr. Sadeghi-Nejad, "do you want to stick needles in your son or daughter every day for years for the sake of an inch or an inch and a half?"

TWO SIDES TO EVERY STORY

If you're a short man seeking salvation through surgery, you've probably heard of the International Center for Limb Lengthening in Baltimore. An affiliate of Sinai Hospital, the ICLL was the first facility of its kind in North America and remains the largest—half of all the limb lengthenings for height are performed here. The bulk of its business, however, deals with correcting functional deformities. "I'm very strict when it comes to doing this surgery on otherwise healthy people," says 47-year-old chief surgeon Dror Paley, M.D., himself 6 feet tall. "In fact, I try to discourage it. The magnitude of what you have to go through is so large, it's not in the realm of having your nose done or your tummy tucked."

Dr. Paley generally will not operate on men over 5'6" (or women over 5'2"), and he requires that all prospective patients first undergo an intensive, 10-hour psychological exam by Windisch. Only about 10 percent go on to have the operation. "You must be careful," says Dr. Paley. "I've had some real nutcases—people who were willing to sell their houses, steal their wives' money, do unbelievable things for a few extra inches."

Depending on the facility and the specifics of the case, those inches typically run between $50,000 and $80,000. When limb lengthening is done on a healthy person, medical insurance won't pay for it. However, if done to correct a leg-length discrepancy, bowlegs, or any other limb deformity, it is usually covered.

Some of those people who can't raise the necessary funds or who don't pass the screening process go elsewhere—like Jack Turner, who ended up in Italy after being "dumped," as he calls it, by Dr. Paley. "The cost turned out to be one-eighth what it was in America," he explains, "and I felt I got better care."

And yet, even though it's been almost 3 years since Turner had his operation, he says he's still at only 80 percent of his former physical ability. "I don't think anyone can break both legs and come back 100 percent," he says. "For instance, I can't run as fast, and I have pain when the weather is damp."

The long-term effects are unknown. Although some doctors insist that dwarves who were lengthened as much as a foot decades ago show no traces of bone weakening or arthritis, other experts remain skeptical. "There's an enormous risk," says Michael Ain, M.D., a 4'3" orthopedic surgeon at Johns Hopkins Hospital in Baltimore. "Nobody really knows what's going to happen to people getting this surgery."

Neither the American Society for Aesthetic Plastic Surgery nor the American Academy of Orthopedic Surgeons (AAOS) endorses cosmetic limb lengthening. Others condemn it outright. "I'm appalled that our society has become so imbued with self-image that patients are willing to put their necks on the line like this. There are just too many risks," says William Tipton, M.D., director of medical affairs for the AAOS. "And the surgeons who are doing these operations on otherwise healthy people should remember this: *Primum non nocere.* That's Latin for 'First, no injury.'"

One of those surgeons is S. Robert Rozbruch, M.D., director of the Institute for Limb Lengthening and Reconstruction at the Hospital for Special Surgery, in New York City. He counters: "Seeing the profound impact this surgery can have on someone has convinced me that, for a very select group of people, it should be brought out of the closet and done more freely."

Paul Steven Miller, for one, thinks limb lengthening is unnecessary. Miller is an attorney and the commissioner of the U.S. Equal Employment Opportunity Commission. He also happens to be a 4'5" dwarf who has experienced height discrimination firsthand. "One law firm told me they feared their clients would think they were running a circus freak show if they hired me," he recounts. Nonetheless, Miller says cosmetic limb lengthening is "silly." "I have a hard time believing it really makes a difference in these people's lives."

THE MENTAL LIFT

With predicted advances in limb lengthening, combined with the recent FDA approval of growth-hormone therapy for short children (see "Booster Shots," on page 281), will Diminutive Man soon take his place next to Cro-Magnon in the Museum of Natural History? Are we entering an era of stature cleansing?

"The way we need to judge this," says David Sandberg, Ph.D., associate professor of psychiatry at the University of Buffalo's school of medicine, "is not by what's happening physically to these patients. Rather, what must be demonstrated is that increased height is actually translating into a better quality of life."

And only the patients themselves can assess that. Among the men we spoke with, sentiments are mixed. "It's kind of like the old P.T. Barnum thing," says Turner, "where you pay a quarter to go look at something that isn't very good. But when you come out, you have to basically say it was great. Not getting 3½ inches was disappointing, but on the other hand, I'm much more comfortable being 5'7" than 5'4½". I can only surmise that it's making subtle differences in my life. Overall, I think it's a great way for men with a height issue to increase their rank in the pecking order, but you're not going to suddenly be dating supermodels."

"Before I had this surgery, I was depressed and very self-conscious," says Mark Pace, D.O., an osteopath in South Florida who was 4'11". "I was afraid to walk into a roomful of children because they would make fun of me, and I could barely talk to women. I had zero confidence. Now, I'm just under 5'3", and the difference is unbelievable. I'm seeing eye-to-eye with people, and I'm actually dating."

"I've gained about $2^1/_2$ inches," says Conran, "and it feels great. In fact, I'm reluctant to let the thrill wear off. I'm almost 5'9". Now, I sure don't consider that tall, but it's not short. It's average, and that's all I ever wanted to be. I wanted to be accepted on my own merits without having my height held against me."

"I can't wait to walk down the streets of New York City, visit my old neighborhood, and see things from a slightly different perspective," adds Jose Rodriguez, who recently got his frames removed and is $2^3/_4$ inches taller. "Those extra inches make you a little more confident, a little more happy, and the day a little brighter."

If you're still skeptical, Rodriguez suggests an experiment. "Take a few books, set them on the floor, and stand on top of them," he says. "You don't think a couple of inches can make a difference, but it's amazing."

NEED TO KNOW

Loosen Your Tie

Finally, an argument for casual Wednesday: According to a new study, wearing a tie can increase your risk of glaucoma, a condition that can lead to irreversible blindness. In a small trial, researchers at the New York Eye and Ear Infirmary found that wearing a tight necktie for just 3 minutes can increase pressure within the eyes enough to raise a person's risk of glaucoma. "The tighter you tie it, the more a tie constricts the jugular vein, increasing pressure in the blood vessels leading to the eyes," says Robert Ritch, M.D., the study author. Dr. Ritch also warns that wearing a constrictive cravat during an eye exam could alter the results, increasing your risk of misdiagnosis. So what's too tight? When you can't stick two fingers between your neck and collar.

Jean Engineering

Jeans are like underwear: They're not comfortable or flattering unless they're suited for your body. Maybe that's why the underwear architects at 2(x)ist are thinking outside the top drawer. The company has introduced Degree Fit Denim—jeans that are sized to match your body type. Instead of your usual 33/32, these have sizes based on your butt and thighs, great for muscular men who want a looser fit around the thighs and a snug fit at the waist. If you've ever worn 2(x)ist underwear, you know how good this company can make your body look. Expect the same in denim. $65 to $175, Macy's and Bloomingdale's.

Can't part with your old jeans? Check out Denim Doctors, who—like many M.D.'s in L.A.—want to make you look good. They will patch, stitch, or even reweave the fabric of your lucky old Levi's until they're good as new. The shop also customizes and sells vintage jeans. Prices range from $15 to $200. The doctors don't make house calls, but they do accept patients by mail. 8044 W. Third St., Los Angeles, CA 90048; (323) 852-0171

No Pain, No Stain

Wrinkles and stains—and inattention to same—are the banes of male style. They are also the cost of living an interesting life. So God bless the hard-working techies at DuPont for developing the fabrics that give us the freedom to avoid blotting, wiping, and ironing. The wrinkle-free revolution swept through a few years ago, to be followed by stain repellency—a case of Teflon falling out of the frying pan and into the attire. Appropriately, the stain-proofing means you won't have to wash your treated clothes too often, and that will be a good thing: The Teflon coating wears down with repeated launderings, and fabric softeners can render it useless. You have to be careful on the drying end, as well. Those anticling dryer sheets contain chemicals that coat the Teflon, turning you back into the stain sponge you were in the early '90s—not a part of your life you want to relive.

Life Shaver

Researchers in the United Kingdom have found that men who shave daily are up to 24 percent less likely to die of a stroke than their less hairy counterparts, who don't need to shave as frequently. But don't invest in Gillette just yet. Researchers attribute the findings to lifestyle differences and hormone levels, not the act of shaving itself.

Oh Soy Smooth

Soy softens. So say researchers at Johnson & Johnson, who are testing it in shaving cream. A study of 18 men found that soy-infused shaving creams can slow the growth of facial hair and make the stubble on the neck less coarse. In addition, soy appears to help eliminate bumps and ingrown hairs. Check the ingredient label to find a soy-based cream.

Hair Today, Gone Tomorrow

Columbia University researchers may have discovered a way to prevent the growth of unwanted hair—like the foliage on your back, for instance. The discovery hinges on a protein called DSG4, which holds cells within a strand of hair together, almost like Velcro. When this protein is eliminated from within a strand of hair, the hair becomes brittle and eventually falls apart. A lotion containing DSG4-inhibiting compounds is currently in development. Clinical trials of the product should begin early next year.

Rudolf's Remedy

A new drug, Finacea, appears to be more effective than existing medications in the treatment of rosacea, an increasingly common disorder characterized by skin redness and inflammation. The finding was unveiled in a study presented at the American Academy of Dermatology's annual meeting.

Centrum for Your Skin

Your insides aren't the only part of your body that can benefit from a daily multivitamin. A recent review of vitamins and skin-care treatments suggests that you can easily eliminate puffiness and dark circles from under your eyes with a lotion containing vitamin K and niacin, says Leslie Baumann, M.D., associate professor of dermatology at the University of Miami. "Also, niacin may help your skin retain more moisture," Dr. Baumann adds. One small study found that people who used niacin cream for just a week reported smoother, moister, less flaky skin, along with a reduction of fine lines and wrinkles. Look for both in drugstores.

Zap Away Zits

Researchers at London's Hammersmith Hospital have found that laser therapy is effective against mild to moderate acne. Pulse-dye lasers, used to treat skin discolorations, employ multiple wavelengths of light that can also prevent the inflammation responsible for persistent acne. In the study, 70 percent of individuals were pimple-free in 3 weeks—half the time it would have taken with oral and topical medications. "Some patients clear after one treatment," says Anthony Chu, M.D., the lead study author. The procedure runs between $300 and $1,000 per treatment. Go to www.usaphotonics.biz and click on "Physician Finder" to locate a doctor near you who performs this procedure.

Give Warts the Cold Shoulder

Who needs medical school? We were able to remove warts without going to a dermatologist, who wanted us to wait 6 weeks for an appointment. Wartner Wart Removal System uses an over-the-counter cryotherapy technique, similar to the liquid nitrogen used by dermatologists, to freeze off warts. With a disposable foam pad that resembles the top of a Q-tip, you apply a mixture of dimethyl ether and propane from a canister, then ice the core of the wart for 10 to 20 seconds. All you feel is a little sting. In our case, the warts were gone in 2 weeks. $20, www.wartner-us.com

PERCENTAGE OF PEOPLE 30 AND UNDER WHO HAVE ACNE: 80

FAST FIXES

Here at *Men's Health,* it's our job to make sure you both look and feel your best. For some men—you know who you are—that's a tall order. If you have more holes in your socks and T-shirts than there are on a golf course, here's a quick course in how to look good for any occasion. Because when our readers look good, so do we.

1. Balance your 'burns. It's happened to the best of us. One sideburn is shorter, so you trim it back, oops, try again, and again, and soon you're the anti-Elvis: no sideburns at all. Or you end up with a crick in your neck from holding your head sideways to hide your asymmetry. Next time, use this trick for making sure they're even: Hold an index finger horizontally at the bottom edge of each sideburn. When you look at your hands in the mirror, you'll be able to tell if one is higher than the other. The ideal length is shortish anyway—no more than three-quarters of the way down your ear.

2. Cut it close. One of our scruffier reporters recently spent 50 minutes in a leather chair for a $45 shave at The Art of Shaving, a high-end "barber spa" with locations in New York City, Miami, and Dallas. "Baby smooth," he judged. The tips he gleaned:

Goop works. Preshave oil (never tried it, right?) warms the skin, softens the beard, and helps your shaving cream adhere and stay moist longer, says Eric Malka, cofounder of The Art of Shaving.

Brush up. Fingers aren't designed to make lather. Use a brush. (Badger hair is best.) Run it under hot water. Circular motion raises the hairs and exfoliates.

Switch directions. For a big-date shave, go with the grain once, reapply cream, and go lightly against the grain. *Men's Health* tried Schick's new four-bladed Quattro razor. Close and easy.

It's the balm. You've removed skin, so help what's left recover with after-shave balm with essential oils and no alcohol. It'll soothe and moisturize. Ignore the commercials—rub it in, don't slap it on.

3. Make perfect scents. At the risk of sounding Brut-al, many of us could use a refresher course on freshening up. Listen to what the experts say about picking cologne.

Amount. "If you're constantly smelling the fragrance, you've applied too much. People should have to get close to you to say, 'Gee, you smell nice,'" says Rochelle Bloom, president of the Fragrance Foundation. A couple of spritzes or splashes is enough.

Location. Pulse points like your neck and wrists will naturally diffuse a scent, Bloom says. Put fragrance on your skin, not on your clothes.

Season. Heat intensifies any fragrance, and scents are stronger when combined with sweat, says Bloom. That's why an aromatic or citrus scent works in the summer; you can go heavier in the winter.

Options. You don't have to use every variation on a fragrance—cologne, aftershave, body wash, deodorant, says Mikel Cirkus, creative director of Firmenich, an aroma manufacturer. One at a time is fine. But make sure the other products don't clash with the scent you choose.

Shortcuts. Body sprays like Axe fall between cologne and deodorant, but use them as a deodorant.

4. Canoodle confidently. We fell for breath strips when Listerine invented them; classier than gum, longer-lasting than drops, no rattling like Tic Tacs. Now everybody makes them. We tried four different brands. Our favorites?

Wrigley's Eclipse Flash. Comes in peppermint, spearmint, and cinnamon. It dissolves fast, lasts long, works well. Chills your mouth, throat, and sinuses. $1.50 for 24 strips

Winterfresh Thin Ice. It dissolves slowly, briefly tastes like licorice, and is a powerful freshener. $1.50 for 24 strips

5. Be a sleeve to fashion. A fraction of an inch often doesn't matter in clothing, except in sleeves. The cuff should reach the wrist bone when your arm is at your side. Too long and you're 14 again, wearing Dad's shirt. Too short and you're a gangly 16, wearing a shirt that fit when you were 14. When you're not wearing a jacket, ill-fitting sleeves can be rolled up. With a suit, you want a half inch of cuff exposed. If the cuff is hiding, unbutton it and you'll gain enough to show, but not so much that the empty buttonhole will be visible. Too long is hard to hide. Best move: Get dress shirts altered. It's worth it.

6. Speak off the cuff. Cuffs come in three basic styles, from least formal to most: the common single-button, a longer three-button model known as a barrel cuff, and the French cuff, which closes with cuff links (called a "double cuff" by the Brits, who refuse to give the French credit for anything). Turnbull & Asser created a lesser-known but increasingly popular fourth style for Terence Young, the director of *Dr. No.* Called the turnback, the cocktail, or the Bond cuff, it's a French cuff that employs two exposed buttons, providing a dressier look with the ease of unbuttoning quickly when it's time for a little boudoir jujitsu with a comely double agent.

7. Get on a roll. The best way to store your ties? Rolled. Start from the skinny end and roll tightly, says Andy Stinson, spokesman for clothing manufacturer Robert Talbott. The tension from rolling will iron out any residual wrinkles.

8. Don't get labeled. We see it unbelievably often: well-dressed guys walking around with tags hanging from their designer coats. This is a style-sucker move that's so obvious it's easy to miss. Designers sew labels with their names on the sleeves of suits and overcoats to identify them on clothing racks in stores. It's easy to think this sleeve tag is meant to stay, but just because it's sewn on doesn't mean it's permanent. Any tag stitched to the exterior of your coat must go—a quick scissor-snip will suffice. Labels on the interior of the coat can stay. Don't wait till your dry cleaner has to tell you.

9. Don't hang out. Nothing ruins the polished look of a suit like the dreaded jacket underhang—that is, when the bottom of your suit jacket or blazer hangs below your coat. There are only two rules for wearing a suit: Always leave the bottom button of the suit coat undone, and make sure your outerwear is longer than your suit coat. A traditional three-quarter-length overcoat is best for shielding you and your suit from the elements. It's also fine—even fashionable—to wear a boxy, hip-length, sporty jacket of wool, down, or leather over a suit. Anything else smacks of that postgraduate time when you didn't have a job, a good coat, or a fashion clue.

10. Lose the belt. When wearing jeans, take off your belt. According to our style editor, Brian Boyé, your jeans ought to hang off your hipbones, not cling for dear life to your underbelly. If you've conquered your gut, you can pull off the beltless look with style.

11. Go to great lengths. The hem of your pants should never bunch up at your ankles or rise above your shoes. The wrong pants length could send the message that you haven't yet recovered from the great Mississippi floods of '93. *Note:* Your pants should "break" (make one little fold) in front, leaving just enough fabric to cover the tops of your shoes. In the back, the hem should fall just above where your heels meet your soles. This keeps your socks hidden while you walk. According to Alan Flusser, author of *Dressing the Man,* jeans and tuxedo trousers should never have cuffs. Short men only look shorter when sporting cuffs, so keep the depth to $1^5/_8$ inch for men under 5'10" and $1^3/_4$" inch for taller men.

12. Leave your wallet at home. There are certain things you never do when you're in a tuxedo. You don't wear brown shoes. You don't stash Twinkies in your cummerbund. And you don't carry a big, fat wallet—it ruins the line and drape of your trousers or causes a bulge in your jacket. One credit card, your bank card, an ID, two business cards, and some big bills will cover all the bases for the wedding, bar mitzvah, Oscars, P. Diddy's housewarming, wherever you're headed. Slip these items into a money clip and be on your way. Consider this option on non-black-tie days, too. It's easier on your rear.

13. Sock it to 'em. Lloyd Boston, host of *The Style Network* and author of *Make Over Your Man,* teaches you the proper way to pull up your socks.

- Patterned and conversation socks are cartoonish. Stick with basic black, navy, camel, and heather gray. If you must wear a pattern, make it a subtle tattersall or check. Athletic socks are only for the gym.

- Always match your socks to your pants, not your shoes.
- For formal settings like the office, buy wool or a wool/Lycra mix; be certain that they're long enough to hide your shins.

14. Follow your nose. A strong chemical odor when you enter a dry cleaner's shop is a warning sign. According to Steven Brinkman, author of *The Men's Clothing Guide,* the EPA's clean-air guidelines mean new equipment should emit less perchloroethylene—the dry cleaner's magic potion. If a shop reeks, the proprietor may not be updating his equipment regularly. Also, make sure he's using the new Teflon-coated irons, which cut the glare left by older irons.

15. Clean up your act. Dry cleaning will make your clothes look crisp, but it's a harsh treatment. Too much of that good thing and your wardrobe is left in tatters. These guidelines will help you balance scents and sensibility.

Khakis. Dry-clean them every other time they're worn. This will not wear out quality slacks and will maintain the precise military crease that's required.

Wool slacks. Clean every third time you wear them. As with khakis, hang them up properly between wearings.

Suits and sport coats. Clean every sixth wearing, if you're the sort of fellow who glows rather than perspires. Every third time if you have that spritz gene.

Sweaters. Have them cleaned once a season, or as needed if you're spill-prone.

OUR FINAL ANSWERS

Shades of White

Do whitening toothpastes work?

—S.G., Miami

Sure, they do, but the change may not be drastic enough for you to actually notice a difference. "A whitening toothpaste will only take off the surface grime from your teeth—it won't completely bleach them—so they'll probably end up just two or three shades whiter, even after weeks of use," says Clifford Whall, Ph.D., director of the American Dental Association's Seal of Acceptance program. That's not enough to blind anyone with your dazzling smile. If you want to see a radical change, have a professional bleach job and your choppers will end up eight or nine shades whiter.

A New Do

How can I get my barber to give me a more stylish haircut?

—H.L., Burlington, Vermont

First, dump your barber and find a stylist. Just saying the word "stylist" makes our testosterone dip, but today there are lots of salons that cater to men. John Allan's in New York City has a full bar, billiard room, and smoking lounge as well as a staff specifically trained to cut men's hair. They'll talk sports and stocks while tickling your scalp and serving you a cocktail. In your town, ask the most fashionable woman you know for some recommendations. Or check out menessentials.com to find a list of recommended hairstylists nationwide.

Remember, stylists speak a different language than barbers. Hairstylist Jonathan Antin, whose clients include Kiefer Sutherland, Tiger Woods, Ricky Martin, and Christian Slater, suggests showing instead of telling. "When a man tries to explain a style he wants, I hand him a magazine and tell him to show me," he says.

If you wear a suit most of the time and use gel in your hair, don't show up at the salon in sweats, with wet hair under a baseball cap. Antin says seeing your usual look will help him create a cut that works well for you and your lifestyle.

Hairy Situation

The older I get, the hairier I grow. How can I get rid of my apelike thatch?

—O.M., Santa Barbara, California

Chewbacca swears by hair inhibitors. "Vaniqa is a prescription cream that inhibits hair growth by blocking the hair-growth enzyme," says Nicholas Perricone, M.D., professor of dermatology at Michigan State University. Any dermatologist can prescribe it for you. You still need to shave, but applying Vaniqa every day lets you shave less often—sometimes up to a month later. "Using Vaniqa cream and a safety razor is the easiest, cheapest, and most effective way to shave your chest," says Dr. Perricone. Other options include wax (grip it and rip it!), depilatories (Nair works well but can irritate the skin), and laser hair removal ($1,000 or more).

Boxers or Briefs?

Once and for all, what kind of underwear do women find sexy?

—H.N., Boston

This is completely body dependent, according to the women we consulted. If you're buffed to *MH*-cover perfection, a pair of Calvin Klein-style boxer briefs will be at your knees—and so will she—in no time. But if you're not, a generous cotton boxer would be your best confidence-builder. Get them in blue, gray, or white—avoid any color you might find in a box of Lucky Charms. Nearly as important is how you wear them. Too many men wear their underwear too high or too tight. Loose and low looks better and more enticing. Also, you may love your tattered, dingy pair, but women don't.

A Tall Order

What can I wear to look taller?

—R.G., San Antonio

A streamlined line equals a taller-looking silhouette. Jackets should be single-breasted with a single vent; two-button is better than three. Pants should be flat-front, never pleated. Long-pointed collars create a lengthening effect, while spread collars can make the neck appear squat. Avoid that. Shoes can have a slightly thicker sole, but trust us, no platforms. Women would rather date a short man than a man in heels.

Suit Yourself

If I buy just one suit, what kind should it be?

—J.O., Fresno, California

The most expensive one you can afford. Buy a black, lightweight wool with a single-breasted, single-vent jacket and flat-front pants. Ermenegildo Zegna (zegna.com) stitches the best in style, and it will probably outlast you.

Not Iron Man Material

Are there any good wrinkle-free clothes, or should I just take an ironing class?

—S.R., Glendale, Arizona

Wool is one of the most forgiving fabrics, and microfiber can stay smooth without steam treatment. Most major clothing companies have come out with lines of wrinkle-resistant cotton shirts in the past 3 years. Here's a hint: Checkered and patterned shirts hide creases—and laziness.

Where There's Smoke, There's Stench

How can I get the smell of smoke out of my jacket after a night of partying?

—K.D., State College, Pennsylvania

Here's a fabric-by-fabric smoke-out system from Heloise, our favorite party girl (especially at cleanup time).

Cotton: Throw it in the dryer on air fluff, along with a fabric-softener sheet to add fragrance. The circulation of air through the machine will speed up the destinking process.

Leather: If you have a smooth, natural-color leather jacket, you can wipe off the scent using a washcloth moistened with apple-cider vinegar. If your coat is dyed black or if it's dyed some color cows don't come in (red, purple), head for a professional leather cleaner.

Suede: A rubdown with a damp washcloth (water only) will do the trick. If the suede is dyed, a little color may come off, but as long as you apply the washcloth evenly, nobody will notice.

Wool: Sprinkle baking soda on the coat, let it sit for half an hour, then vacuum it off. And whatever you do, keep your smoky clothes out of the closet, or your entire wardrobe will smell like Keith Richards.

Get Quality Time

Why are high-end watches so damn high-end? I'd really love to buy one but don't want to be played for a sucker by some tinker in Switzerland.

—N.H., Shreveport, Louisiana

The drugstore watch-versus-boutique timepiece debate is sort of like a comparison of a minivan with a 2003 Nissan 350Z. Both cars will get you to work on time, but which would you prefer to drive? And it's not just the look. High-end mechanical watches require lots of human contact and craftsmanship, says Jim Lubic, executive director of the American Watchmakers-Clockmakers Institute. That costs money. Aside from their aesthetic value, luxury watches are handmade from better materials than machine-manufactured ones. These include heavier cases; scratch-resistant crystals (not plastic); gold wheels (not brass); and sharper, crisper timekeeping pieces made of higher-quality metal. In addition, luxury watches (which should have the term "certified chronometer" printed on their faces) are sent to Switzerland to undergo rigorous timekeeping tests, which drive the prices even higher.

But then, you expect to be paid for the quality you put into your job, right? So do the watchmakers. And when your son passes the watch on to your grandson at his college graduation, the thousand bucks you spent will be long forgotten. But your reputation as a guy who did things right won't be.

Sole Searching

How many pairs of shoes do I need?

—S.J., Big Spring, Texas

The women we talked to insisted they "need" close to 50 pairs of shoes; most men can get away with five: flip-flops—leather or rubber—to wear with shorts; athletic shoes (Nike, New Balance) for sports; funky sneakers (Puma, Adidas) to wear with jeans or khakis; formal loafers (Tod's, Cole Haan) to wear with jeans and slacks; and black lace-up dress shoes (Bruno Magli) for the office and formal occasions. The site 123shoes.com is a painless way to shop.

THE STORE WHERE CONSUMERS MOST OFTEN SHOP FOR SHOES: WAL-MART

INDEX

Underscored references indicate boxed text. **Boldfaced** page references indicate photographs.

F

Q

R

S

PHOTO CREDITS

Front cover: Blake Little
Back cover (top): Blake Little
Back cover (bottom): Barbe Ondrea
Page 1: Svend Lindbaek
Pages 12 to 15: Beth Bischoff
Pages 20 to 21: Beth Bischoff
Page 32: Beth Bischoff
Page 37: Sally Ullman
Page 93: Diego Uchitel
Pages 102 to 105: Beth Bischoff
Page 117: Augustus Butera
Page 149: Hilmar
Page 175: Blake Little
Pages 185 to 187: Darryl Estrine
Page 203: David Sacks/Getty Images
Page 235: Stefan Nyvang
Page 265: Peter Berson